Parkinson's Disease and Nonmotor Dysfunction

CURRENT CLINICAL NEUROLOGY

Daniel Tarsy, MD, SERIES EDITOR

Parkinson's Disease and Nonmotor Dysfunction, edited by ***Ronald F. Pfeiffer and Ivan Bodis-Wollner,*** *2005*

Thrombolytic Therapy for Acute Stroke, Second Edition, edited by ***Patrick D. Lyden,*** *2005*

Movement Disorder Emergencies: *Diagnosis and Treatment,* edited by ***Steven J. Frucht and Stanley Fahn,*** *2005*

Inflammatory Disorders of the Nervous System: *Pathogenesis, Immunology, and Clinical Management,* edited by ***Alireza Minagar and J. Steven Alexander,*** *2005*

Neurological and Psychiatric Disorders: *From Bench to Bedside,* edited by ***Frank I. Tarazi and John A. Schetz,*** *2005*

Multiple Sclerosis: *Etiology, Diagnosis, and New Treatment Strategies,* edited by ***Michael J. Olek,*** *2005*

Seizures in Critical Care: *A Guide to Diagnosis and Therapeutics,* edited by ***Panayiotis N. Varelas,*** *2005*

Vascular Dementia: *Cerebrovascular Mechanisms and Clinical Management,* edited by ***Robert H. Paul, Ronald Cohen, Brian R. Ott, Stephen Salloway,*** *2004*

Atypical Parkinsonian Disorders, edited by ***Irene Litvan,*** *2005*

Handbook of Neurocritical Care, edited by ***Anish Bhardwaj, Marek A. Mirski, and John A. Ulatowski,*** *2004*

Handbook of Stroke Prevention in Clinical Practice, edited by ***Karen L. Furie and Peter J. Kelly,*** *2004*

Clinical Handbook of Insomnia, edited by ***Hrayr P. Attarian,*** *2004*

Critical Care Neurology and Neurosurgery, edited by ***Jose I. Suarez,*** *2004*

Alzheimer's Disease: *A Physician's Guide to Practical Management,* edited by ***Ralph W. Richter and Brigitte Zoeller Richter,*** *2004*

Field of Vision: *A Manual and Atlas of Perimetry,* edited by ***Jason J. S. Barton and Michael Benatar,*** *2003*

Surgical Treatment of Parkinson's Disease and Other Movement Disorders, edited by ***Daniel Tarsy, Jerrold L. Vitek, and Andres M. Lozano,*** *2003*

Myasthenia Gravis and Related Disorders, edited by ***Henry J. Kaminski,*** *2003*

Seizures: *Medical Causes and Management,* edited by ***Norman Delanty,*** *2002*

Clinical Evaluation and Management of Spasticity, edited by ***David A. Gelber and Douglas R. Jeffery,*** *2002*

Early Diagnosis of Alzheimer's Disease, edited by ***Leonard F. M. Scinto and Kirk R. Daffner,*** *2000*

Sexual and Reproductive Neurorehabilitation, edited by ***Mindy Aisen,*** *1997*

Parkinson's Disease and Nonmotor Dysfunction

Edited by

Ronald F. Pfeiffer, MD

Department of Neurology, University of Tennessee Health Science Center, Memphis, TN

and

Ivan Bodis-Wollner, MD, DSc

Departments of Neurology and Ophthalmology, State University of New York, Downstate Medical Center, Brooklyn, NY

HUMANA PRESS TOTOWA, NEW JERSEY

999 Riverview Drive, Suite 208
Totowa, New Jersey 07512

humanapress.com

This publication is printed on acid-free paper. ∞
ANSI Z39.48-1984 (American Standards Institute) Permanence of Paper for Printed Library Materials.

Production Editor: C. Tirpak
Cover design by Patricia F. Cleary

Cover Illustration: From Figs. 1 and 2, Chapter 12, "Cardiovascular Autonomic Dysfunction," by David S. Goldstein.

For additional copies, pricing for bulk purchases, and/or information about other Humana titles, contact Humana at the above address or at any of the following numbers: Tel: 973-256-1699; Fax: 973-256-8314; E-mail: humana@humanapr.com, or visit our Website: http://humanapress.com

e-ISBN 1-59259-859-5

Printed in the United States of America. 10 9 8 7 6 5 4 3 2 1

Library of Congress Cataloging-in-Publication Data

Parkinson's disease and nonmotor dysfunction / edited by Ronald F. Pfeiffer
and Ivan Bodis-Wollner.
p. ; cm. -- (Current clinical neurology)
Includes bibliographical references and index.
ISBN 1-58829-316-5 (alk. paper)
1. Parkinson's disease.
[DNLM: 1. Parkinson Disease--complications. 2. Autonomic Nervous System
Diseases--etiology. 3. Behavioral Symptoms--etiology. 4. Sensation
Disorders--etiology. 5. Sleep Disorders--etiology. WL 359 P24654 2005] I.
Pfeiffer, Ronald. II. Bodis-Wollner, Ivan, 1937- III. Title. IV. Series.

RC382.P2577 2005
616.8'33--dc22

2004025976

Series Editor's Introduction

Parkinson's Disease and Nonmotor Dysfunction fills a major gap in the current rapidly growing body of knowledge concerning Parkinson's disease. Drs. Pfeiffer and Bodis-Wollner have correctly perceived that many nonmotor features of Parkinson's disease are given insufficient attention in the medical literature. Unfortunately, they are often also given insufficient attention by the practicing neurologists who see these patients. As recently pointed out, there is clearly much more to Parkinson's disease than depletion of the nigrostriatal dopamine system *(1)*. Parkinson's disease (not just multiple system atrophy) is a multisystem disorder, both pathologically and in its clinical manifestations. This is clearly true for the various motor system abnormalities, which are not fully corrected by dopamine replacement therapy strategies, but also for the nonmotor system abnormalities that are the subject of this volume.

Although recently there has been increased awareness of the cognitive, psychiatric, and sleep disorders commonly associated with Parkinson's disease, many of their manifestations remain under-recognized and their importance in managing patients is underestimated. Even less attention is paid to the myriad of other nonmotor disturbances that plague these patients. For example, among the autonomic disorders, although orthostatic hypotension is well recognized, it is usually attributed to dopaminergic medications rather than to effects of the underlying disease. Urologic disorders are also very familiar in these patients, but may not be properly understood or well managed. Beyond this, there is much less awareness of the less common and less obvious autonomic disorders which are herein reviewed chapter by chapter. Their link to Parkinson's disease is usually unappreciated and there is frequently an unfortunate tendency to attribute the symptoms they produce to advancing age. Finally, unusual sensory and painful phenomena, dysphagia, fatigue, and visual deficits are other less common features of this remarkably varied disease that readers of this book may become acquainted with as signs of Parkinson's disease for the first time.

This book highlights the fact that management of Parkinson's disease requires a multidisciplinary approach. This may not always require referral to a consultant but at least requires awareness of the spectrum of nonmotor symptoms. Some of these symptoms may be more subtle than others. Understandably, many will not be forthcoming in the typical initial encounter in which more troublesome motor symptoms usually dominate the visit. Some need to be elicited by careful inquiry on the part of the medical caregiver. Symptom questionnaires may be especially useful in gathering symptoms that can be returned to in subsequent visits. Knowledge and understanding of Parkinson's disease is growing exponentially. This volume establishes the baseline of current knowledge and undoubtedly will stimulate further fruitful inquiry in the field.

1. Lang AE, Obeso JA. Challenges in Parkinson's disease: restoration of the nigrostriatal dopamine system is not enough. Lancet 2004; 3:309–316.

Daniel Tarsy, *MD*
Parkinson's Disease & Movement Disorders Center
Beth Israel Deaconess Medical Center
Harvard Medical School
Boston, MA

Preface

The idea that Parkinson's disease (PD) is characterized only by such motor features as tremor, rigidity, bradykinesia, and postural instability is deeply embedded not only in the minds of patients and their family members, but also in the training and practice of many physicians. However, even a quick perusal of the amazingly perceptive clinical description that James Parkinson put to paper in 1817 reveals that from the beginning, various features not reflective of motor dysfunction were recognized and described as being part of PD. It has only been relatively recently that attention has been refocused on these nonmotor features, and the realization has grown that nonmotor features are frequently present in PD and can be the source of considerable discomfort and disability for affected individuals. In fact, it is not at all infrequent that these nonmotor features play a dominant role in the clinical picture.

The growing recognition that nonmotor features are an important component of PD has, in turn, led to the realization that these aspects of the condition have often received insufficient attention in the current medical and lay literature. This volume on *Parkinson's Disease and Nonmotor Dysfunction* is an attempt to at least partially correct that deficiency and provide a source of detailed information describing and explaining these nonmotor features that can be readily accessed by the practicing physician. To this end, a truly outstanding group of experienced researchers and clinicians has been assembled to provide this in-depth review of nonmotor dysfunction in PD, which has been subdivided into five diverse domains.

Behavioral abnormalities are problems encountered in the management of PD, particularly in individuals with more advanced disease, which are both distressingly frequent and frequently distressing. They may be intrinsic components of the disease process itself (depression and dementia), treatment-induced complications (psychosis and postsurgical behavioral changes), or a combination of both (anxiety, obsessionality). Whatever their derivation, behavioral abnormalities can seriously impact and impair quality of life for both patients and family members.

Autonomic dysfunction is often mistakenly considered to be a feature of multiple system atrophy and not PD. In reality, individuals with PD can, and frequently do, display various features indicative of autonomic dysfunction. Gastrointestinal, urogenital, cardiorespiratory, thermoregulatory, and other aspects of autonomic function may become impaired in PD, not simply as consequences of medication-induced derangements, but as part of the disease process itself. These autonomic features often develop in the later stages of the illness but may also appear early, occasionally even before the classic motor components become evident.

Sleep-related dysfunction can be a source of considerable consternation, not only to patients but also to their family members, who often suffer the indirect, and sometimes the direct (at least in the setting of rapid eye movement sleep behavior disorder), consequences of the patient's sleep disturbance. As with behavioral and autonomic dysfunction, sleep-related disturbances can be either disease-related or medication-induced and may occur both early and later in the course of PD.

Sensory dysfunction is perhaps the least well-known or recognized and also the most purely nonmotor facet of nonmotor dysfunction in PD. Abnormalities of primary sensory function (vision and olfaction) occur, as do more complex sensory phenomena, as exemplified by the visuo-cognitive deficits and the various pain syndromes and disorders of sensation that may plague the patient with PD.

Finally, a section of this volume is devoted to several problems (oculomotor dysfunction and fatigue) that tread on, or perhaps cross over, the line between motor and nonmotor dysfunction in PD. However, they are included here because they often are not covered extensively in the more traditional discussions of the motor features of PD.

It is our hope that this collection of contributions by a truly tremendous contingent of authors will serve to increase awareness of the contributions that nonmotor features may make to the collective clinical picture experienced by the patient with PD. Early recognition of these features will lead, we hope, to more prompt and effective treatment of them, a goal that can be firmly shared and appreciated by both patient and physician alike.

Ronald F. Pfeiffer, MD
Ivan Bodis-Wollner, MD, DSc

Contents

Contributors

ANDREA ANTAL, PhD • Department of Clinical Neurophysiology, Georg-August University of Göttingen, Göttingen, Germany
IVAN BODIS-WOLLNER, MD, DSc • Departments of Neurology and Ophthalmology, State University of New York, Downstate Medical Center, Brooklyn, NY
DARYL BOHAC, PhD • Department of Psychiatry, University of Nebraska Medical Center, Omaha, NE
MARIE-ANDRÉE BRUNEAU, MD, FRCP(C), MSc • Department of Psychiatry, University of Montreal, Montréal, Québec, Canada
WILLIAM J. BURKE, MD • Department of Psychiatry, University of Nebraska Medical Center, Omaha, NE
CHERYL M. CARLUCCI, MD • Department of Neurology, University of South Florida, Tampa, FL
CYNTHIA COMELLA, MD • Department of Neurological Sciences, Rush University Medical Center, Chicago, IL
STEWART A. FACTOR, DO • Department of Neurology, Albany Medical College, Albany, NY
HUBERT H. FERNANDEZ, MD • Department of Clinical Neurosciences, Brown University School of Medicine, Providence, RI
BLAIR FORD, MD, FRCP(C) • Department of Neurology, Columbia University, New York, NY
JOSEPH H. FRIEDMAN, MD • Department of Clinical Neurosciences, Brown University School of Medicine, Providence, RI
STEVEN J. FRUCHT, MD • Department of Neurology, Columbia University, New York, NY
SARAH FURTADO, MD, PhD, FRCP(C) • Department of Clinical Neurosciences, University of Calgary, Calgary, Alberta, Canada
CAROL EWING GARBER, PhD • Department of Cardiopulmonary and Exercise Sciences, Bouvé College of Health Sciences, Northeastern University, Boston, MA
NIR GILADI, MD • Department of Neurology, Tel-Aviv Sourasky Medical Center, Tel-Aviv, Israel
DAVID S. GOLDSTEIN, MD, PhD • Clinical Neurocardiology Section, National Institute of Neurological Disorders and Stroke, National Institutes of Health, Bethesda, MD
TANYA GUREVICH, MD • Department of Neurology, Tel-Aviv Sourasky Medical Center, Tel-Aviv, Israel
DAVID HARDESTY, MD • Department of Neurology, Columbia University, New York, NY
ROBERT A. HAUSER, MD • Department of Neurology, University of South Florida, Tampa, FL
PATRICIA KAVANAGH, MD, MBA • Department of Neurology, Columbia University College of Physicians & Surgeons, New York, NY
CHRISTOPHER KENNARD, MBBS, PHD, FRCP, FMedSci • Division of Neuroscience and Psychological Medicine, Imperial College, London, England, UK
AMOS D. KORCZYN, MD • Department of Neurology, Tel-Aviv University Medical School, Tel-Aviv, Israel
MARK S. LEDOUX, MD, PhD • Departments of Neurology and Anatomy & Neurobiology, University of Tennessee Health Science Center, Memphis, TN
NORMAN A. LEOPOLD, DO • Department of Neurology, Drexel University School of Medicine, Philadelphia, PA
JOHN A. LUCAS, PhD • Department of Psychiatry and Psychology, Mayo Clinic in Jacksonville, Jacksonville, FL

KAREN MARDER, MD, MPH • Department of Neurology, Columbia University College of Physicians & Surgeons, New York, NY
ERIC S. MOLHO, MD • Department of Neurology, Albany Medical College, Albany, NY
MARIA L. MORO-DE-CASILLAS, MD • Department of Neurology, University Hospitals of Cleveland and Case Western Reserve University School of Medicine, Cleveland, OH
PARASHKEV NACHEV, MA, BM, BCh, MRCP(UK) • Division of Neuroscience and Psychological Medicine, Imperial College, London, England, UK
RONALD F. PFEIFFER, MD • Department of Neurology, University of Tennessee Health Science Center, Memphis, TN
DAVID E. RILEY, MD • Department of Neurology, University Hospitals of Cleveland and Case Western Reserve University School of Medicine, Cleveland, OH
LAURIE M. RILLING, PhD • Department of Psychiatry and Psychology, Mayo Clinic in Jacksonville, Jacksonville, FL
ROBERT L. RODNITZKY, MD • Department of Neurology, Roy J. and Lucile A. Carver University of Iowa College of Medicine, Iowa City, IA
HOLLY A. SHILL, MD • Department of Neurology, Barrow Neurological Institute, Phoenix, AZ
TANYA SIMUNI, MD • Department of Neurology, Northwestern University Feinberg School of Medicine, Chicago, IL
CARLOS SINGER, MD • Department of Neurology, University of Miami School of Medicine, Miami, FL
JANICE SMOLOWITZ, RN, EdD, ANP • Department of Clinical Nursing, Columbia University, New York, NY
SUZANNE STEVENS, MD • Departments of Neurology and Psychology, Rush University Medical Center, Chicago, IL
DANIEL TARSY, MD • Department of Neurology, Beth Israel-Deaconess Medical Center and Harvard Medical School, Boston, MA
RYAN J. UITTI, MD • Department of Neurology, Mayo Clinic in Jacksonville, Jacksonville, FL
DARYL VICTOR, MD • Department of Neurology, Columbia University, New York, NY
CHERYL WATERS, MD, FRCP(C) • Department of Neurology, Columbia University, New York, NY
STEVEN P. WENGEL, MD • Department of Psychiatry, University of Nebraska Medical Center, Omaha, NE
ZBIGNIEW K. WSZOLEK, MD • Department of Neurology, Mayo Clinic in Jacksonville, Jacksonville, FL

I Behavioral Dysfunction in Parkinson's Disease

1
Depression

William J. Burke, Steven P. Wengel, and Daryl Bohac

SUMMARY

Depression is the most common psychological disturbance that affects people with Parkinson's disease (PD). Despite an increasing amount of research devoted to this topic, uncertainty still exists concerning many aspects of depression in PD. Significant questions remain regarding some very basic issues, including how best to diagnose depression in PD, how frequently depression complicates PD, the risk factors for developing depression, and how to best treat depression. This chapter provides a current perspective on what is known about depression in PD, reviewing its epidemiology, clinical features, neuropsychological features, and treatment. Rather than providing a comprehensive overview, the focus here is on updating the major themes of research in this field.

Key Words: Parkinson's disease; depression; dysthymia; mania; mesocortical limbic pathway; selective serotonin reuptake inhibitor; electroconvulsive therapy.

1. INTRODUCTION

The most common psychological problem that affects those with Parkinson's disease (PD) is depression. However, doubt still remains with several factors of depression in PD, despite the growing research pertaining to this topic. This chapter provides the present knowledge about depression in PD, describing its epidemiology, clinical and neuropsychological features, and treatment.

2. DEPRESSION IN PD

2.1. *Prevalence*

Even ostensibly simple questions can be difficult to answer concerning the understanding of depression in PD. How frequently depression occurs in persons with PD is a striking example. Depending on the population studied and method used, reported rates of depression have varied enormously. An overall depression rate of 43% is one of the most commonly cited figures *(1)*. Approximately half of these cases involve patients with major depressive disorder, and the other half involves minor depression or dysthymia. Studies that have reported high rates have generally used specialty populations, in contrast to community-based samples, where lower rates have been found.

Tandberg et al. *(2)* carefully assessed depressive symptoms in patients with PD as part of a wider prevalence study of PD. They found that 7.7% of community-dwelling patients met Diagnostic and Statistical Manual of Mental Disorders (DSM-III) criteria *(3)* for major depressive disorder (MDD). In addition to examining categorical depression, they also obtained information on depressive symptoms using the Montgomery-Åsberg depression rating scale (MADRS; *4*). According to MADRS, only 5.1% of patients were moderately to severely depressed, but 45.5% had mild depres-

From: *Current Clinical Neurology*
Parkinson's Disease and Nonmotor Dysfunction
Edited by: R. F. Pfeiffer and I. Bodis-Wollner © Humana Press Inc., Totowa, NJ

sive symptoms. Also, the rate of major depression was strongly impacted by cognitive impairment as defined by the Mini-Mental State Exam (MMSE) score *(5)*. Rates of MDD were 3.6% in patients with an MMSE score greater than 20 but increased to 25.6% in patients whose MMSE score was below 20. Interestingly, rates were also higher in those with possible PD (18.8%) versus those with probable PD (4.6%). The authors attribute these figures to a higher rate of dementia in those with possible PD and suggest that the higher rates in the cognitively impaired indicate more widespread cerebral involvement *(2)*.

The low rates of depression found by Tandberg et al. are similar to those from another study that used structured interviews to analyze all cognitively intact patients with PD in the community who reported depressive symptoms in the General Health Questionnaire (GHQ; *6,7*). Although depressive symptoms in the GHQ occurred in 34.2% of patients with PD only 2.7% met criteria for MDD.

A bimodal distribution has been suggested for the onset of depression in PD *(8–10)*. One peak seems to follow diagnosis and may be related to left hemisphere dysfunction, whereas the second peak occurs late in the course of PD and may be associated with impaired activities of daily living *(8)*. Some evidence also suggests that depression in PD is more common in younger patients *(11)*, females *(12,13)*, and in those with more bradykinesia and rigidity (as opposed to tremor dominance; *14–16*).

2.2. Diagnostic Difficulties

An issue that contributes to the diverse findings in the frequency and severity of depression is the process of diagnosis. DSM-IV criteria *(17)* can be difficult to apply to patients with PD because only symptoms that are not a result of a general medical condition or direct physiological effect of a substance (e.g., medication) are counted. In PD, this presents obvious problems, particularly when deciding about the DSM-IV "somatic" symptoms, such as psychomotor change and sleep, appetite/weight, and energy disturbance. If the "exclusive" directions of DSM-IV are followed, many patients will end up without a mood disorder diagnosis despite appearing to meet criteria for major depression.

The difficulty inherent in assigning causality has led to alternative approaches like counting symptoms as present or absent (regardless of presumed causality—an "inclusive approach"), focusing only on the more "psychological symptoms" of depression or including additional nonsomatic symptoms to supplement the mood assessment.

Leentjens et al. *(18)* addressed this subject by viewing the sensitivity of individual depressive symptoms and their relative contribution to the diagnosis of depression in patients with PD. They examined the individual items of the Hamilton *(19)* and MADRS in a discriminate analysis. Not surprisingly, nonsomatic symptoms were the most discriminating, but somatic symptoms also had meaningful contributions. Specifically, reduced appetite and awakening in early morning were relatively low-prevalence symptoms that proved useful in supporting a diagnosis of depression, whereas other somatic symptoms were not.

It is also important to consider the impact of dementia on the diagnosis of depression, because rates of depression may be higher in the cognitively impaired patient with PD. Dementia can complicate the evaluation process in several ways. First, as discussed previously, several symptoms of dementia overlap with depression. DSM symptoms that tend to lose specificity when confronted with mild cognitive impairment include loss of interest, decreased energy, psychomotor changes, and decreased concentration. Also, as cognitive impairment progresses, it becomes increasingly difficult to recognize a depressive disorder because of the difficulty in accessing the individual's internal affective state.

Depression itself has been proposed as a preliminary symptom of PD. This association is supported by a retrospective study that compares the number of contacts with a general practitioner between persons who developed PD and a control group. There were substantially more visits to the general practitioner in the 2 years preceding diagnosis in the developing PD group, and many of these visits were for mood disorders *(20)*. In another study, patients with a diagnosis of MDD were shown to have more than a twofold risk of receiving a diagnosis of PD when compared to a control group of patients with osteoarthritis *(21)*.

With the preponderance of clinical studies that show elevated rates of depression in patients with PD, a critical issue arises in whether these rates are higher in patients with PD in comparison to those with other chronic illnesses. If depression is more common in patients with PD, a pathophysiological link between the conditions is implied.

Several medical illnesses have been associated with depression, yet often the nature of the relationship is unclear. Krishnan et al. *(22)* described the difficulty in establishing causal relationships in comorbid illnesses. They suggested that this effort is particularly difficult in later life because the lifetime prevalence of all conditions is steady or increases with age. As such, there is a tendency to find a correlation between virtually all conditions. This "pseudo-correlation" is particularly observed in disorders where frequency increases with age, such as PD, Alzheimer's disease, and cardiovascular disease. Consequently, many of these associations may be only a statistical artifact and not clinically relevant *(22)*.

A recent study using the Danish Psychiatric Central Register and Danish National Hospital Register attempted to answer the question of whether patients with PD are at an increased risk of developing depression when compared to those with other medical illnesses *(23)*. These authors determined the rates of initial admissions for depression in patients with PD, diabetes, and osteoarthritis. They found an increased incidence of depression in patients with PD versus those with the other conditions who had comparable degrees of disability. The risk of receiving a diagnosis of depression was highest in the 6-months of follow-up diagnosis of PD but remained elevated 1 year later, although to a lesser extent. The authors conclude that these findings support the theory that depression is not simply a psychological reaction to PD but that a common pathophysiology underlies these conditions *(23)*. A major limitation of this study is that it captures only a small portion of patients with PD who have depression severe enough to warrant hospitalization.

2.3. Risk Factors

Many attempts have been made to identify risk factors for the development of depression in PD. However, these efforts generally have failed to consider factors known to predispose people to depression in general. Accordingly, Leentjens et al. *(24)* first considered general risk factors for depression (e.g., age, sex, prior history of depression, family history of depression, and somatic comorbidity) in a PD population and found that these five risk factors predicted 75% of depression in their sample using a multivariate model. When disease-specific markers were then included in the model, only the right-sided onset of PD improved the model. Thus, established risk factors for depression generally may also be markers of depression in PD.

2.4. Etiology

Significant attention has been given to attributing depression to either psychological or biological sources. This is a hollow effort, if only because biology of necessity underlies psychology. However, Brown and Jahanshahi *(10)* provided a summary of the role of psychosocial factors that may contribute to depression in PD. They concluded that certain patients are more vulnerable to depression, including: (a) those who have an early age of onset; (b) patients in the earliest stages of disease; (c) those with more advanced disease; (d) and those with more rapidly progressive deterioration. Although only a weak association has been generally reported between depression in PD and severity of illness, they suggest a crucial related factor is the rate at which disability progresses. Those patients whose disability progresses slowly enough for them to adapt may show slight depression or recover from a prior depression. Those with a more rapid progression may fail to adapt as easily and are then at higher risk of developing depression.

These authors also raise the question of why patients with apparently similar levels of physical illness and disability have distinctively different affective states. Factors that seem to explain some of this variability are the availability and quantity of social support, as well as the strategies that individuals use to cope with stress. Patients who have good social support, who are satisfied with that support, and who have good self-esteem and active coping mechanisms appear to be at lower risk for depression *(10,25)*.

2.5. Pathology

Regarding the contribution of biology to depression in PD, it is worth noting the fascinating case of a 65-year-old woman with a 30-year history of PD who developed acute depression during high-frequency deep-brain stimulation (DBS) *(26)*. This woman went from a euthymic state to one of acute depression when her left basal ganglia was stimulated 2 mm below the site where stimulation relieved the signs of PD. The authors suggest that stimulation may have affected the activity of nigra γ-aminobutyric acid (GABA)ergic neurons innervating the ventral nuclei of the thalamus with projections to the prefrontal and orbitofrontal cortexes. This is an interesting region because disruption of connections between the basal ganglia and frontal cortex has been reported to have a role in stroke-related depression, and disruption of these pathways by vascular disease has been proposed as an etiology for late-life depression *(27)*.

Other neuropathological findings that may contribute to depression in PD are the degeneration of dopaminergic, serotonergic, noradrenergic, and cholinergic nuclei in the brainstem *(28)*. Neuronal loss in the locus coeruleus in PD may be even more severe than in the substantia nigra *(29)*. A specific pathway that may be an important factor is the mesocortical limbic pathway, which arises in the ventromedial tegmental area and projects to areas critical for effect, such as the cingulate, entorhinal, and orbitofrontal cortex, as well as the subcortical portions of the limbic forebrain *(30,31)*. This pathway has been shown to be disrupted in patients with depression and PD. Additionally, positron emission tomography studies have demonstrated hypometabolism in the cingulate and frontal cortex in depressed PD patients when compared with controls *(32)*.

3. THE INTERPLAY OF MOOD AND COGNITION IN PARKINSON'S DISEASE

3.1. Background

Cognitive impairments in PD are common and vary in severity. The most commonly affected areas are free recall of previously learned information, visuospatial skills, and executive functions, such as problem-solving, planning, and flexibility *(32)*. The overlap in the effects of depression and PD on cognitive functioning is substantial. Consequently, the ability of the clinician to pinpoint the independent impact can be challenging.

3.2. Depression and Cognition

The depressed patient often presents in a hesitant manner and may appear to give up easily while undergoing cognitive testing *(34,35)*. For example, an initial response to questions designed to tap into the patient's knowledge about common objects, events, and people might be "I don't know." However, when encouraged to try answering the question, the depressed patient will often provide a correct response. Moreover, depressed patients are often inconsistent in their responses. They may appropriately answer the first three items from the same test described previously, miss the next one, answer the following two questions correctly, miss the next two, and so on. This style of responding often leads to depressed patients scoring lower than normal controls on cognitive measures.

Rosenstein *(36)* offered these general guidelines regarding the cognitive functioning of the depressed patient: (a) memory and attention, although often slightly below expectation, are usually not in the impaired range; (b) language functioning is nearly always normal, as are intellectual functioning and visuospatial functioning; (c) psychomotor functions are often within normal limits, but slightly below expectation; (d) and finally, the efficiency of executive functions appears to be reduced in the depressed patient. For example, how easily patients can shift cognitive sets may be slowed, but their performances are often still within normal limits.

3.3. PD and Cognition

Cognition is quite variable in PD. Some patients may present with dementia that can easily be quantified with neuropsychological tests; others may have little or no cognitive impairment on routine neuropsychological tests; however, most will present with a pattern of cognitive impairment that does not rise to the level of dementia *(37)*. Moreover, a number of mediating variables that also can influence cognitive functioning occur in patients with PD. These variables include the age of the patient, as well as the age of onset, motor symptom severity, side of onset, and medication effects *(38)*. Generally, a higher incidence of cognitive impairment and dementia can be expected with a later age of onset.

Overall, patients with PD demonstrate various areas of impaired neurocognitive functioning. Memory performance is characterized by inconsistent learning throughout trials and impaired free recall following delay, combined with normal recognition memory. In fact, the ability of the patient with PD is often near normal for verbal learning, but free retrieval of the previously learned information is inefficient. In contrast, when procedural learning or implicit memory is assessed, patients with PD demonstrate poor ability to acquire and retain new skills.

Attention and concentration abilities are impaired in the PD patient. However, with most measures of simple memory (e.g., digit span forward) they perform normally. It is when attentional complexity is increased that deficits may appear, and this is likely related to decreased executive functioning in the patient with PD. Complex attention is mediated by frontal systems. Bondi et al. *(39)* have shown that nondemented patients with PD have frontal system impairments, including problems with cognitive flexibility, planning, temporal ordering, and verbal fluency.

Language abilities are largely intact, but if deficits do occur, it is often in the area of verbal fluency. As disease severity increases, complex language comprehension may become impaired, perhaps secondary to slowed speed of information processing. Because language skills often are well-retained over the course of disease, verbal intellectual functioning remains largely stable. In contrast, performance-based intellect, with its emphasis on speed of performance and visuospatial analysis, is frequently impaired relative to verbal IQ.

3.4. PD and Depression

Mild depression or dysthymia probably does not significantly impact cognition in PD. However, as the severity of depression increases, the likelihood that it will impact cognition increases. Recently, Norman et al. *(40)* demonstrated that depressed patients with PD perform worse with measures of memory when compared to nondepressed patients with PD. Moreover, depressed patients with PD had memory impairment similar to depressed patients without PD. Thus, the authors postulated that the memory dysfunction noted in their patients was owing to depression alone.

The relationship between depression and PD and its influence on cognition is not well-understood. Nevertheless, depression and PD do appear to have individual, as well as overlapping, influences on cognitive functioning. In the case of the nondemented patient with PD who becomes depressed, the additive effect of depression on executive functioning alone, much less memory, may lead one to suspect the patient has developed dementia. However, it is more likely that the cognitive dysfunction associated with PD alone is now exacerbated by the depression. A patient with mildly impaired cognitive flexibility prior to the onset of depression may now appear moderately impaired. Additionally, memory functioning may be significantly worse because of encoding and consolidation problems; consequently, the ability to even recognize previously learned information is reduced. Thus, timely treatment of depression in the patient with PD may help to reduce the risk of developing excess disability, thereby helping to maintain a better quality of life.

4. MOOD EFFECTS OF PD TREATMENT

4.1. Depression

Conflicting reports exist for the effects of antiparkinsonian drugs on depressive symptoms. One explanation for this is that most studies of these agents have been designed to monitor the effects of drugs on motor symptoms instead of mood. Since the 1970s, levodopa has been reported to cause affective changes; both improvement and worsening of depressive symptoms have been noted. Some estimate the prevalence of levodopa-induced depressive symptoms is approximately 12% *(41)*. Alternatively, levodopa has also been reported to produce mild improvement in depressive symptoms, possibly from improvement in motor symptoms rather than a true antidepressant effect *(41)*. Other agents, including bromocriptine and pergolide, have also been associated with depressive symptoms in patients with PD. Overall, Factor and colleagues conclude that "depression in PD patients more accurately reflects an issue of comorbidity rather than one of medication-induced side effects" *(41)*.

Subthalamic DBS (STN-DBS) has been reported to cause depressive symptoms in 6 of 24 consecutive patients with PD *(42)*. Three of the six patients became transiently suicidal. In five of the six patients, depressive symptoms began within the first month postoperatively. All six required treatment with antidepressants (AD).

4.2. Mania

Dopaminergic agents have been reported to cause manic symptoms, such as extreme optimism, spending sprees, and euphoria. Originally reported to occur in 1.5% of levodopa-treated patients *(41)*, manic symptoms have also been reported in patients treated with other dopaminergic agents. Bromocriptine has been reported to produce mania in patients with PD, particularly at higher doses, and also in patients without PD, such as postpartum women taking the drug to suppress lactation *(41)*. Manic symptoms were reported to begin within the first week of treatment and resolved upon discontinuation of the drug. Selegiline has also been implicated in producing these symptoms *(41)*. Unlike depressive symptoms, manic symptoms do not seem to occur in untreated patients with PD, but appear to be a consequence of the treatment of PD symptoms.

Interestingly, although DBS has been implicated in causing depressive symptoms (*see* Subheading 4.1.), there have been cases of mania associated with this treatment as well *(43)*. Three of 15 consecutive patients undergoing STN-DBS developed manic symptoms after stimulation was initiated, and in the three cases, mania resolved after the stimulation was changed from the lower two electrodes to the higher pair of electrodes. The authors suggest that DBS may have triggered mania through stimulation of midbrain projections to the orbitofrontal or anterior cingulate striato-pallido-thalamo-cortical circuits.

5. TREATMENT OF DEPRESSION IN PD

5.1. Maximize Antiparkinsonian Therapy

Many patients with PD report that their mood symptoms fluctuate in concert with their motor symptoms. That is, when "off" motorically, they may experience fairly abrupt dysphoric episodes. In this case, the most appropriate treatment is to optimize PD therapy first rather than adding an antidepressant *(44,45)*. In fact, one author suggested that "optimized dopaminergic therapy is a prerequisite for a successful management of depression—particularly in patients with fluctuating PD" *(46)*.

5.2. Use of Antidepressant Drugs

As in other depressive syndromes, the depression associated with PD appears to respond to conventional AD drugs. However, there still has not been a randomized, placebo-controlled trial demonstrating treatment efficacy in PD *(47)*. As the locus ceruleus and raphe nuclei are affected by the disease, levels of norepinephrine and serotonin may decrease as the illness progresses. Therefore, the use of agents to ameliorate the deficiency states of these neurotransmitters seems reasonable. However, several caveats apply when treating depressed patients with PD. First, they may be susceptible to motor side effects of agents that do not ordinarily affect the motor systems of patients with PD. Second, patients with PD may be very sensitive to side effects that other patients might not find objectionable, such as anticholinergic side effects and orthostatic hypotension. Lastly, there are several important drug–drug interactions that need to be noted when using ADs in patients with PD. These issues will be discussed in the following sections.

5.3. Selective Serotonin Reuptake Inhibitors

Selective serotonin reuptake inhibitors (SSRIs) are frequently prescribed for patients with PD as first-line therapy. As a class, SSRIs have numerous attractive features. Dosing is fairly straightforward, with once-daily administration usually being adequate. Additionally, titration is often unnecessary, because the starting dose may also be the therapeutic dose for many patients. SSRIs virtually never cause orthostatic hypotension and rarely produce anticholinergic side effects, with the exception of paroxetine. However, they may have an antagonistic effect on dopamine *(44)*. Case reports have been published of patients with PD, who experience a decline of motor symptoms when an SSRI was added to their regimen, although this is a relatively uncommon phenomenon. In an open trial of paroxetine, Ceravolo and colleagues *(48)* found no reduction of motor scores overall, but did describe 1 of 33 subjects who experienced a worsening of tremor while taking paroxetine. This reaction was completely reversed upon discontinuation of the drug. Also uncommon, but concerning, is the possibility of inducing the "serotonin syndrome" if an SSRI is prescribed to a patient already taking selegiline *(49)*. Symptoms of the serotonin syndrome include myoclonus, delirium, tremors, fever, hyperreflexia, and diaphoresis *(46)*.

5.4. Mirtazapine

Mirtazapine is a non-SSRI AD that is an antagonist of α-2 noradrenergic autoreceptors and serotonin-2 and -3 receptors, appearing to be well-tolerated in patients with PD. At lower doses (<30 mg/day), it has prominent sedative and appetite-stimulating effects. Mirtazapine is usually given at bedtime owing to sedation. However, a recent case series reported four patients with PD who developed sleep-related behavioral problems, including nocturnal confusion, talking during sleep, and hallucinations while taking mirtazapine *(50)*. In three of these patients, the dose prescribed was 30 mg at bedtime; the fourth patient was taking 15 mg at bedtime. These symptoms resolved when mirtazapine was discontinued.

5.5. Bupropion

Bupropion is a novel AD whose therapeutic mode of action is unknown. Although not proven, it is hypothesized to have pro-dopaminergic effects. It is usually well-tolerated in patients with PD and does not produce orthostatic hypotension. In fact, it may raise blood pressure in some patients. It tends to be more "activating" than many other antidepressants and may therefore ameliorate fatigue. It is usually dosed twice a day, with the time of the second administration adjusted to avoid causing or aggravating insomnia.

5.6. Venlafaxine

Venlafaxine has a dual mechanism of action. At doses up to 150 mg per day, it functions much like an SSRI. At higher doses, it also acts as a norepinephrine reuptake inhibitor. Like most antidepressants, no controlled trials have been done with venlafaxine in patients with PD. In clinical practice, it appears to be well-tolerated in this population.

5.7. Tricyclic Antidepressants

Once the mainstay of treatment for depression, tricyclic antidepressants (TCAs) have had a great decrease in use since the advent of newer ADs. However, they still play a role, particularly for those patients who have not responded to several adequate trials of other ADs. Of the available TCAs, nortriptyline is preferred because of its lower risk of orthostatic hypotension and anticholinergic side effects. It may be started at 10 to 25 mg at bedtime, with gradual titration up to 75 mg per day based on clinical response and serum levels. Orthostatic hypotension is still a potential side effect; patients with PD are more vulnerable to this, as a consequence of both the disease itself and dopaminergic therapy. Patients should be counseled to consume adequate fluids and exercise special care when rising from a chair or a bed.

5.8. Testosterone

A case series described five men with PD who complained of fatigue, depression, anxiety, and sexual dysfunction. They were found to have low levels of free testosterone but responded to topical testosterone gel *(51)*.

5.9. Electroconvulsive Therapy

Electroconvulsive therapy (ECT) has been reported to improve not only mood but motor symptoms in depressed PD patients *(52)*. It also decreases "off" time in patients with PD who have severe on–off phenomenon who are not depressed *(53)*. These beneficial effects are transient, typically lasting several weeks. Thus, for the motor improvement to be maintained, ECT would need to be administered at least monthly. Although effective for depressive symptoms in this population, ECT may cause delirium in susceptible individuals. It may also contribute to an increase in dyskinesia or even psychotic symptoms in patients with PD, perhaps from an increase in permeability of the blood–brain barrier. If either of these symptoms are seen during a course of ECT in a patient with PD, the antiparkinsonian medication doses should be reduced by approximately one-third.

5.10. Psychosocial Treatment

Although ADs are effective and often necessary for treating depression in patients with PD, psychosocial interventions should not be neglected. Psychotherapy can be very helpful for cognitively intact patients with PD, and may be the most helpful for those demonstrating depressive symptoms at the time of diagnosis *(46)*. Because PD is a chronic, progressive illness, helping patients develop coping strategies and providing support is beneficial. Involving the spouse in the treatment plan is recommended, as the spouse is often the key support person for the patient. Support groups should be strongly recommended as they may provide an excellent form of encouragement for both the patient and family.

REFERENCES

1. Cummings JL. Depression and Parkinson's disease: a review. Am J Psychiatry 1992;149:443–454.
2. Tandberg E, Larsen JP, Aarsland D, Cummings JL. The occurrence of depression inParkinson's disease. A community-based study. Arch Neurol 1996;53:175–179.
3. American Psychiatric Association. Diagnostic and Statistical Manual of Mental Disorder, 3rd ed. American Psychiatric Association, Washington, DC, 1980.
4. Montgomery SA, Asberg M. A new depression scale designed to be sensitive to change. Br J Psychiatry 1979;134:382–389.
5. Folstein MF, Folstein SE, McHugh PR. "Mini-Mental State": a practical method for grading the cognitive state of patients for the clinician. J Psychiatr Res 1975;12:189–198.
6. Goldberg DP, William P. A User's Guide to the General Health Questionnaire. NFER-Nelson, Windsor, 1988.
7. Hantz P, Caradoc-Davies G, Caradoc-Davies T, et al. Depression in Parkinson's disease. Am J Psychiatry 1994;151:1010–1014.
8. Starkstein SE, Preziosi TJ, Bolduc PL, Robinson RG. Depression in Parkinson's disease. J Nerv Ment Dis 1990;178:27–31.
9. Celesia GG, Wanamaker WM. Psychiatric disturbances in Parkinson's disease. Dis Nerv Syst 1976;37:123–125.
10. Brown R, Jahanshahi M. Depression in Parkinson's disease: a psychosocial viewpoint. Adv Neurol 1995;65:61–84.

11. Starkstein SE, Berthier ML, Bolduc PL, et al. Depression in patients with early versus late onset Parkinson's disease. Neurology 1989;39:1441–1445.
12. Gotham AM, Brown RG, Marsden CD. Depression in Parkinson's disease: a quantitative and qualitative analysis. J Neurol Neurosurg Psychiatry 1986;49:381–389.
13. Brown RC, MacCarthy B. Psychiatric morbidity in patients with Parkinson's disease. Psychol Med 1990;20:77–87.
14. Huber SJ, Paulson GW, Shuttleworth EC. Depression in Parkinson's disease. Neuropsychiatry Neuropsychol Behav Neurol 1988;1:47–51.
15. Jankovic J, McDermott M, Carter J, et al. Parkinson Study Group. Variable expression of Parkinson's disease: a baseline analysis of the DATATOP cohort. Neurology 1990;40:1529–1534.
16. Brown GL, Wilson WP. Parkinsonism and depression. South Med J 1972;65:540–545.
17. American Psychiatric Association. Diagnostic and Statistical Manual of Mental Disorders, 4th ed. American Psychiatric Association, Washington, DC, 1994.
18. Leentjens AFG, Marinus J, Van Hilten JJ, et al. The contribution of somatic symptoms to the diagnosis of depressive disorder in Parkinson's disease: a discriminant analytic approach. J Neuropsychiatry Clin Neurosci 2003;15:74–77.
19. Hamilton M. A rating scale for depression. J Neurol Neurosurg Psychiatry 1960;23:56–62.
20. Gonera EG, van't Hof M, Berger HJ, et al. Symptoms and duration of the prodromal phase in Parkinson's disease. Mov Disord 1997;12:871–876.
21. Nilsson FM, Kessing LV, Bolwig TC. Increased risk of developing Parkinson's disease for patients with major affective disorder-a register study. Acta Psychiatr Scand 2001;104:380–386.
22. Krishnan KR, Delong M, Kraemer H, et al. Comorbidity of depression with other medical diseases in the elderly. Biol Psychiatry 2002;52:559–588.
23. Nilsson FM, Kessing LV, Sorensen TM, et al. Major depressive disorder in Parkinson's disease: a register-based study. Acta Psychiatr Scand 2002;106:202–211.
24. Leentjens AFG, Lousberg R, Verhey FJR. Markers for depression in Parkinson's disease. Acta Psychiatr Scand 2002;106:196–201.
25. MacCarthy B, Brown RG. Psychosocial factors in Parkinson's disease. Br J Clin Psychol 1989;28:41–52.
26. Bejjani BP, Damier P, Arnulf I, et al. Transient acute depression induced by high-frequency deep-brain stimulation. N Engl J Med 1999;340:1476–1480.
27. Alexopoulos G, Kiosses D, Klimstra S, Kalayam B, Bruce M. Clinical presentation of the "depression-executive dysfunction syndrome" of late life. Am J Geriatr Psychiatry 2002;10:98–106.
28. Oertel WH, Hoglinger GU, Caraceni T, et al. Depression in Parkinson's disease. Adv Neurol 2001;86:373–383.
29. Zarow C, Lyness SA, Mortimer JA, Chui HC. Neuronal loss is greater in the locus coeruleus than nucleus basalis and substantia nigra in Alzheimer and Parkinson Diseases. Arch Neurol 2003;60:337–341.
30. Price KS, Farley IJ, Hornykiewicz O. Neurochemistry of Parkinson's disease: relationbetween striatal and limbic dopamine. Adv Biochem Psychopharmacol 1978;19:293–300.
31. Javoy-Agid F, Agid Y. Is the mesocortical dopaminergic system involved in Parkinson's disease? Neurology 1980;30:1326–1330.
32. Baxter LR, Jr., Schwartz JM, Phelps ME, et al. Reduction of prefrontal cortex glucose metabolism common to three types of depression. Arch Gen Psychiatry 1989;46:243–250.
33. Huber SJ, Bornstein RA. Neuropsychological evaluation of Parkinson's disease. In: Huber SJ, Cummings JL, eds. Parkinson's Disease: Neurobehavioral Aspects. Oxford University Press, New York, 1989, pp. 32–45.
34. desRosiers G. Primary or depressive dementia: Mental status screening. Int J Neurosci 1992;64:33–67.
35. LaRue A. Aging and Neuropsychological Assessment. Plenum, New York, 1992, pp. 259–289.
36. Rosenstein LD. Differential diagnosis of the major progressive dementias and depression in middle and late adulthood: A summary of the literature of the early 1990s. Neuropsychol Rev 1998;8:109–167.
37. Mahurin RK, Feher EP, Nance ML, et al. Cognition in Parkinson's disease and related disorders. In: Parks RW, Zec RF, Wilson RS, eds. Neuropsychology of Alzheimer's Disease and Other Dementias. Oxford University Press, New York, 1993, pp. 308–349.
38. Levin BE, Katzen HL. Early cognitive changes and nondementing behavioral abnormalities in Parkinson's disease. Adv Neurol 1995;65:85–95.
39. Bondi MW, Kaszniak AW, Bayles KA, Vance KT. Contributions of frontal system dysfunction to memory and perceptual abilities in Parkinson's disease. Neuropsychology 1993;7:89–102.
40. Norman S, Troster AI, Fields JA, Brooks R. Effects of depression and Parkinson's disease on cognitive functioning. J Neuropsychiatry Clin Neurosci 2002;14:31–36.
41. Factor SA, Molho ES, Podskalny GD, Brown D. Parkinson's disease: drug-induced psychiatric states. Adv Neurol 1995;65:115–138.
42. Berney A, Vingerhoets F, Perrin A, et al. Effect on mood of subthalamic DBS for Parkinson's disease: a consecutive series of 24 patients. Neurology 2002;59:1427–1429.

43. Kulisevsky J, Berthier ML, Gironell A, et al. Mania following deep brain stimulation for Parkinson's disease. Neurology 2002;59:1421–1424.
44. Mendis T, Suchowersky O, Lang A, Gauthier S. Management of Parkinson's disease: a review of current and new therapies. Can J Neurol Sci 1999;26:89–103.
45. Lieberman A. Managing the neuropsychiatric symptoms of Parkinson's disease. Neurology 1998;50:S33–S38.
46. Poewe W, Seppi K. Treatment options for depression and psychosis in Parkinson's disease. J Neurol 2001;248(Suppl 3):III12–III21.
47. Aarsland D, Cummings JL. Depression in Parkinson's disease. Acta Psychiatr Scand 2002;106:161–162.
48. Ceravolo R, Nuti A, Piccinni A, et al. Paroxetine in Parkinson's disease: effects on motor and depressive symptoms. Neurology 2000;55:1216–1218.
49. Ritter JL, Alexander B. Retrospective study of selegiline-antidepressant drug interactions and a review of the literature. Ann Clin Psychiatry 1997;9:7–13.
50. Onofrj M, Luciano AL, Thomas A, et al. Mirtazapine induces REM sleep behavior disorder (RBD) in Parkinsonism. Neurology 2003;60:113–115.
51. Okun MS, McDonald WM, DeLong MR. Refractory nonmotor symptoms in male patients with Parkinson disease due to testosterone deficiency: a common unrecognized comorbidity. Arch Neurol 2002;59:807–811.
52. Burke WJ, Peterson J, Rubin EH. Electroconvulsive therapy in the treatment of combined depression and Parkinson's disease. Psychosomatics 1988;29:341–346.
53. Wengel SP, Burke WJ, Pfeiffer RF, et al. Maintenance electroconvulsive therapy for intractable Parkinson's disease. Am J Geriatr Psychiatry 1998;6:263–269.

2
Anxiety

Hubert H. Fernandez and Tanya Simuni

SUMMARY

Anxiety disorders in Parkinson's disease (PD) have been found to exceed prevalence rates in the geriatric population. Anxiety occurs more frequently in PD than in most other medical illnesses of comparable disability. Thus, anxiety may be etiologically related to the neurobiological changes that accompany PD and not simply a behavioral reaction to chronic disability. The anxiety disorder in PD tends to be panic, phobic, or generalized anxiety disorder. It can be a manifestation of an "off" state, can be worsened by motor fluctuations, or can occur independently from—and even precede—motor manifestations. Anxiety in PD may be directly related to dopaminergic deficit or may be the result of imbalance in other neurochemical pathways. The neurotransmitters primarily implicated in the pathogenesis of anxiety are norepinephrine, serotonin, and γ-aminobutyric acid, as well as some neuropeptides.

The key to successful management of anxiety in PD is its early recognition. A "team approach" to treatment that includes pharmacological and nonpharmacological measures, such as education, counseling, and stress-reduction strategies, is most beneficial, particularly in a complex illness where motor and behavioral dysfunction are often intertwined and tend to affect each other.

Well-designed studies that address the pharmacological management of anxiety in PD are needed. Nonetheless, based on clinical experience, the effective agents for primary anxiety disorders seem comparably efficacious in PD-related anxiety.

Key Words: Anxiety; generalized anxiety disorder; panic; phobia; epidemiology; pathology; pharmacology.

1. INTRODUCTION

1.1. *Definitions*

According to the Diagnostic and Statistical Manual of Mental Disorders (DSM)-IV classification, anxiety disorders are classified into the following categories: panic disorder with agoraphobia, panic disorder without agoraphobia, agoraphobia without panic disorder, specific phobia, social phobia, obsessive-compulsive disorder (OCD), posttraumatic stress disorder, acute stress disorder, generalized anxiety disorder (GAD), anxiety disorder owing to a general medical condition, substance-induced anxiety disorder, and anxiety disorder not otherwise specified *(1)*.

A *panic attack* is a discrete period of the sudden onset of intense apprehension, fearfulness, or terror that are often associated with feelings of impeding doom. During these attacks, symptoms like shortness of breath, palpitations, chest pain, choking or smothering sensations, and fear of "going crazy" or losing control are present. In a *panic disorder,* there is persistent concern over recurrent unexpected panic attacks.

Agoraphobia is anxiety about, or avoidance of, places or situations from which escape might be difficult (or embarrassing).

From: *Current Clinical Neurology*
Parkinson's Disease and Nonmotor Dysfunction
Edited by: R. F. Pfeiffer and I. Bodis-Wollner © Humana Press Inc., Totowa, NJ

In *specific phobia,* the anxiety is provoked by exposure to a specific feared object or situation, often leading to avoidance behavior, whereas *social phobia* is provoked by exposure to certain types of social or performance situations.

Obsessive-compulsive behavior is characterized by obsessions that cause marked anxiety or distress and/or by compulsions that serve to neutralize anxiety.

Posttraumatic stress disorder is characterized by the re-experiencing of an extremely traumatic event, accompanied by symptoms of increased arousal and avoidance of stimuli associated with the trauma. These symptoms are similar in *acute stress disorder,* but they occur immediately in the aftermath of an extremely traumatic event.

Generalized anxiety disorder is characterized by at least 6 months of persistent anxiety and worry.

2. EPIDEMIOLOGY

Most non-Parkinson's disease (PD) studies have shown that anxiety disorders are less common in the elderly when compared with younger adults. The Epidemiologic Catchment Area study found the overall prevalence of anxiety disorders to be 5.5% in people over the age of 65 years, in comparison with 7.3% in subjects of all ages *(2)*. Bland et al. *(3)* found the 6-month prevalence rates of all anxiety disorders to be 3.5% in people over the age of 65 living independently, 5.5% in people 65 or older living in institutions, and 6.5% in subjects of all ages.

In contrast, anxiety disorders in PD have been found to exceed prevalence rates in the geriatric population and occur more frequently than in any other medical illness of comparable disability (*see* Table 1). It is also of interest that anxiety disorders in psychiatric patients generally begin by young adulthood. Therefore, the onset of anxiety at a late age in PD, and its higher prevalence when compared to the geriatric population and other chronic illnesses, suggests that anxiety may be etiologically related to the neurobiological changes that accompany PD and not just a behavioral reaction to chronic disability.

3. CLINICAL FEATURES

3.1. Types of Anxiety Disorders Found in PD

GAD, panic disorder, social phobia, phobic disorder, agoraphobia, and OCD all have been described with PD *(6,8,11)*. The types of anxiety disorders in PD appear to be clustered in the panic, phobic, and GAD areas *(6,8)*. Vazquez et al. *(10)* described only panic disorder, whereas Schiffer et al. *(13)* reported the presence of panic and GAD. Lauterbach and Duvoisin *(11)* described anxiety disorders in familial Parkinsonism and noted a lower rate of panic disorder (7.9%) and higher rates of social phobia (5.3%) and OCD (13.2%) in their cohort.

In addition, there are two types of OCD-like behaviors recently described in PD: pathological gambling and punding. Pathological gambling is classified under *impulse control disorders* in the DSM-IV and is characterized by "failure to resist the impulse to gamble despite personal, family, or vocational consequences" *(1)*. In most reports, the behavior appears after the onset of PD *(16–18),* more often in the "on" state *(16)* or during an increase in levodopa or dopamine agonist dose *(17,18)* and resolves with atypical antipsychotic agents or reduction of anti-PD medications *(18)*. Thus, overstimulation of mesolimbic dopamine receptors from dopaminergic drug use appears to be the most accepted explanation for this behavior.

Punding was initially observed among amphetamine and cocaine abusers, but has now been described in PD as well *(19,20)*. It is a stereotyped motor behavior in which there is an intense fascination with repetitive handling and examining of mechanical objects, such as picking at oneself, taking apart watches and radios, or sorting and arranging common objects, such as lining up pebbles or rocks. Although punding may be considered a form of compulsion, it usually is not perceived by the patient as relieving a sense of inner tension, as is usually the case in OCD. Similarly to pathological gambling, punding usually occurs after chronic dopaminergic therapy and is relieved by reduction of anti-PD medications *(20)*.

Table 1
Prevalence of Anxiety in Parkinson's Disease

Author(s)	Result	Control	Instrument/ method
Menza et al., 1994 *(4)*	104 patients with PD had a mean anxiety scale of 25.2 when compared to 20.9 for medical controls ($n = 61$) ($p < 0.001$)	Medical control of equal disability	Zung self-rating anxiety scale
Gotham et al., 1986 *(5)*	Patients with PD scored higher than healthy control, but the same as those with arthritis	Chronic arthritis and healthy control	Spielberger anxiety index
Stein et al., 1990 *(6)*	9/24 (38%) patients with PD had anxiety	Patients who have PD without anxiety	Schedule for affective disorders, schizophrenia and DSM-IIIR
Starkstein et al., 1993 *(7)*	40% of patients had anxiety	None	DSM-III
Menza et al., 1993 *(8)*	12/42 (29%) patients with PD but only 1/21 (5%) control had anxiety	Chronic debilitating osteoarthritis	DSM-IIIR; Zung self-rating anxiety scale
Hillen and Sage, 1996 *(9)*	4/130 patients with PD with motor fluctuations experienced panic in the "off" state	None	Patient interview
Vasquez et al., 1993 *(10)*	31/131 (24%) levodopa-treated PD experienced panic attacks	None	Hamilton scale for anxiety; DSM-IIIR
Lauterbach and Duvoisin, 1991 *(11)*	Lifetime prevalence of generalized anxiety disorder = 5.3%; panic disorder = 7.9%; social phobia = 5.3%; agoraphobia = 15.8%; OCD = 13.2 %	None	DSM-III
Rubin et al., 1986 *(12)*	16/210 patients with PD reported marked episodic anxiety; 8/16 had panic-disorder	None	Standardized questionnaire and DSM-IIIR
Schiffer et al., *(13)*	75% of depressed patients with PD ($n = 16$) met criteria for generalized anxiety disorder versus 10% in depressed multiple sclerosis ($n = 20$)	Multiple sclerosis	DSM = III
Ringman et al., 2002 *(14)*	Anxiety found in 67% of patients with PD ($n = 40$) compared to 13% of controls ($n = 80$)	Patients with non-neurological illnesses	Neuropsychiatric inventory
Shulman et al., 2002 *(15)*	39% had anxiety (19% recognized by neurologist) ($n = 101$)	None	Beck Anxiety Inventory

Despite the obvious clinical features of anxiety, physicians tend to focus on the motor disability in PD, frequently neglecting to address the nonmotor manifestations of the disease. Similarly, patients with PD tend to attribute all their symptoms to suboptimal motor control, making it difficult to recognize neurobehavioral aspects of disability unless structured questionnaires are administered. Shulman et al. *(15)* demonstrated a significant discrepancy between the prevalence of anxiety based on validated patients self-reported scales (39%) in comparison to the diagnosis identified by the physician (19%). The same was true for depression and sleep disturbance.

3.2. Anxiety and Motor Performance

Most studies have observed anxiety symptoms to appear after the diagnosis of PD has been established *(6,10,21)*. However, one study reported the onset of anxiety preceding the appearance of Parkinsonism in 12 of 28 patients *(11)*.

Although most studies found no significant difference in PD severity between those with and without anxiety *(6,8)*, the relationship between anxiety and motor fluctuations is intriguing. It has long been recognized that symptoms like panic, flushing, and sweating can be principal nonmotor manifestations during the "off" state *(22)*. Moreover, pervading anxiety disorders are reported to occur more often among PD patients who experience "on–off" motor fluctuations, and symptoms tend to worsen during the "off" state *(6,10,21)*. One study showed that anxiety significantly improved from "off" to "on" and worsened again in the "on" state when dyskinesias appeared *(23)*, whereas others failed to consistently show a relationship between anxiety and motor state *(24)*. Therefore, it appears that anxiety itself can be a manifestation of an "off" state, can decline with motor fluctuations, or can occur independently from, and even precede, motor manifestations.

3.3. Anxiety and Medications

Studies of the relationship between anxiety and anti-PD medications have produced conflicting results. Although one group of investigators found panic attacks to be more common among levodopa-treated patients *(10)*, others have reported: (a) no difference in levodopa dose between anxious and nonanxious patients *(6)*; (b) 44% of patients with PD experienced anxiety prior to levodopa therapy *(21)*; and (c) no correlation between levodopa dose and anxiety levels *(8)*. Similar conflicting findings have been reported with pergolide *(8,25)*.

3.4. Anxiety and Laterality of PD

To determine whether anxiety in PD might be primarily a psychological reaction to chronic disability, investigators reviewed laterality of PD symptoms; the hypothesis was that patients with right-sided Parkinsonism (affecting their dominant side) would be expected to be more anxious. The opposite was found: anxiety in PD was associated mainly with left-sided symptoms *(2,12,26)*.

3.5. Depression, Dementia, and Anxiety

Depression occurs in up to 40% of patients with PD. Although anxiety in PD can occur in the absence of depression, there appears to be a special relationship between the two psychiatric disorders in PD *(10,26)*. Menza et al. *(8)* found that 92% of patients with PD with anxiety also had depression, and 67% of depressed patients with PD carried a diagnosis of anxiety. Similarly, Henderson et al. *(21)* found depression in combination with panic and/or anxiety occurred more frequently among patients with PD, when compared with healthy spousal controls. Depression in PD has often been described as "atypical" *(13)* with greater anxiety and less self-punitive ideation *(27)*.

The relationship between anxiety and dementia in PD remains unclear. Two studies hypothesized that anxiety may occur less frequently among demented patients with PD *(6,28)*, but others found no correlation between the two disorders *(10,26,29)*. A major drawback is that the majority of epidemiological studies of anxiety in PD have failed to comment on the cognitive status of their cohort *(13,21)* or deliberately excluded patients with significant cognitive impairment *(6,8)*.

4. NEUROBIOLOGY

The etiology of anxiety in PD is not well-understood and, unfortunately, has not been systematically studied. The notion that the higher prevalence of anxiety in PD versus the general population is based on the impact of chronic illness on the patient's psychological state is not supported by the data demonstrating higher frequency of GAD and panic attacks in PD when compared to patients with multiple sclerosis or other debilitating medical conditions (e.g., osteoarthritis) *(6,8)*. As mentioned previously, one study demonstrated that anxiety symptoms may precede the onset of PD motor features *(11)*. A recent study demonstrated that premorbid anxiety can be a risk factor for PD where a cohort of 35,815 male health care professionals was followed prospectively for 12 years *(30)*. By the end of the follow-up period, 189 subjects had developed PD. After adjustment for age, smoking, and caffeine intake, the relative risk of PD was 1.5 times higher in the group with the highest level of anxiety in comparison with the lowest *(30)*. Thus, available data generally support the hypothesis that anxiety in PD is the result of neurochemical and neuroanatomical changes of the disease itself, rather than a psychological reaction to a chronic condition.

4.1. Neuroanatomy

The alterations in basal ganglia (BG) motor circuitry in PD have been well-studied and delineated *(31)*. However, the pathology of PD extends beyond the "motor" BG. The neuroanatomical structural circuits that PD and anxiety may potentially have in common involve the nucleus accumbens, which modulates output of the striatal motor system based on ventral tegmental and temporal lobe limbic inputs *(32)*. The shell of the nucleus accumbens is closely linked to, or continuous with, the anterior extension of the amygdala *(33)*. Thus, both structures provide circuitry linkage between the BG motor system and limbic structures, thereby possibly generating an anxiety-type response *(34)*.

4.2. Neurochemistry

The neurochemical substrate of anxiety in PD is complex. Clearly, the principal neurochemical abnormality in PD is dopamine deficiency. Anxiety in PD may be directly related to dopaminergic deficit or the possible result of imbalance in other neurochemical pathways directly or indirectly affected by PD. The primary neurotransmitters implicated in pathogenesis of anxiety are norepinephrine (NE), serotonin, γ-aminobutyric acid (GABA), as well as some neuropeptides *(35)*.

4.2.1. Dopamine

Some evidence suggests that dopamine deficiency may be directly related to anxiety, specifically social phobias and panic disorder *(36,37)*. Indeed, in a study of levodopa infusion in patients with motor fluctuations, higher serum levodopa levels correlated with lower anxiety scores *(38)*. Anxiety scores were lowest during the "on" state and highest during motor "off" states *(38)*. No escalation of anxiety was found with dyskinesias, although other authors have noted a negative impact of dyskinesias, at least on mood *(23)*. Nonetheless, it is unlikely that dopamine deficiency is the sole neurochemical reason for anxiety in PD, because the majority of studies have not demonstrated any difference in the degree of motor disability between patients who have PD with and without anxiety *(6,8)*.

4.2.2. Norepinephrine

Dopamine deficiency can also lead to imbalance in other neurochemical pathways. One of the major neurotransmitters implicated in the development of anxiety is NE *(34)*. Dopamine inhibits the rate of firing of the locus ceruleus. Therefore, dopaminergic deficiency can bring dysregulation of NE *(10,29)*. PD itself may have an impact on NE pathways, and loss of catecholaminergic cells in the locus ceruleus has been demonstrated in PD *(39,40)*. The noradrenergic pathways emanating from the locus ceruleus are also affected, specifically the dorsal ascending noradrenergic pathway that projects from the locus ceruleus to the cerebral cortex, amygdala, hippocampus, and septum. Another postulated mechanism in the development of primary anxiety disorder is the inhibition of presynaptic α-2-adrenergic receptors *(35)*. In animal models, inhibition of these receptors presynaptically results in increased NE activity and anxiety behavior *(35)*. Yohimbine, an α-2-adrenergic receptor antagonist, has been shown to cause panic attacks in patients with panic disorder, but not in healthy controls *(41)*. The number of α-2-adrenergic receptors decreases in subjects with PD both centrally and peripherally *(8,42)*. Richard et al. *(43)* demonstrated that yohimbine challenge in subjects with PD who had a history of anxiety produced panic attacks at a rate comparable to psychiatric patients with primary panic disorder. All patients with PD, irrespective of history of anxiety, demonstrated sensitivity to yohimbine-induced somatic symptoms, whereas none of the controls did *(43)*. This data supports the role of impairment of NE pathways in PD-related anxiety disorders.

4.2.3. Serotonin

Another neurotransmitter implicated in primary anxiety disorders is serotonin. A functional polymorphism in the promoter region of the serotonin transporter gene has been recently linked to anxiety *(44)*. Patients with PD who carried the short allele of the serotonin transporter scored higher on anxiety scales than noncarriers, pointing to potential common genetic mechanisms of primary anxiety and anxiety in PD *(46)*. Evidence also shows degeneration of serotoninergic systems in PD. Studies have demonstrated loss of neurons in the median and dorsal raphe nuclei *(47)*. PD is associated with reduced concentration of serotonin in the basal ganglia nuclei as well as frontal cortex and reduced density of binding sites for serotonin-reuptake inhibitors in the putamen *(48)*.

4.2.4. γ-Aminobutyric Acid

The potential role of GABA in anxiety is supported by animal data. Animals exposed to prolonged stress had a reduction in $GABA_A$ receptor binding in the frontal cortex, hippocampus, and hypothalamus *(49)*. More importantly, the efficacy of benzodiazepines, which are $GABA_A$ agonists, supports involvement of the GABAergic system in anxiety treatment in the development of anxiety disorders *(50)*. The exact role of GABA dysfunction in anxiety in PD has not been established. Autopsy data from PD brains demonstrate conflicting evidence, with increased concentration of GABA in the putamen and pallidum but reduced concentration in the cortex *(51)*.

4.2.5. Glutamate

Glutamate could be an influence in PD-related anxiety. PD is associated with the disinhibition of glutamatergic output from the subthalamic nucleus, resulting in excessive glutamatergic stimulation of the BG motor nuclei and possibly, mesolimbic structures as well *(31)*. Glutamate receptors mediate excitatory neurotransmission, which is activated by stress *(51)*. *N*-methyl-D-aspartate receptor (NMDA) antagonists have been shown to have anxiolytic effects in animal models of anxiety *(52)*. However, studies of NMDA antagonists in human subjects have been halted by the impact of those agents on memory and cognition.

4.2.6. Neuropeptides

Various neuropeptides have also been implicated in primary anxiety disorders. Cholecystokinin and corticotropin-releasing factor seem to be anxiogenic, whereas neuropeptide-Y and substance-P are anxiolytic *(35)*. Pharmacological agents acting on those neuropeptides may prove to be more efficacious than existing strategies for the treatment of anxiety, although their role in parkinsonian anxiety remains to be determined.

4.3. Neuroimaging

Functional imaging studies are becoming a valuable tool in the investigation of neuroanatomical and neurophysiological substrates of different psychiatric disorders. Positron emission tomography studies in GAD have indicated decreased glucose metabolism in the basal ganglia *(53)*. GAD was not associated with asymmetry in cerebral metabolism, contrary to panic disorders, which seem to be associated with right-brain metabolic abnormalities *(53)*. There are no functional imaging studies that address cerebral metabolism in PD-related anxiety. However, a clinical study reviewing the impact of laterality of PD symptoms on anxiety demonstrated a strong correlation of anxiety to left-body Parkinsonism *(26)*. The same association was evident for depressive symptoms.

5. TREATMENT

The key to successful management of anxiety in PD is early recognition. Once anxiety is identified, a "team approach" to treatment is the most beneficial. Nonpharmacological management, including education, counseling, and stress-reduction strategies, should be an integral part of any neurobehavioral disorder. However, the majority of patients will still require pharmacological intervention.

Studies that assess the pharmacological management of anxiety in PD are necessary, and PD motor symptoms should be adequately treated. Although most studies find no correlation between PD disability and incidence of anxiety, there is a clear correlation of anxiety with the "off" state for the subset of patients with motor fluctuations *(38)*.

Several animal studies have addressed the role of dopamine agonists in anxiety. Ropinirole demonstrated anxiolytic properties in rat, mouse, and marmoset models of anxiety, but these were not PD animal models *(54)*. An investigational D2-selective dopamine agonist, U-95666E (sumanirole), was shown to have both antiparkinsonian and anxiolytic effects in the 6-hydroxydopamine (OHDA) rat model of PD *(55)*. Clinical trials of available dopamine agonists in PD have not reviewed anxiety as an end-point. However, the incidence of treatment-induced anxiety is higher with dopamine agonists when compared with levodopa *(56,57)*. Pramipexole has an antidepressant effect in primary depression, but its impact on anxiety has not been studied *(58,59)*.

5.1. Benzodiazepines

The majority of patients with PD who experience anxiety require anxiolytic therapy in combination with dopaminergic medications. Benzodiazepines can be effective for the management of GAD, panic disorders, and social phobias but are not effective in OCD *(60)*. There is no adverse interaction between benzodiazepines and dopaminergic therapy, but the potential additive sedative effect of both agents can lead to the escalation of daytime somnolence, disruption of the sleep–wake cycle, and falling. Cognitively impaired patients can experience further deterioration of cognition when taking benzodiazepines and are at risk for developing hallucinations. These agents should be avoided in the elderly, especially in patients with PD on polypharmacy. Benzodiazepines should be limited to short-term use if at all possible. Chronic use should be considered only when all alternative strategies to treat anxiety have failed.

5.2. Selective Serotonin Receptor Inhibitors

Selective serotonin receptor inhibitors (SSRIs) are becoming the preferred agents for the management of virtually any type of anxiety. SSRIs have a favorable side-effect profile and display limited drug–drug interaction. SSRIs are widely used in PD for depression and associated anxiety. Data exists on the efficacy of SSRIs in PD-related depression. Although in a comprehensive review of the subject, Tom and Cummings *(61)* concluded that data are limited and more studies are necessary. No studies address the efficacy of these agents in PD-related anxiety. Overall, SSRIs are safe to use in PD; however, there are several issues of which physicians need to be aware.

1. Concomitant use of SSRIs and monoamine oxidase inhibitors (MAOI) can lead to the development of the serotonin syndrome (SS). Nonselective MAOIs are contraindicated in patients taking levodopa owing to the risk of hypertensive crisis. Selegiline, which continues to be widely used in PD for its putative neuroprotective benefit, as well as its mild symptomatic dopaminergic effect, is a selective monoamine oxidase (MAO)-B inhibitor. Selegiline does not produce MAO-A inhibition at the recommended dose of 10 mg per day. However, at higher doses, it becomes a nonselective MAOI *(62)*. The selegiline package insert has a warning against its concomitant use with either tricyclic antidepressants (TCA) or SSRIs, because of the potential for central nervous system toxicity that occurs with the SS, which is characterized by alterations of mental status, motor, and autonomic function. Despite this theoretical concern, both the manufacturer's information and a survey of a large group of movement disorders specialists suggest it is a rare phenomenon *(63,64)*.
2. There are case reports of motor worsening or new-onset drug-induced Parkinsonism in the setting of SSRI use, specifically fluoxetine *(65,66)*. Whether this reflects some unique property of fluoxetine or is a falsely elevated incidence as a consequence of its wide use is unclear.
3. SSRIs can interact with agents metabolized by the cytochrome P450 system. Although some dopamine agonists can inhibit P450 enzymes, this interaction is of limited clinical significance. Among dopamine agonists, pramipexole does not inhibit P450 enzymes *(67)*. SSRIs vary in their degree of P450 inhibition: sertraline causes relatively less inhibition than fluoxetine and paroxetine *(68)*.

Until formal clinical trials address the issues of efficacy and safety of SSRIs in PD, the choice of a particular SSRI for the management of anxiety in PD should be based on the side-effect profile of the particular agent, the patient's tolerance, and comorbidities.

5.3. Tricyclic Antidepressants

TCAs act by blocking NE and serotonin uptake, as well as producing long-term increases in receptor sensitivity *(69)*. TCAs have a role in the management of PD-related pain, sleep dysfunction, and hypersalivation. However, their use in PD is limited by anticholinergic side effects. TCAs also carry a relatively high risk of causing or worsening confusion. The TCA, amoxapine, should not be used in PD because it is partly a dopamine receptor-blocking agent and can worsen Parkinsonism *(70)*.

5.4. Bupropion and Buspirone

Bupropion is a monocyclic antidepressant with indirect dopamine agonist properties *(69)*. Bupropion improves depression in some patients with PD *(71)* and may also have a positive effect on PD motor symptoms. The most troublesome potential side effect is seizures, yet the risk is primarily confined to individuals with pre-existing epilepsy. The effect of bupropion on PD anxiety has not been systematically evaluated, but its overall "stimulating" properties may limit its use.

Buspirone, which is pharmacologically related to bupropion, also has dopamine agonist properties. It can be effective for GAD but is less likely to help panic or social phobia *(72)*. Based on its mechanism of action, buspirone has been studied in PD. The drug was well-tolerated in doses up to 60 mg per day, but did not produce either antiparkinsonian or anxiolytic effects *(73)*. At higher doses (100 mg/day), it caused a decline in motor function and worsening of anxiety *(73)*. Another study that primarily analyzed the impact of buspirone on dyskinesias in PD did not demonstrate an anxiolytic effect at a dose of 20 mg per day *(74)*.

5.5. Other Therapies

5.5.1. Mirtazapine

Mirtazapine is a newer antidepressant that acts via indirect enhancement of serotonin 5-HT_1 receptors, as well as by direct inhibition of α-2 presynaptic adrenergic receptors. Data has shown mirtazapine to be effective in GAD *(75)* and potentially may be a good treatment option for patients with PD who experience anxiety and sleep dysfunction owing to its sedative effect at low doses. Mirtazapine was noted to have a tremor-suppressing effect in a case-report series *(76)*. However, that observation awaits clarification in prospective placebo-controlled studies.

5.1.2. Surgery

Surgery assumes an increasing role in PD management. Despite the extensive body of literature regarding the impact of surgical interventions on the cognitive and mood status of patients with PD *(77,78)*, information on its effect on anxiety is limited and mixed. Generally, surgical protocols exclude patients with a high degree of anxiety unless sufficiently treated because of concern that these patients will be unable to go through a lengthy and stressful surgical procedure performed while they are awake. There are isolated reports of reduced anxiety with pallidal stimulation, thalamotomy, and pallidotomy. Higginson et al. *(79)* reported on the impact of surgery on anxiety in 39 patients with advanced PD who underwent either ablative or deep-brain stimulation (DBS) procedures. Surgical targets included globus pallidus (Gpi) (24 pallidotomies; 10 GPi DBS) and nucleus ventralis intermedius (VIM) nucleus of the thalamus (4 DBS; 1 thalamotomy). The prevalence of anxiety decreased from 72% (28 of 39 patients) before surgery to 49% (19 of 39 patients) after surgery based on the Beck Anxiety Inventory scale. The side of surgery had no impact on the degree of anxiety reduction. Investigators concluded that surgical intervention in PD is associated with the reduction of anxiety. Although the study had significant methodological limitations, at the very least it provides confirmation that surgical intervention does not usually worsen symptoms of anxiety in PD. Another study reviewed the effect of bilateral subthalamic nucleus (STN)-DBS on anxiety in a cohort of 20 patients followed postoperatively for 12 months. Anxiety scores improved postoperatively in 50% of the patients, remained unchanged in 37%, and worsened in 12% *(80)*. Neurobehavioral benefit was sustained at 12-month follow-up.

In contrast, one study reported persistence and slight worsening of GAD after STN-DBS *(81)*. Interestingly, a large proportion of patients with postoperative anxiety attributed their symptoms to the fear of failure of stimulators *(81)*. Additional data in the form of prospective, blinded studies that address the efficacy of different surgical targets is necessary.

6. CONCLUSION

There is a remarkable paucity of organized data on the choice of pharmacological management of anxiety in PD, and well-designed studies are necessary. However, based on current clinical experience, agents that are effective in the management of primary anxiety disorders are also efficacious in PD-related anxiety.

REFERENCES

1. American Psychiatric Association. Diagnostic and Statistical Manual of Mental Disorders, 4th ed. American Psychiatric Association, Washington, DC, 1994.
2. Regier DA, Boyd JH, Burke JD Jr., et al. One month prevalence of mental disorders in the United States: based on five epidemiologic catchment area sites. Arch Gen Psychiatry 1988;45:977–986.
3. Bland RC, Newman SC, Orn H. Prevalence of anxiety disorders in the elderly in Edmonton. Acta Psychiatr Scand Suppl 1988;338:57–63.
4. Menza MA, Mark MH. Parkinson's disease and depression: the relationship to disability and personality. J Neuropsychiatry Clin Neurosci 1994;6:165–169.
5. Gotham AM, Brown RG, Marsden CD. Depression in Parkinson's disease: a quantitative and qualitative analysis. J Neurol Neurosurg Psychiatry 1986;49:381–389.
6. Stein M, Heuser IJ, Juncos JL, Uhde TW. Anxiety disorders in patients with Parkinson's disease. Am J Psychiatry 1990;147:217–220.
7. Starkstein SE, Robinson RG, Leiguardia R, et al. Anxiety and depression in Parkinson's disease. Behav Neurol 1993;6:151–154.
8. Menza MA, Robertson-Hoffman DE, Bonapace AS. Parkinson's disease and anxiety: comorbidity with depression. Biol Psychiatry 1993;34:465–470.
9. Hillen ME, Sage JI. Nonmotor fluctuations in patients with Parkinson's disease. Neurology 1996;47:1180–1183.
10. Vazquez A, Jimenez-Jimenez FJ, Garcia-Ruiz P, Garcia-Urra D. Panic attacks in Parkinson's disease. A long-term complication of levodopa therapy. Acta Neurol Scand 1993;87:14–18.
11. Lauterbach EC, Duvoisin RC. Anxiety disorders in familial Parkinsonism. Am J Psychiatry 1991;148:274.
12. Rubin AJ, Kurlan R, Schiffer R, et al. Atypical depression and Parkinson's disease. Ann Neurol 1986;20:150.
13. Schiffer RB, Kurlan R, Rubin A, Boer S. Evidence for atypical depression in Parkinson's disease. Am J Psychiatry 1988;145:1020–1022.
14. Ringman JM, Diaz-Olavarrieta C, Rodriguez Y, et al. The prevalence and correlates of neuropsychiatric symptoms in a population with Parkinson's disease in Mexico. Neuropsychiatry Neuropsychol Behav Neurol 2002;15:99–105.
15. Shulman LM, Taback RL, Rabinstein AA, Weiner WJ. Non-recognition of depression and other non-motor symptoms in Parkinson's disease. Parkinsonism Relat Disord 2002;8:193–197.
16. Molina JA, Sainz-Artiga MJ, Fraile A, et al. Pathologic gambling in Parkinson's disease: a behavioral manifestation of pharmacologic treatment? Mov Disord 2000;15:869–872.
17. Gschwandtner U, Aston J, Renaud S, Fuhr P. Pathologic gambling in patients with Parkinson's disease. Clin Neuropharmacol 2001;24:170–172.
18. Seedat S, Kesler S, Niehaus DJ, Stein DJ. Pathological gambling behaviour: emergence secondary to treatment of Parkinson's disease with dopaminergic agents. Depress Anxiety 2000;11:185–186.
19. Friedman JH. Punding on levodopa. Biol Psychiatry 1994;36:350–351.
20. Frenadez HH, Friedman JH. Punding on L-dopa. Mov Disord 1999;14:836–838.
21. Henderson R, Kurlan R, Kersun JM, Como P. Preliminary examination of the comorbidity of anxiety and depression in Parkinson's disease. J Neuropsychiatry Clin Neurosci 1992;4:257–264.
22. Marsden CD, Parkes JD. "On-off" effects in patients with Parkinson's disease on chronic levodopa therapy. Lancet 1976;1:292–296.

23. Menza MA, Sage J, Marshall E, et al. Mood changes and "on-off" phenomena in Parkinson's disease. Mov Disord 1990;5:148–151.
24. Richard IH, Justus AW, Kurlan R. Relationship between mood and motor fluctuations in Parkinson's disease. J Neuropsychiatry Clin Neurosci 2001;13:35–41.
25. Lang AE, Quinn N, Brincat S, et al. Pergolide in late-stage Parkinson's disease. Ann Neurol 1982;12:243–247.
26. Fleminger S. Left-sided Parkinson's disease is associated with greater anxiety and depression. Psychol Med 1991;21:629–638.
27. Cummings JL. Depression and Parkinson's disease: a review. Am J Psychiatry 1992;149:443–454.
28. Iruela LM, Ibanez-Rojo V, Palanca I, Caballero L. Anxiety disorders and Parkinson's disease (letter). Am J Psychiatry 1992;149:719–720.
29. Lauterbach EC. The locus ceruleus and anxiety disorders in demented and nondemented familial Parkinsonism. Am J Psychiatry 1993;150:994.
30. Weisskopf MG, Chen H, Schwarzschild MA, et al. Prospective study of phobic anxiety and risk of Parkinson's disease. Mov Disord 2003;18:646–651.
31. Alexander GE, DeLong MR, Strick PL. Parallel organization of functionally segregated circuits linking basal ganglia and cortex. Annu Rev Neurosci 1986;9:357–381.
32. Mogenson GJ, Jones DL, Yim CY. From motivation to action: functional interface between the limbic system and the motor system. Prog Neurobiol 1980;14:69–97.
33. Heimer L, Alheid GF, de Olmos JS, et al. The accumbens: beyond the core-shell dichotomy. J Neuropsychiatry Clin Neurosci 1997;9:354–381.
34. Schiffer RB. Anxiety disorders in Parkinson's disease: insights into the neurobiology of neurosis. J Psychosom Res 1999;47:505–508.
35. Jetty PV, Charney DS, Goddard AW. Neurobiology of generalized anxiety disorder. Psychiatr Clin North Am 2001;24:75–97.
36. Pitchot W, Ansseau M, Gonzalez Moreno A, et al. Dopaminergic function in panic disorder: comparison with major and minor depression. Biol Psychiatry 1992;32:1004–1011.
37. Potts NL, Davidson JR. Social phobia: biological aspects and pharmacotherapy. Prog Neuropsychopharmacol Biol Psychiatry 1992;16:635–646.
38. Maricle RA, Nutt JG, Valentine RJ, Carter JH. Dose-response relationship of levodopa with mood and anxiety in fluctuating Parkinson's disease: a double-blind, placebo-controlled study. Neurology 1995;45:1757–1760.
39. German DC, Manaye KF, White CL, III, et al. Disease-specific patterns of locus coeruleus cell loss. Ann Neurol 1992;32:667–676.
40. Patt S, Gerhard L. A Golgi study of human locus coeruleus in normal brains and in Parkinson's disease. Neuropathol Appl Neurobiol 1993;19:519–523.
41. Charney DS, Woods SW, Heninger GR. Noradrenergic function in generalized anxiety disorder: effects of yohimbine in healthy subjects and patients with generalized anxiety disorder. Psychiatry Res 1989;27:173–182.
42. Cash R, Ruberg M, Raisman R, Agid Y. Adrenergic receptors in Parkinson's disease. Brain Res 1984;322:269–275.
43. Richard IH, Szegethy E, Lichter D, et al. Parkinson's disease: a preliminary study of yohimbine challenge in patients with anxiety. Clin Neuropharmacol 1999;22:172–175.
44. Ohara K, Nagai M, Suzuki Y, et al. Association between anxiety disorders and a functional polymorphism in the serotonin transporter gene. Psychiatry Res 1998;81:277–279.
45. Menza MA, Palermo B, DiPaola R, et al. Depression and anxiety in Parkinson's disease: possible effect of genetic variation in the serotonin transporter. J Geriatr Psychiatry Neurol 1999;12:49–52.
46. Halliday GM, Blumbergs PC, Cotton RG, et al. Loss of brainstem serotonin- and substance P-containing neurons in Parkinson's disease. Brain Res 1990;510:104–107.
47. Raisman R, Cash R, Agid Y. Parkinson's disease: decreased density of 3H-imipramine and 3H-paroxetine binding sites in putamen. Neurology 1986;36:556–560.
48. Drugan RC, Skolnick P, Paul SM, Crawley JN. A pretest procedure reliably predicts performance in two animal models of inescapable stress. Pharmacol Biochem Behav 1989;33:649–654.
49. Rickels K, Case WG, Downing RW, Winokur A. Long-term diazepam therapy and clinical outcome. JAMA 1983;250:767–771.
50. Agid Y, Cervera P, Hirsch E, et al. Biochemistry of Parkinson's disease 28 years later: a critical review. Mov. Disord 1989;4(Suppl 1):S126–S144.
51. Krystal JH, D'Souza DC, Petrakis IL, et al. NMDA agonists and antagonists as probes of glutamatergic dysfunction and pharmacotherapies in neuropsychiatric disorders. Harv Rev Psychiatry 1999;7:125–143.
52. Trullas R, Jackson B, Skolnick P. Anxiolytic properties of 1- aminocyclopropanecarboxylic acid, a ligand at strychnine-insensitive glycine receptors. Pharmacol Biochem Behav 1989;34:313–316.
53. Wu JC, Buchsbaum MS, Hershey TG, et al. PET in generalized anxiety disorder. Biol Psychiatry 1991;29:1181–1199.
54. Rogers DC, Costall B, Domeney AM, et al. Anxiolytic profile of ropinirole in the rat, mouse and common marmoset. Psychopharmacology (Berlin) 2000;151:91–97.

55. Sethy VH, Ellerbrock BR, Wu, H. U-95666E: a potential anti-parkinsonian drug with anxiolytic activity. Prog. Neuropsychopharmacol Biol Psychiatry 1997;21:873–883.
56. Parkinson Study Group. Pramipexole vs levodopa as initial treatment for Parkinson disease: A randomized controlled trail. JAMA 2000;284:1931–1938.
57. Rascol O, Brooks DJ, Korczyn AD, et al. A five-year study of the incidence of dyskeinesia in patients with early Parkinson's disease who were treated with ropinirole or levodopa. 056 Study Group. N Engl J Med 2000;342:1484–1491.
58. Corrigan MH, Denahan AQ, Wright CE, et al. Comparison of pramipexole, fluoxetine, and placebo in patients with major depression. Depress Anxiety 2000;11:58–65.
59. Lattanzi L, Dell'Osso L, Cassano P, et al. Pramipexole in treatment-resistant depression: a 16-week naturalistic study. Bipolar Disord 2002;4:307–314.
60. Connor KM, Davidson JR. Generalized anxiety disorder: neurobiological and pharmacotherapeutic perspectives. Biol Psychiatry 1998;44:1286–1294.
61. Tom T, Cummings JL. Depression in Parkinson's disease. Pharmacological characteristics and treatment. Drugs Aging 1998;12:55–74.
62. Heinonen EH, Myllyla V. Safety of selegiline (deprenyl) in the treatment of Parkinson's disease. Drug Safety 1998;19:11–22.
63. Richard IH, Kurlan R, Tanner C, et al. Serotonin syndrome and the combined use of deprenyl and an antidepressant in Parkinson's disease. Parkinson Study Group. Neurology 1997;48:1070–1077.
64. Ritter JL, Alexander B. Retrospective study of selegiline-antidepressant drug interactions and a review of the literature. Ann Clin Psychiatry 1997;9:7–13.
65. Steur EN. Increase of Parkinson disability after fluoxetine medication. Neurology 1993;43:211–213.
66. Jimenez-Jimenez FJ, Tejeiro J, Martinez-Junquera G, et al. Parkinsonism exacerbated by paroxetine. Neurology 1994;44:2406.
67. Wynalda MA, Wienkers LC. Assessment of potential interactions between dopamine receptor agonists and various human cytochrome P450 enzymes using a simple in vitro inhibition screen. Drug Metab Dispos 1997;25:1211–1214.
68. Stoudemire A. New antidepressant drugs and the treatment of depression in the medically ill patient. Psychiatr Clin North Am 1996;19:495–514.
69. Artigas F, Nutt DJ, Shelton R. Mechanism of action of antidepressants. Psychopharmacol Bull 2002;36(Suppl 2):123–132.
70. Vernier P, Pollak P, Groslambert R, Gavend M. Parkinsonian syndrome secondary to amoxapine. Presse Med 1984;13:1007.
71. Goetz CG, Tanner CM, Klawans HL. Bupropion in Parkinson's disease. Neurology 1984;34:1092–1094.
72. Small GW. Recognizing and treating anxiety in the elderly. J. Clin Psychiatry 1997;58(Suppl 3):41–47.
73. Ludwig CL, Weinberger DR, Bruno G, et al. Buspirone Parkinson's disease, and the locus ceruleus. Clin Neuropharmacol 1986;9:373–378.
74. Bonifati V, Fabrizio E, Cipriani R, Vanacore N, Meco G. Buspirone in levodopa-induced dyskinesias. Clin Neuropharmacol 1994;17:73–82.
75. Kasper S. Clinical efficacy of mirtazapine: a review of meta-analyses of pooled data. Int Clin Psychopharmacol 1995;10(Suppl 4):25–35.
76. Pact V, Giduz T. Mirtazapine treats resting tremor, essential tremor, and levodopa-induced dyskinesias. Neurology 1999;53:1154.
77. Pillon B, Ardouin C, Damier P, et al. Neuropsychological changes between "off" and "on" STN or GPi stimulation in Parkinson's disease. Neurology 2000;55:411–418.
78. Saint-Cyr JA, Trepanier LL, Kumar R, et al. Neuropsychological consequences of chronic bilateral stimulation of the subthalamic nucleus in Parkinson's disease. Brain 2000;123:2091–2108.
79. Higginson CI, Fields AJ, Troster AI. Which symptoms of anxiety diminish after surgical interventions for Parkinson disease? Neuropsychiatry Neuropsychol Behav Neurol 2002;14:117–121.
80. Daniele A, Albanese A, Contarino MF, et al. Cognitive and behavioural effects of chronic stimulation of the subthalamic nucleus in patients with Parkinson's disease. J Neurol Neurosurg Psychiatry 2003;74:175–182.
81. Houeto JL, Mesnage V, Mallet L, et al. Behavioural disorders, Parkinson's disease and subthalamic stimulation. J Neurol Neurosurg Psychiatry 2002;72:701–707.

3
Obsessionality

Marie-Andrée Bruneau

SUMMARY

This chapter examines the fascinating issue of obsessionality in Parkinson's disease (PD). Initially described is the concept of obsessionality and current notions about the pathophysiology of obsessive-compulsive disorder (OCD). Also defined are the perseverations and their possible confusion with obsessive-compulsive symptoms (OCS). Particular features of obsessionality in some neurological illnesses are provided, and factors related to obsessionality in PD are reviewed. Both the Parkinsonian personality and similarities that may link bradyphrenia and obsessional slowness are discussed, and finally, descriptive studies of obsessionality in PD are reviewed. OCS in neurological illnesses, including PD, may be clinically identical to idiopathic OCD, but descriptions usually outline certain differences. OCS in neurological disease processes often are associated with movement disorders and cognitive dysfunction, primarily of the dysexecutive type. However, the issue regarding whether the etiopathology, phenomenology, and treatment response of OCS in neurological illnesses are similar to those of idiopathic OCD remains.

Key Words: Parkinson's disease; obsessionality; obsessive-compulsive disorder; perseveration; basal ganglia; frontal lesions.

1. INTRODUCTION

Parkinson's disease (PD) is one of the most intriguing neuropsychiatric disorders, giving the clinician a striking demonstration of the intricate intertwining of motor, cognitive, and behavioral functions within the brain. PD has been associated with many comorbid psychiatric disorders, such as depression and psychosis, which are discussed in Chapters 1, 2, and 5 of this book. However, one has to question if psychiatric syndromes in neurological diseases may be compared to primary psychiatric illnesses and, if so, share the same pathophysiology, clinical expression, and response to treatment.

This chapter discusses obsessionality in PD by first reviewing the concept of obsessionality and describing current notions about the pathophysiology of obsessive-compulsive disorder (OCD). Perseverations and their possible confusion with obsessive-compulsive symptoms (OCS), along with obsessionality in neurological illnesses and their particular features, are discussed. Finally, concepts linking obsessionality and PD and descriptive studies of OCS in PD are addressed. This chapter aims to clarify the reader's knowledge of how OCS and PD could be related and also relate new issues that need to be analyzed in future research.

2. THE CONCEPT OF OBSESSIONALITY

Obsessionality is usually associated with OCD or obsessive-compulsive personality disorder (OCPD). OCD is defined in the fourth edition of the Diagnostic and Statistical Manual of Mental Disorders (DSM-IV; *1*) as recurring obsessions and compulsions "severe enough to be time-consuming ...

From: *Current Clinical Neurology*
Parkinson's Disease and Nonmotor Dysfunction
Edited by: R. F. Pfeiffer and I. Bodis-Wollner © Humana Press Inc., Totowa, NJ

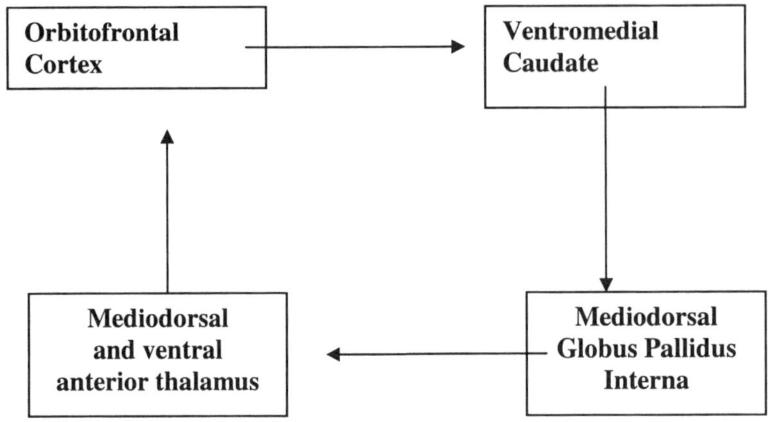

Fig. 1. Orbitofrontal circuit.

or cause marked distress or significant impairment" while people recognize that their reactions are irrational or disproportionate and egodystonic (i.e., aspects of a personality that are viewed as disgusting, unacceptable, or incompatible with the rest of the personality).

Obsessions are recurrent intrusive thoughts, impulses, or images that the patient attempts to ignore, or suppress. Examples of topics are contamination, aggressive, sexual, pathological doubt or need for symmetry. Compulsions are repetitive behaviors or mental acts (e.g., washing, counting, or checking) that the patient feels driven to perform to reduce the anxiety associated with obsessions or according to rules that must be rigidly applied.

OCPD is a pervasive pattern of preoccupation with orderliness, perfectionism, mental and interpersonal control at the expense of flexibility, openness, and efficiency *(1)*. Coincident aspects of OCD and OCPD are the need for order and symmetry, hoarding behaviors, and a certain mental inflexibility.

3. PATHOPHYSIOLOGY OF OCD

The pathophysiology of OCD has been studied in recent years using imagery, provocation, and treatment studies. Striatal dysfunction has been described as being at the root of this illness *(2,3)*. The striatum integrates complex neural networks related to motor, cognitive, and motivational functions. Thus, it is responsible for motor planning and integration, learning and reinforcement, and behavioral integration and selection. In OCD, this striatal filter becomes dysfunctional and allows unselected impulses to move to the orbitofrontal and cingulate cortex. Hyperactive orbitofrontal and cingulate cortico–subcortical circuits (*2,3;* Figs. 1 and 2) run in continuous loops and are postulated to give rise to OCS.

The striatum is also responsible for maintaining balance between the excitatory and inhibitory influences on thalamocortical pathways via dopaminergic modulation of the direct and indirect loops (Fig. 3; *4*). In a simplified way, the direct loop is operative until the desired action is completed; the indirect path suppresses the behavior, permitting a change of behavioral sets. The premise in OCD is that direct influences are prominent because the indirect loop is dysfunctional. If there is a loss of indirect influences, the patient becomes stuck in a "what if?" set. The excessive reverberation of instinctual impulses to the orbitofrontal and cingulate cortex maintains danger avoidance responses. The orbitofrontal cortex is, in fact, responsible for emotional reactions associated with survival stimuli (e.g., reproduction, violence, hygiene, and order), and it becomes hyperactive to control these free-running impulses *(5,6)*.

It remains unclear why this indirect loop becomes dysfunctional in OCD. One hypothesis is that some striatal neurons (striosomes) are very sensitive to hypoxic insults. If they are injured, the influence of the direct pathway becomes excessively prominent. The origin of such hypoxic insults could be varied *(5,6)*. In idiopathic OCD, a prenatal hypoxic insult associated with a possible genetic predis-

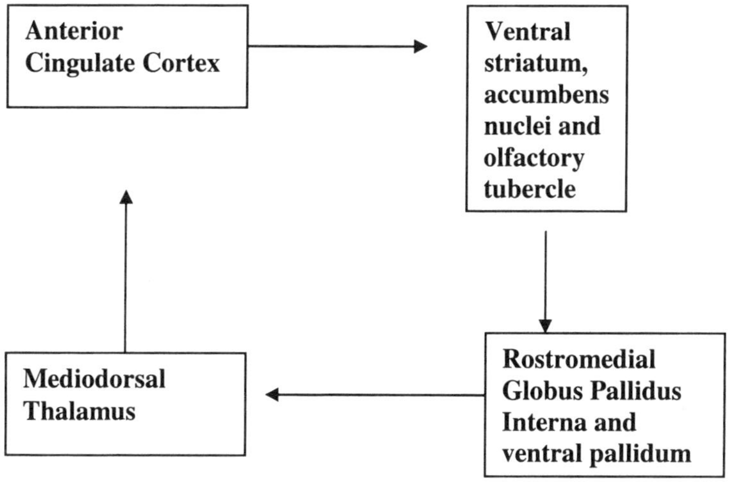

Fig. 2. Cingulate circuit.

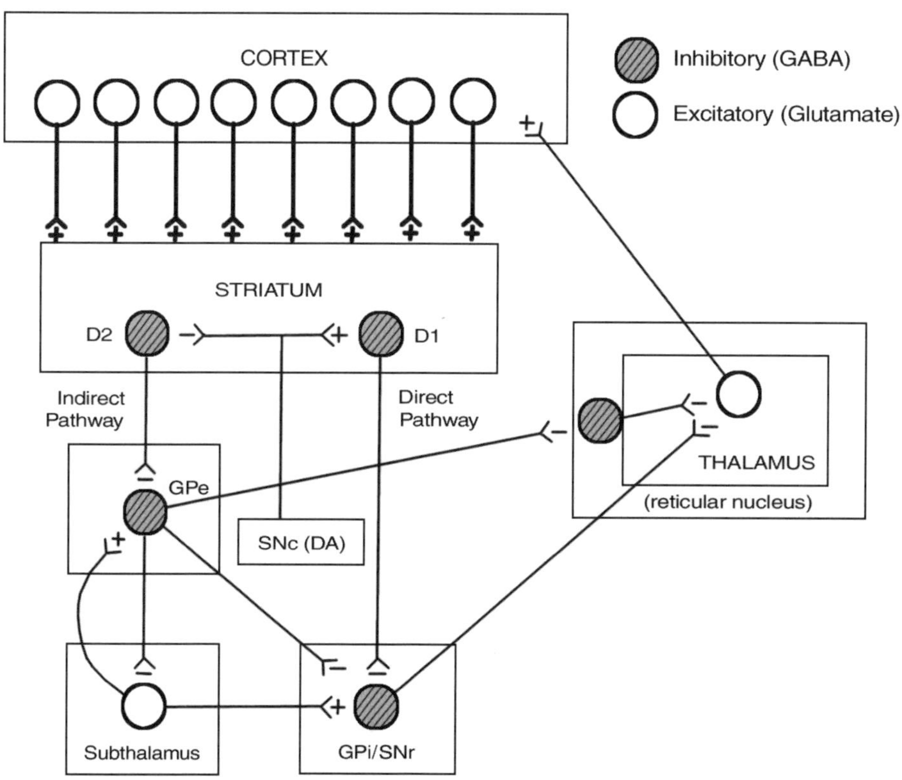

Fig. 3. Direct and indirect dopaminergic pathways. SN, substancia nigra; GPi, globus pallidus internal; GPe, globus pallidus external; D2, dopaminergic receptors type 2; D1, dopamineric receptors type 1.

position has been postulated. About 10% of patients with OCD have family members with OCD, and this reaches 15 to 30% when considering OCS. Twin studies show a 60 to 90% monozygotic concordance when compared to 20 to 50% for dizygotic twins *(7)*. However, any kind of insult (ischemic,

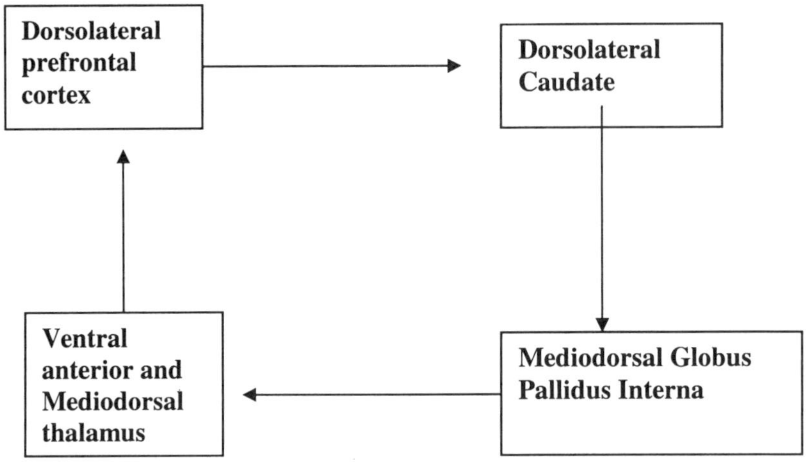

Fig. 4. Dorsolateral circuit.

infectious, or traumatic) to these neurons could give rise to the same symptomatology and explain the pathophysiology of "neurological" OCD, i.e., OCD appearing after a neurological insult.

In short, conscious executive processing (frontal) and implicit-automatic processing (basal ganglia) function in parallel in a normal brain. If the basal ganglia filter is dysfunctional, the frontal cortex becomes overloaded with information that is usually treated automatically (or unconsciously). This kind of information then intrudes into conscious knowledge, which leads to obsessions. Behavioral selection is then confined to compulsive actions.

Treatment of OCD by serotonergic medications or by psychosurgery changes the balance between direct and indirect pathways by reducing the global excitatory tonus of the system and consequently reducing excitatory thalamocortical projections *(5,6)*.

4. THE CONCEPT OF PERSEVERATIONS

Perseveration is defined as the inappropriate continuation of an act or thought after its proper context has passed, or as the pathological repetition of the same response to different stimuli *(8)*. Cummings *(9)* declared that perseverations might represent OCS in neurological patients with cognitive dysfunction. Indeed, perseverations have a stereotypical and repetitive aspect that resembles OCS. Perseveration involves self-regulation difficulty and mental inflexibility—aberrations usually associated with executive dysfunction. Executive functions include task planning, problem solving, mental flexibility, self-control, and inhibition. These functions are processed by the dorsolateral cortico–subcortical pathway (Fig. 4; *4*), whereas OCS are associated with hyperactivity of orbitofrontal and cingulate pathways *(2,3)*. Yet, executive dysfunction has been described in some, although not all, neuropsychological studies in OCD *(10–12)*. Based on neuropsychological studies, it is difficult to distinguish between OCS and perseveration in neurological illnesses, yet perseverations are usually associated with cognitive dysfunction, devoid of anxiety, and do not seem to be driven by the same emotional aspects associated with OCD *(8)*.

5. OCS IN NEUROLOGICAL ILLNESSES

OCS have been described in some neurological illnesses. Frontal lobe lesions are associated with perseverative behaviors *(13)*. In some cases, stereotypies similar to OCS are described. An example of early frontal lobe degeneration is frontotemporal dementia (FTD). A diagnosis of FTD supposes mental inflexibility, perseverative, and stereotypical behavior or speech as supportive features *(14)*. Therefore, as many as 78% of patients with FTD display OCS, and these may be the symptoms leading to diagnosis *(15)*. Descriptions range from classical OCD (counting, checking, cleaning, and symmetry compulsions) to verbal and motor stereotypies. OCS in FTD are associated with coincident executive dysfunction. Patients with FTD display less distress, resistance, and insight, and their obsessions are less likely to be associated with compulsions in comparison to the typical patient with OCD *(15)*.

Pathological processes that involve basal ganglia, particularly the caudate nucleus, are, not surprisingly, associated with OCD. The most elegant description of OCD relating to basal ganglia lesions of various etiologies (e.g., ischemic, infectious, and toxic) has been published by Laplane et al. *(16,17)*. They described OCD linked with lesions commonly localized to the caudate, putamen, or pallidum; the descriptions ranged from classical OCD to motor or verbal stereotypies without a cognitive counterpart. For example, some patients could not stop stirring soup or turning lights on and off. Punding and sucking behaviors were also described. The absence of anxiety or distress with compulsions is striking in these descriptions. No clearly evident obsessions could be found to account for the compulsive behavior. OCS were often associated with movement disorders and executive dysfunction.

Sydenham's chorea, a poststreptococcal infectious movement disorder involving antineuronal antibodies directed against basal ganglia, is associated with OCD in 60 to 80% of cases *(18)*. OCD occurs only in relationship to the chorea, never with the poststreptococcal rheumatic arthritis alone, which supports the concept that central nervous system involvement is necessary for the expression of this symptomatology. Some descriptions of OCD in Huntington's disease *(19)*, a neurodegenerative genetic disorder affecting the caudate nuclei, are also recorded in the literature. Moreover, OCD is strongly linked with Tourette's syndrome (TS) to the extent that some authors view OCD as a differential expression of the putative *TS* gene *(20)*. The pathophysiology of *TS* is believed to involve dopaminergic striatal hyperinnervation, which then gives rise to hyperactive cortico–subcortical pathways via thalamic disinhibition (Figs. 1 and 2). Sensory-motor loop hyperactivity therefore may be responsible for tics, whereas orbitofrontal and cingulate loops hyperactivity may produce OCD *(21)*. However, the phenomenological distinction between complex tics and compulsions remains a difficult task. Tics are usually preceded by a sensory urge; compulsions may be driven by a cognitive urge (obsession?). Performance of tics and completion of compulsive behaviors both provide relief to the patient with *TS*.

The neurological illness associated with OCD that is possibly the most similar to PD is Von Economo's encephalitis *(22)*. Von Economo's encephalitis, or encephalitis lethargica, was pandemic between 1917 and 1929, affecting up to 5 million people worldwide. Its etiology has never been determined, although an infectious pathogen was suspected. Its pathology entailed basal ganglia, substantia nigra, and mesencephalic inflammation. Patients first presented with flu-like symptoms and then developed neurological symptoms—most prominently lethargy or hypersomnolence. Movement disorders (Parkinsonism, choreoathethosis, and myoclonus) also occurred in some patients, along with psychotic features (e.g., delusions, hallucinations, and catatonia).

The postencephalitic syndrome, appearing months to years after the acute infection, was associated with Parkinsonism in 30 to 60% of cases and neuropsychiatric features in 50 to 100%. It also was associated with a subcortical type of dementia with prominent executive dysfunction. Most interestingly, OCS appeared in conjunction with oculogyric crises. Case reports depicted stereotyped compulsive movements without obsessions; counting, touching, or symmetry compulsions; sexual or aggressive obsessions; sensations of "forced thought"; and coprolalia and palilalia *(23)*. These crises could last from a few minutes to hours and were sometimes associated with tics and acute mood changes.

6. OCD IN PD

6.1. *Basal Ganglia Illnesses*

Similarly to OCD, PD involves basal ganglia dysfunction. Degeneration of the dopamine-containing neurons of the substantia nigra, with consequent loss of dopaminergic input to the basal ganglia, leads to the clinical presentation of PD *(24)*. Dopaminergic neuronal loss and its effect on the nigrostriatocortical circuit are illustrated clinically primarily by hypokinetic and cognitive syndromes. The disruption of dopaminergic transmission makes the indirect pathway predominant with a global thalamocortical inhibition and resulting hypokinetic symptoms (rigidity and bradykinesia). Cognitive dysfunction in PD originally was believed to be related to dorsolateral striatocortical circuit dysfunction *(25)*, also the consequence of the loss of monoaminergic afferents, primarily dopaminergic but also possibly noradrenergic, serotonergic, and cholinergic. Although Parkinsonism can be associated with the Alzheimer's type of cognitive dysfunction (PD + Alz) and Lewy body dementia, the usual type of cognitive dysfunction related to PD is a subcortical type of dementia. Findings include bradyphrenia, visuospatial deficits, encoding memory difficulties with preserved recognition, diminution of verbal fluency, and executive dysfunction, including mental rigidity and perseverations *(26)*. As discussed earlier, perseverations may be confused with OCS in some reports.

6.2. Parkinsonian Personality

Obsessionality in PD carries various idiosyncratic notions. A premorbid Parkinsonian personality with obsessional features (perfectionism, preoccupation with control, and mental rigidity) has been described in PD, the so-called "Parkinsonian personality" *(27,28)*. Analogies can be made between this description and Cloninger's hypodopaminergic personality with reduced novelty seeking *(29)*, and it can be questioned whether these characteristics represent early signs of central hypodopaminergism associated with executive dysfunction. Executive dysfunction may impede the adaptation to new settings, because patients have difficulty changing strategies or cognitive sets. Such individuals may also be less likely to engage in novelty-seeking behavior, because they may have problems dealing with new situations. To further complicate matters, it must be recognized that the retrospective quality of such descriptions is subject to recollection bias, which itself might be influenced by the actual symptomatology.

6.3. Obsessional Slowness and Bradyphrenia

Some authors have compared the obsessional slowness encountered with severe forms of OCD to Parkinsonian bradyphrenia *(30,31)*. They suggest that obsessional slowness represents difficulty in initiating action and suppressing perseverative behaviors. Patients with OCD are excessively meticulous and disintegrate their sequences of action until perfection is reached, resulting in slowness of execution. In bradykinesia, spontaneity of movement is lost, and movements disintegrate into multiple cautious and slowed action sequences. Bradyphrenia and obsessional slowness in thought processes may, therefore, share common ground *(32)*.

6.4. Prevalence Studies of OCS in PD

Despite that clinical wisdom implies that PD can be associated with OCS, only four studies reviewed the prevalence of OCS in PD from 1984 to 2002. Tomer et al *(33)* studied OCS in 30 patients with PD using the Leyton Obsessional Inventory (LOI). The LOI is divided into "symptoms" questions (recurring thoughts, checking, dirt and contamination, order and routine, and so forth) and "trait" questions (stubbornness, pedantry, hoarding, and so on). Of these 30 patients, 17 suffered from OCS, and 19 had an obsessional trait. A significant correlation was found between LOI results and the results on the Beck Depression Inventory. Müller et al. *(34)* reviewed OCS in 20 PD patients using the Maudsley Obsessive-Compulsive Inventory (MOCI) and the Hamburg Obsessive-Compulsive Inventory. Patients with PD scored higher than controls only on the "ordering" subscale. Maia et al. *(35)* measured OCS in 100 patients with PD using the Yale-Brown Obsessive-Compulsive Scale (YBOCS) and found OCS in 17 patients with a mean YBOCS of 17.1; only 5 patients met criteria for OCD. No differences in OCS between PD and controls could be demonstrated. Alegret et al. *(36)* reported on 72 patients with PD, finding higher MOCI and LOI scores in patients with PD than in controls. However, these scores did not reach a pathological level. Alegret et al. found higher proportions of "checking," "doubting," and "cleaning" OCS in their subjects with PD. Patients' MOCI scores correlated with the severity and duration of their illness. Alegret et al. linked OCS to neurochemical changes associated with PD progression. Yet, they did not discuss the possibility that dysexecutive difficulties in relation to dysfunction of the nigrostriatofrontal circuitry could be confused with OCS.

Taken as a whole, these four studies suggest the presence of OCS in PD. However, rarely do these symptoms reach diagnostic values for OCD. Furthermore, different screening instruments, a small number of patients, and the absence of a control group in some studies render these results difficult to interpret. Based on this literature, there is no clear epidemiological view of OCS in PD, nor is it known whether OCS in PD might be related to side effects of medication or to affective or cognitive symptoms. Also unknown is whether OCD in basal ganglia "neurological" illnesses, such as PD, is truly similar to "idiopathic" OCD.

6.5. OCS in PD: Perseverations?

To address these issues, we studied OCS in 35 patients with PD and 35 paired controls *(37)* with the hypothesis that OCS are present and significant in PD and may represent early manifestations of an emerging dysexecutive syndrome.

Our primary outcome measure was the YBOCS score *(38)*. The YBOCS is the gold-standard instrument to evaluate OCS and has been well-validated in psychiatric populations, containing a list of obsessions and compulsions used to probe for possible OCS in a given patient. The maximum score is 40, where a score of more than 8 indicates OCS, and more than 16 indicates OCD. We used the Wisconsin Card Sorting Test (WCST) to measure perseverations. In this test, the patient must sort cards using a variety of criteria (i.e., form, number, and color; *39*). The patient must discover the sorting rule, which will change after a certain number of correct answers. We used the WCST because of its sensitivity to executive dysfunction. Subjects were divided in two groups according to YBOCS scores (<8 = negligible OCS/>8 = presence of OCS). Mann-Whitney-U tests were performed on reported variables. A Chi-square test was done to evaluate the possible relationship between OCS and levodopa treatment (comparing the presence/absence of OCS and levodopa treatment) in patients with PD.

Patients with PD had statistically significantly higher scores on the YBOCS than controls. Early perseverative errors in the WCST were more frequent in patients with PD and OCS when compared to those without. No differences were found between subjects who had PD with or without OCS in terms of anxiety, depression, motor symptoms, demographic variables, or Mini-Mental State Exam scores *(40)*. The presence or absence of OCS could not be predicted by levodopa therapy. No variables discriminated between the two control groups based on the presence or absence of OCS.

Confirming our hypothesis that OCS are present to a significant extent in PD, our group of patients with PD showed higher YBOCS scores than controls. However, the mean YBOCS score did not qualify for an OCD diagnosis. Thus, although OCS measures are higher in patients with PD than in controls, they should not be viewed as representing an obsessional pathology *per se*. We found that our patients with PD were more prone to OCS of the ordering, symmetry, or checking type, and that these symptoms were egosyntonic (i.e., denoting aspects of a personality viewed as acceptable and consistent with that person's total personality).

Our findings also suggest a link between higher obsessionality and perseverative symptoms. The need for symmetry and sameness could be explained by a difficulty in changing strategies to adapt to a continually evolving environment (early executive dysfunction). Checking could compensate for encoding memory difficulties. Supporting this hypothesis, a recent study in PD reported a beneficial effect of subthalamic stimulation on dorsolateral prefrontal function *as well as* on obsessive-compulsive traits *(41)*. Dysexecutive difficulties may have influenced retrospective studies of a possible premorbid Parkinsonian personality. It has been proposed that this premorbid mental rigidity could designate an early sign of hypodopaminergism, affecting the processing of information by the frontal cortex *(27)*.

7. "NEUROLOGICAL" OCS

In summary, OCS in neurological illnesses like PD may be clinically identical to idiopathic OCD. However, typical descriptions reflect certain differences. OCS in neurological illnesses are primarily associated with compulsions; obsessions are less well-defined. Compulsions may range from pure motor stereotypies to more complex behaviors. Order and symmetry preoccupations, repetitive movements, and forced thought are often described. Anxiety is not overwhelming in the majority of cases, and patients consider these OCS to bé egosyntonic. Therefore, they make less effort to resist these urges. OCS often correlate with movement disorders and cognitive dysfunction, mostly dysexecutive in character. Some overlap, or communication between different cortico–subcortical loops could explain why motor (motor pathway), cognitive (cingulate and dorsolateral pathways), and OCS (cingulate and orbitofrontal pathways) occur simultaneously *(4)*.

The question remains whether the etiopathology of OCS in neurological illnesses is similar to idiopathic OCD. Whether the phenomenology varies depending on type and location of the causal lesion, or whether cognition is preserved or not, is also in question. This raises the possibility that measuring obsessions and compulsions separately may lead to a better definition of the concept. In this regard, DSM-IV criteria used in defining obsessional illnesses are not helpful. Carefully designed treatment studies of OCS in neurological illnesses are also lacking. It would be helpful to know if these symptoms can be alleviated by pharmacotherapy or psychotherapy in the same manner as in idiopathic OCD.

Accurate definitions of OCS and perseveration should be proposed to distinguish both concepts. Both compulsion and perseveration involve inhibition difficulties. However, perseverations are devoid of emotion and motivation usually involved in compulsions (i.e., compulsions without obsessions?). If OCS and perseverations are considered to be part of the same pathophysiological spectrum, some contradiction remains in the fact that executive dysfunction (perseveration) is associated with dorsolateral hypofunction, whereas OCS are associated with orbitofrontal and cingulate hyperactivity. One hypothesis is that perseverations in neurological illnesses have been mistakenly labeled as OCS in some reports. An alternative hypothesis is that both disorders may occur simultaneously. Yet another hypothesis is that orbitofrontal hyperactivity may lead to relative dorsolateral hypofunction, where the frontal cortex is unable to analyze stimuli other than the one that predominates. Carefully designed imagery studies may help to provide answers.

8. CONCLUSION

OCS in neurological disorders demonstrate differences from those present in idiopathic OCD and are interconnected with executive dysfunction and movement disorders. Patients also display less anxiety and resistance. Studies of obsessionality in PD and the parkinsonian personality suggest similarities between obsessional slowness and bradyphrenia. We have found that patients with PD score higher than controls on an OCS scale. Patients suffering from PD with OCS, in comparison to those without, are more susceptible to early perseverative errors, which suggests that OCS in PD may have been mistaken in prior studies for early executive dysfunction. The description of OCS in neurological illnesses should be revised to designate actual OCD from perseverations associated with executive dysfunction.

ACKNOWLEDGMENTS

Grateful thanks to Dr. Paul Lespérance, Sylvain Chouinard, Pierre Blanchet, Hélène Masson, and Martin Thibodeau, without whom this research and discussion could not have been possible.

REFERENCES

1. American Psychiatric Association. Diagnostic and Statistical Manual of Mental Disorders, 4th ed. American Psychiatric Association, Washington, DC, 1994.
2. Baxter LR. Brain imaging as a tool in establishing a theory of brain pathology in obsessive compulsive disorder. J Clin Psychiatry 1990;51(Suppl 2):22–25.
3. Baxter LR. Neuroimaging studies of obsessive-compulsive disorder. Psychiatr Clin North Am 1992;15:871–884.
4. Mega MS, Cummings JL. Frontal-subcortical circuits and neuropsychiatric disorders. J Neuropsychiatry Clin Neurosci 1994;6:358–370.
5. Saxena S, Bota RG, Brody AL. Brain-behavior relationships in obsessive-compulsive disorder. Semin Clin Neuropsychiatry 2001;6:82–101.
6. Graybiel AM, Rauch SL. Toward a neurobiology of obsessive-compulsive disorder. Neuron 2000;28:343–347.
7. Wolff M, Alsobrook JP, Pauls DL. Genetic aspects of obsessive-compulsive disorder. Psychiatr Clin North Am 2000;23:535–544.
8. Kaplan HI, Sadock BJ. Synopsis of Psychiatry: Behavioral Sciences/Clinical Psychiatry, 8th ed. in *Typical Signs and Symptoms of Psychiatric Illness Defined*. Lippincott Williams and Wilkins, Baltimore, MD, 1998, p. 282.
9. Cummings JL. Behavioral and psychiatric symptoms associated with Huntington's disease. Adv Neurol 1995;65:179–186.
10. Purcell R, Maruff P, Kyrios M, et al. Cognitive deficits in obsessive-compulsive disorder on tests of frontal-striatal function. Biol Psychiatry 1998;43:348–357.
11. Abruzzese M, Ferri S, Scarone S. The selective breakdown of frontal functions in patients with obsessive-compulsive disorder and in patients with schizophrenia; a double dissociation experimental finding. Neuropsychologia 1997;35:907–912.
12. Cavedini P, Ferri S, Scarone S, et al. Frontal lobe dysfunction in obsessive-compulsive disorder and major depression: a clinical-neuropsychological study. Psychiatry Res. 1998;78:21–28.
13. Lovell MR, Franzen MD. Neuropsychological assessment. In: Silver JM, Yudofsky SC, Hales RE, eds. Neuropsychiatry of Traumatic Brain Injury, 1st ed. American Psychiatric Press, Washington, 1994, pp. 133–160.
14. Neary D, Snowden JS, Gustafson L, et al. Frontotemporal lobar degeneration: a consensus on clinical diagnosis criteria. Neurology 1998;51:1546–1554.
15. Ames D, Cummings JL, Wirshing WC, et al. Repetitive and compulsive behavior in frontal lobe degenerations. J Neuropsychiatry Clin Neurosci 1994;6:100–113.
16. Laplane D, Levasseur M, Pillon B, et al. Obsessive-compulsive and other behavioural changes with bilateral basal ganglia lesions. Brain 1989;112:699–725.
17. Laplane D. Obsessions et compulsions par lésions des noyaux gris centraux. Rev. Neurol. 1994;150:594–598.
18. Swedo SE, Rapoport JL, Cheslow DL, et al. High prevalence of obsessive-compulsive symptoms in patients with Sydenham's chorea. Am J Psychiatry 1989;145:246–249.
19. Shoulson I. Huntington's disease: cognitive and psychiatric features. Neuropsychiatry Neuropsychol Behav Neurol 1990;3:15–22.
20. Robertson MM. Tourette syndrome, associated conditions and the complexities of treatment. Brain 2000;123:425–462.
21. Leckman JF, Peterson BS, Pauls DL, et al. Tic Disorders. Psychiatr Clin North AM 1997;20:839–861.
22. Cheyette SR, Cummings JL. Encephalitis Lethargica: lessons for contemporary neuropsychiatry. J Neuropsychiatry Clin Neurosci 1995;7:125–134.
23. Ward CD. Encephalitis Lethargica and the development of neuropsychiatry. Psychiatr Clin North Am 1986;9:215–224.
24. Cornford ME, Chang L, Miller BL. The neuropathology of Parkinsonism: an overview. Brain Cogn 1995;28:321–341.
25. Dubois B, Pillon B. Cognitive deficits in Parkinson's disease. J Neurol 1997;244:2–8.
26. Taylor AE, St-Cyr JA. The neuropsychology of Parkinson's disease. Brain Cogn 1995;28:281–296.
27. Menza MA, Golbe LI, Cody RA, et al. Dopamine-related personality traits in Parkinson's disease. Neurology 1993;43:505–508.
28. Hubble JP, Koller WC. The parkinsonian personality. Adv Neurol 1995;65:43–48.
29. Cloninger RC. A systematic method for clinical description and classification of personality variants. Arch Gen Psychiatry 1987;44:573–588.
30. Hymas N, Lees A, Bolton D, et al. The neurology of obsessional slowness. Brain 1991;114:2203–2233.
31. Lees A. The concept of bradyphrenia. Rev. Neurol. 1994;150:823–826.
32. Ratnasuriya RH, Marks IM, Forshaw DM, et al. Obsessive slowness revisited. Br J Psychiatry 1991;159:273–274.
33. Tomer R, Levin BE, Weiner WJ. Obsessive-compulsive symptoms and motor asymmetries in Parkinson's disease. Neuropsychiatry Neuropsychol Behav Neurol 1993;6:26–30.
34. Müller N, Pytz A, Kathmann N, et al. Characteristics of obsessive-compulsive symptoms in Tourette's syndrome, obsessive-compulsive disorder, and Parkinson's disease. Psychiatry Res 1997;70:105–114.
35. Maia AS, Pinto AS, Barbosa ER, et al. Obsessive-compulsive symptoms, obsessive-compulsive disorders, and related disorders in Parkinson's disease. J Neuropsychiatry Clin Neurosci 2003;15:371–374.

36. Alegret M, Junque C, Valldeoriola F, et al. Obsessive-compulsive symptoms in Parkinson's disease. J Neurol Neurosurg Psychiatry 2001;70:394–396.
37. Bruneau M-A, Lespérance P, Chouinard S. Obsessionality in Parkinson's disease. J Neuropsychiatry Clin Neurosci, in press.
38. Mollard E, Cottraux J, Bouvard M. French version of the Yale-Brown Obsessive-Compulsive Scale. L'Encéphale 1989;15:335–341.
39. Heaton RK, Chelume GJ, Talley JL, et al. Wisconsin Card Sorting Test Manual. Psychological Assessment Resources, Odessa, FL, 1993.
40. Folstein MF, Folstein SE, McHugh PR. "Mini-Mental State": a practical method for grading the cognitive state of patients for the clinician. J Psychiatr Res 1975;12:189–198.
41. Alegret M, Junque M, Valldeoriola F, et al. Effects of bilateral subthalamic stimulation on cognitive function in Parkinson's disease. Arch Neurol 2002;58:1223–1227.

4
Dementia

Patricia Kavanagh and Karen Marder

SUMMARY

With an estimated prevalence of 20 to 40%, cognitive impairment and dementia are common in Parkinson's disease (PD). The relative risk for incident dementia has ranged from 1.7 to 5.9 when compared with age-matched controls without PD. Postmortem studies have not found distinct associations between PD, PD with dementia, dementia with Lewy bodies, and Alzheimer's disease. The varying syndromes may represent a spectrum, where individuals exhibit differences in the type, sequence, or time-course of degeneration of neuronal circuits. Dementia in PD is clinically associated most frequently with older age and more severe motor symptoms, which may have a combined effect.

Environmental and genetic risk factors have been proposed, but they have yet to be demonstrated consistently. Early features of dementia in PD are executive dysfunction, impaired verbal fluency, and visuospatial disturbances, making it clinically distinct from Alzheimer's disease. As memory impairment is a late phenomenon, cognitive impairment may be advanced before dementia is diagnosed. Depression, medication-induced psychosis, and apathy are more common in cognitively impaired individuals and may herald dementia. Dementia in PD is an independent risk factor for morbidity and mortality, and treatment should begin with the reduction or elimination of anticholinergic medications and amantadine, followed by the reduction of dopaminergic medications. Cholinesterase inhibitors may help to preserve function in the early and moderate stages. Effects of deep-brain stimulators (DBS) on cognitive decline are not yet well-understood, and further research is needed.

Key Words: Parkinson's disease (PD); dementia; cognitive impairment; executive dysfunction; cholinesterase inhibitors.

1. INTRODUCTION

Cognitive impairment and dementia are frequently associated with Parkinson's disease (PD), although this relationship was not described originally. In his 1817 description of paralysis agitans, James Parkinson stated that "...the senses and intellect (are) uninjured" *(1)*. But later observers debated this point. In 1973, Martin et al. *(2)* proposed that intellectual impairment be recognized as a feature of PD, based on an observational study of 100 consecutive cases of PD. Parkinson's disease dementia (PDD) is linked most clearly with age and severity of motor symptoms *(3–7)*. PDD can be clinically distinguished from Alzheimer's disease (AD) by more prominent impairment of executive function, verbal fluency, and visuospatial skills early in the disease *(8,9)*. Dementia is associated with increased morbidity and mortality *(10–12)*. Dementia, independent of severity of extrapyramidal symptoms (EPS), had a twofold increased risk of mortality over a mean follow-up of 3.9 years *(11)*. No specific pathological substrate or specific therapy for PDD has been identified; however, early recognition of dementia is important in PD to help patients and families plan for their needs.

From: *Current Clinical Neurology*
Parkinson's Disease and Nonmotor Dysfunction
Edited by: R. F. Pfeiffer and I. Bodis-Wollner © Humana Press Inc., Totowa, NJ

2. EPIDEMIOLOGY

2.1. Prevalence

Prevalence estimates for dementia in PD range from less than 10% to more than 80% *(13–15)*. This wide range reflects varying diagnostic criteria for both PD and dementia, methods of evaluation, and use of both hospital- and community-based samples. Studies where diagnostic criteria for dementia are limited to Diagnostic and Statistical Manual of Mental Disorders, Revised 3rd edition (DSM-III-R) definition *(16)*, evaluation is based on a neuropsychological battery, and the sample is community-based rather than hospital-based, have yielded a prevalence of 17.6 to 41% *(4,5,17)*. Use of the Mini-Mental State Exam (MMSE), rather than a full neuropsychological battery, produced prevalence estimates within this range in community-based samples and DSM-III-R criteria *(18,19)*.

2.2. Incidence

Incidence rates in community- and hospital-based series range from 42.6 to 112.5 per 1000 person-years of observation *(3,5,7,20–22)*; the two highest rates were from community-based samples *(5,7)*.

The relative risk (RR) of incident dementia among patients with PD when compared to age-matched controls without PD in community-based samples ranges from 1.7 (95% confidence interval [CI] 1.1–2.7) to 5.9 (95% CI 3.9–9.1). Whereas the incidence of PDD was similar in the two studies *(5,7)*, there was a higher incidence of dementia in the control population of the first study *(5)*, which resulted in a lower RR.

2.3. Incidence and Prevalence as a Measure of Dementia

Because dementia is associated with increased mortality *(11,12,23)*, incidence may be more useful than prevalence as a measure of PDD frequency. Nursing home residents with a possible higher prevalence of dementia *(4)* have not been included in some studies *(21)* and may not be proportionally represented in others.

In a longitudinal study of 210 patients, patients with PD were evaluated for differences between those who followed-up and those who failed to return. There was a significant association between failure to follow-up and poorer performance on neuropsychological testing, suggesting that even incidence studies may underestimate the true occurrence of PDD *(24)*.

3. PATHOLOGY

The hallmarks of idiopathic PD are neuronal loss in the substantia nigra (SN) with Lewy bodies (LB) in some of the surviving neurons. In a clinicopathological study of PD by Hughes et al. *(25)*, all cases with nigral LB also had cortical LB. However, the cognitive status of the individuals studied is not noted.

Cognitive impairment in PD has been associated with increased pathology in the medial SN *(29)*, ventral tegmental area, and locus ceruleus (LC) *(27)*, along with the basal forebrain *(28,29)*. A study that examined the LC, SN, and nucleus basalis found the greatest neuronal loss to be in the LC of both AD and PD cases (demented and nondemented;[*30*]). Another study reported that dementia in PD without concurrent AD was linked with significantly lower LC neuronal counts *(27)*.

Taken as a whole, the clinicopathologic studies indicate that symptomatic individuals have a wide range of pathology without distinct associations between specific syndromes and pathology. PD, PD with dementia, dementia with LB (DLB), and AD appear to occur along a spectrum, and the varying clinical manifestations may represent differences in the type of neuronal circuits impaired, sequence, or time-course of degeneration.

The heterogeneous pathology in PDD can be organized into three broad types: those with senile plaques and neurofibrillary tangles, suggestive of concomitant AD; those with severe subcortical neuronal loss and LB inclusions, especially in the medial SN, suggesting that extensive PD pathology alone may cause dementia *(26)*; and finally, those with findings that suggest DLB may be a cause of PDD. A prospective clinicopathological study examined brains of subjects with DLB, PDD, and PD without dementia. Cortical Lewy body densities could not separate cases of DLB from PDD, but high density of parahippocompal LBs was both sensitive and specific for dementia *(31)*.

3.1. *Contribution of AD Pathology*

A wide range of AD pathology has been reported. In a series of 31 cases in which patients met criteria for clinical dementia and idiopathic PD, pathological changes consistent with coexistent AD were found in 29%, DLB in 10%, and vascular changes in 6%. In the remaining subjects, there was no concomitant pathology to account for dementia, which implies that the neuronal changes of PD may cause dementia *(32)*. In a series of 507 cases of PD, investigators *(33)* found that of the 153 (30.2%) who were demented, 78.4% met criteria for AD, and an additional 6.5% had changes suggestive of AD. Results showed that 8% had evidence of cerebrovascular disease, and 5.2% had no pathology other than PD. Other investigators, noting that AD is characterized by reactive gliosis and increased expression of heat shock proteins, found reactive gliosis and increased expression of the heat shock proteins, hsp27 and αB-crystallin, in PDD specimens in comparison to those of nondemented PD subjects *(34–37)*. These findings imply that PDD may represent a stage in PD that shares biochemical changes with AD, although it is unclear whether it is a different disease or a common response to different insults.

3.2. *PD With Concomitant Pathology*

Clinicopathological studies have demonstrated a relationship between PDD and more severe changes in the medial SN *(26)*, ventral tegmental area and LC *(27)*, and basal forebrain *(28,29)* when compared to PD without dementia. Loss of neurons in the nucleus basalis of Meynert without concomitant AD has been observed in idiopathic PD *(38,39)*.

In one study, dementia in PD correlated with α-synuclein immunostaining cortical LB more closely than with AD-type pathological changes *(40)*. The degree of cognitive impairment in PD is associated with the total number of cortical LB and the amount of neurofibrillary tangles in the temporal cortex *(41)*. As indicated, a small percentage of PDD cases involve no other pathology than PD.

3.3. *Relationship of PDD to DLB*

The consensus guidelines for DLB diagnosis require progressive cognitive decline observed within 12 months of the onset of motor symptoms *(42)*. The requirement for dementia to occur within the narrow time-frame may not be sensitive for DLB, because the duration from motor symptoms to dementia may be longer in some individuals ultimately found to have LB pathology. In one study, subjects with clinically diagnosed PD with onset of dementia at least 4 years after onset of motor symptoms, who had become unresponsive to levodopa, were compared with nondemented controls with PD. Of 13 individuals with dementia, 12 had findings of diffuse or transitional LBD as the primary pathological substrate for dementia (1 had progressive supranuclear palsy). Mean and median LB counts were increased nearly 10-fold in neocortex and limbic areas. Alzheimer pathology was modest, but there was a significant correlation with neocortical LB and senile plaques, as well as neurofibrillary tangles *(43)*.

4. RISK FACTORS

PDD has been related to older age *(3–5,7)*. In one community-based series, the prevalence of dementia in PD increased from 0 for those under 50 to 787.1 per 100,000 for those over age 80 *(17)*. Severity of extrapyramidal motor symptoms (EPS), particularly bradykinesia, has been consistently associated with incident dementia *(5,7,20,22,44,45)*. Dementia has been found to be more frequent among patients at baseline who had masked facies and hypokinesia when compared with those who presented primarily with tremor or rigidity *(46)*. Hallucinations before baseline and akinetic-dominant or mixed tremor/akinetic PD have been identified as risk factors for dementia *(47)*.

Older age and more severe EPS may have a combined effect. When patients were grouped by age and severity of motor impairment, the incidence of dementia increased with both age and motor impairment. By age 80, if Unified Parkinson's Disease Rating Scale (UPDRS) was less than 25, cumulative incidence was 0.07, but when UPDRS was greater than 25, the cumulative incidence was 0.12 *(5)*. In another study, the combination of older age (>72) and more severe EPS (UPDRS > 25) increased the risk of incident dementia 10-fold (RR 9.7, 95% CI, 3.9–24.4). Older age combined with low EPS, or severe EPS combined with younger age, was not associated with a significant increase in dementia risk *(6)*. This suggests that the risk of incident dementia is the result of combined, rather than separate, effects of age and severity of EPS.

In some studies with PDD *(20,21,48)*, age at onset of PD is a factor but not others *(5,22,47)*. Some studies have shown men to be at an increased risk for PDD *(17,22,49–51)*, whereas other studies have not demonstrated such an association *(7,44,52)*.

Lower educational attainment correlates with dementia in PD *(51)*. In a cohort of 180 nondemented patients with PD and controls, current smoking, but not smoking history, was found to be associated with incident dementia in PD (RR = 4.5, 95% CI, 1.2–16.4; *[53]*). The same study found no link between incident PDD and history of head injury, hypertension, or diabetes mellitus. Pesticides, organophosphates, toluene, xylene, rural living, and well-water exposure have not been associated with increased risk of dementia in PD *(49,51)*. An inverse relationship has been observed between postmenopausal hormone replacement therapy and PDD (odds ratio [OR] 0.22, 95% CI, 0.05–1.0), but hormone replacement therapy was not shown to affect the risk of PD itself *(54)*.

Family history of dementia may increase the risk of dementia in PD. In a pilot case–control study, patients with PDD were six times as likely to have a first-degree relative with dementia when compared with nondemented patients with PD *(49)*. In another study, siblings of patients with PDD were three times as likely (RR 3.2, 95% CI, 1.1–9.4) as siblings of normal subjects to have AD. For siblings of patients with PDD older than 65, the RR of AD was 4.9 (CI 1.1–21.4) in comparison with siblings of normal subjects over 65 *(55)*. However, a recent large case-control study found no increased risk of dementia in first degree relatives of subjects with Parkinson's disease without dementia *(56)*.

5. GENETIC RISK FACTORS

Several genetic risk factors for AD have been examined in demented patients with PD. APOE e4 has not been found to be associated with PDD by most investigators *(57–60)*. However, one investigator found APOE e4 allele more than twice as frequently in PDD subjects as in normal controls. Nondemented patients with PD did not differ significantly from controls *(61)*. A meta-analysis of 10 studies examining APOE as a risk factor for dementia in PD estimated OR of 1.78 (95% CI: 1.22–2.60) for APOE e4 *(65)*. Recent work suggests a correlation with APOE e2 and the dementia of PD *(63,64)*, although findings are not consistent *(62)*.

In a few families in Southern Italy and Greece, PD has been associated with mutations in the gene for α-synuclein; some individuals were demented. A recent clinicopathological study of familial PD with dementia found α-synuclein triplication *(65)*. A study of another kindred with autosomal dominant DLB demonstrated a novel mutation *(66)*. Intracellular aggregations of α-synuclein have been also found in a range of neurodegenerative diseases, but these have not been indicated to be related to genetic mutations in idiopathic PD or PDD *(67)*. The overrepresentation of the H1 haplotype of tau has been reported in progressive supranuclear palsy *(68,69)*, frontotemporal degeneration *(70)*, and idiopathic PD *(71)*. A specific association of the H1 haplotype and PDD has not yet been reported.

Although one study suggested that the estrogen receptor gene is a susceptibility gene for PDD (but not PD, [72]), the *Pvu*II polymorphism was not linked with PDD in a clinicopathological study *(73)*. Generally, toxin exposures have not been demonstrated as significant factors, but increased risk of PDD among patients with the CYP2D6 29B+ allele and pesticide exposure has been reported *(74)*.

6. PSYCHIATRIC COMORBIDITY

Depression and medication-induced psychosis may be more common in demented individuals with PD. In a community-based study, 22% of patients with PDD had major depression versus 2.3% of nondemented patients ($p < 0.001$; *[19]*). A Hamilton Depression Rating Scale (HDRS; *[75]*) score greater than 10 was associated with incident dementia in PD (RR 3.55; 95% CI, 1.6–7.9) in another series *(5)*. In a longitudinal study, patients with major depression had greater cognitive decline than mildly or nondepressed patients ($r = -0.42$, $p < 0.01$; *[76]*). At follow-up, the mean HDRS of patients who had become demented had improved from 10.6 to 7.1. It is possible that major depression is associated with a more aggressive form of PD that includes progression to dementia and that pre-existing depression may interact with PD to produce a more rapid evolution to dementia. The improved Hamilton scores may alternatively reflect that depression is more difficult to assess independently in a demented patient.

Psychosis and confusional states may predict cognitive impairment. Although confusion or psychosis may be induced by levodopa, an inverse correlation between duration on levodopa therapy and organic mental syndrome was observed in 203 patients. Patients who developed confusion and psychosis had older onset, more severe EPS, and were treated with levodopa earlier in their course *(77)*. In another study, incident dementia was associated with baseline depression (OR = 6.1, 95% CI = 1.4–26.9) and confusion or psychosis from levodopa (OR = 2.9, 95% CI = 1.5–6.0; *[45]*).

Apathy in PD may exist with or without depression, but it may be independently associated with dementia. As measured by tests, including the MMSE and Cambridge examination of cognition in the elderly (CAMCOG), patients suffering from PD with high apathy were more impaired, especially in executive function. Apathy was better correlated with cognitive impairment than with depression *(78)*.

7. NEUROPSYCHOLOGICAL FEATURES OF COGNITIVE IMPAIRMENT AND DEMENTIA IN PD

DSM-IV *(79)* requires memory impairment for a diagnosis of dementia. This requirement may lead to underdiagnosis, because memory impairment in early PDD may be mild relative to other aspects of cognitive decline. When dementia presents before motor symptoms, other causes, such as AD or DLB, should be considered. Parkinsonism with dementia may also occur in progressive supranuclear palsy, olivopontocerebellar degeneration, or vascular dementia, yet cognitive impairment may be a late phenomenon.

Cognitive impairment in PD can present along a spectrum and may be unrecognized in its early stages because of more prominent motor impairment. Attention is impaired and may fluctuate *(80)*. Early PDD characteristically involves impaired executive function (i.e., planning, initiating, sequencing, and monitoring tasks, and set shift). Visuomotor and visuospatial skills are relatively impaired. Verbal fluency is usually impaired, but other language functions are relatively unaffected, as is orientation. When compared to nondemented PD cases, patients with PDD demonstrate disturbed organization during memory encoding and retrieval, deficits in verbal fluency, attention, and vigilance *(80)*.

7.1. Premorbid State

Baseline cognitive impairment may portend the development of dementia in PD. Only three longitudinal studies have examined the neuropsychological impairments associated with incident dementia in nondemented PD patients *(8,9,21)*. In a nondemented cohort of 164 patients with PD followed for a mean of 3.7 years, impaired verbal memory and executive function were associated with the development of dementia *(9)*. When patients questionably demented at baseline were excluded, total immediate recall and delayed recall were still associated with later dementia.

Table 1 summarizes key premorbid neuropsychological impairments and their RR of incident dementia.

Table 1
Neuropsychological Impairments Associated With Incident Dementia in Parkinson's Disease

Author	Year	Abnormal test	Relative risk
Levy[a,b] *(9)*	2002	Immediate recall	0.92 (0.87–0.97)
		Delayed recall	0.73 (0.59–0.91)
		Selective reminding	0.87 (0.77–0.99)
		Identities and Oddities	0.85 (0.73–0.98)
Mahieux[c] *(21)*	1998	Picture completion	4.99 (1.0–24.1)
		Interference-Stroop	3.8 ($p = 0.08$)
		Verbal fluency	2.7 (0.8–9.1)
Jacobs[b,c] *(8)*	1995	Letter fluency	3.3 (1.0–10.8)
		Category fluency	6.01 (1.25–28.84)

[a] Higher scores are associated with reduced risk of dementia.

[b] These studies were conducted in essentially the same cohort of community dwellers in northern Manhattan. Jacobs followed the cohort for mean of 2.7 (±1.03) years, and Levy for a mean of 3.7 (±2.3) years.

[c] Higher scores are associated with increased risk of dementia.

Table 2
Neuropsychological Impairments in Parkinson's Disease, Dementia, and Alzheimer's Disease

	PD	PDD	AD
Executive function	++	+++	+++
Attention	0	++	++
Vigilance	0/+	++	++
Orientation	0	0	++
Reaction time	+	+	+
Visuospatial function	++	++	++
Memory			
Free recall-immediate	+	++	++
Free recall-delayed	+	++	+++
Delayed recognition	0	0/+	+++
Language			
Naming	0	0/+	+++
Verbal fluency	++	+++	++

7.2. Progression of Dementia

As dementia progresses, existing deficits worsen, but memory loss may become more prominent. In one study, subjects demonstrated poorer performance on visual confrontation naming (Boston Naming Test) and delayed recall memory *(81)*. It is not understood whether this represents progression of cognitive impairment specific to PD or the onset of another dementing disorder like AD.

7.3. PDD Compared to AD

The dementia of PD has distinct characteristics and is marked by a different pattern of impairment from AD *(8,20,82)*. Patients with PDD have impaired immediate memory as in AD; however, cued recall and recognition memory remain commensurate with immediate recall, whereas on successive tests, patients with AD retain less information with each trial. The memory deficit in AD can be thought of as impaired encoding or consolidating information. The memory deficit of PD may be a retrieval deficit and could reflect loss of executive function, specifically the ability to systematically search memory. Similarly, the impaired verbal fluency of PDD may represent loss of systematic retrieval and generation of language compared to AD. There is relative preservation of delayed recall and delayed recognition memory, naming and orientation *(83)*. Relative impairments are summarized in Table 2.

7.4. Role of Neurotransmitters

As indicated, the cognitive impairment of PD has been hypothesized to correlate with the dopaminergic compromise of subcorticofrontal circuits. Impaired visuospatial and executive function were observed in patients with 1-methyl-4-phenyl-1,2,3,6-tetra-hydropyridine (MPTP)-induced Parkinsonism when compared to age and education matched controls *(84)*. In one study, patients with PD off levodopa therapy or never treated were impaired on complex choice reaction times; patients on levodopa did not differ significantly from normal controls. This suggests that processing concurrent cognitive information requires intact dopaminergic circuits *(85)*. Arguably, as neurodegeneration proceeds, a cholinergic deficit emerges, supported by pathological findings of degeneration in the nucleus basalis of Meynert. The disrupted cellular function represented by cortical LB may also have a role.

Depression in PD may reflect spread of pathology beyond the dopaminergic pathways. Cerebrospinal (CSF) 5-hydroxyindoleacetic acid (5-HIAA) has been shown to be decreased in PD with major depression *(86,87)*; another report documented reduced CSF 5-HIAA in PDD *(88)*, which argues that serotonergic degeneration plays a role in both the depression and dementia of PD.

7.5. Clinical Significance of Neuropsychological Impairment

Cognitive impairment may be overlooked in PD. Diagnostic criteria for dementia emphasize memory impairment, which may be subtle and could possibly only manifest on complex memory tasks. Incipient dementia can be mistakenly attributed to bradykinesia, depression, apathy, or confusion. Formal neuropsychological testing may aid the diagnosis and management of PD *(89)*.

8. IMAGING STUDIES

Single-photon emission computed tomography (SPECT), positron emission tomography (PET), magnetic resonance spectroscopy (MRS), functional magnetic resonance imaging, and volumetric MRI have been used to study the neuroanatomical changes in PDD in cross-sectional studies. Several studies where demented patients with PD were compared with nondemented PD patients and normal controls have found patterns of abnormal activity in the patients with PDD. Nondemented patients with PD were not significantly different from controls *(90–93)*. One investigator compared 13 demented and 13 nondemented patients with PD to 10 unaffected controls using SPECT. Regional cerebral blood flow in nondemented subjects with PD was not significantly different from controls. Of the 13 demented patients, 4 demonstrated bilateral frontal hypoperfusion; 8 had frontoparietal hypoperfusion, and 1 had parietal hypoperfusion alone *(91)*. However, a study of nondemented PD patients found temporoparietal hypometabolism with both MRS and PET, suggesting that both glycolytic and oxidative pathways are impaired in PD *(94)*.

Patients with PDD when compared with nondemented patients with PD of similar motor disability showed decreased dopamine uptake in the anterior cingulate gyrus, ventral striatum, and right-caudate nucleus when measured with 18F-dopa PET *(95)*. This finding supports the hypothesis that dementia in PD is associated with greater impairment of mesolimbic and caudate dopaminergic function.

As all studies published to date have been cross-sectional, the disease stage of subjects at the time of evaluation is unknown. Prospective studies that assess patients with PD periodically with neuropsychological testing and functional imaging might help to identify the biological correlates of clinical progression to dementia.

9. TREATMENT

9.1. Cognitive Complications of PD Therapy

Treatment of PD may be linked with confusion and psychosis, and patients who develop these signs should be assessed for cognitive impairment. Often, the patient and physician, and in later stages, the caregiver, must choose between better motor control and better cognitive function. The antiparkinsonian agents, particularly levodopa, dopamine agonists, and amantadine, may cause or exacerbate hallucinations. When a patient has symptoms or signs of dementia, it is advisable to reduce or eliminate medications with pure or high anticholinergic activity. Amantadine, which often increases confusion in demented patients, may be reduced or eliminated. Finally, dopaminergic agents should be reduced to the lowest tolerable dose. Moreover, patients may become unresponsive to levodopa with the development of dementia; these medications may no longer be useful.

9.2. Pharmacological Treatments of PDD

No pharmacotherapy is established for either the prevention or symptomatic treatment of dementia of PD. A randomized crossover study of patients suffering from PD with later onset of cognitive impairment, treated with donepezil for 20 weeks, showed a mean increase in the MMSE score of 2.1 (standard deviation [SD] 2.7), a significant effect when compared to placebo ($p < 0.013$; [*96*]). In an open study of 11 patients with PDD who were treated with tacrine (7) and donepezil (4), there was significant cognitive improvement as measured by Alzheimer's Disease Assessment Scale (ADAS)-cog and a trend toward improvement as measured by MMSE and Global Deterioration Scale without motor worsening *(97)*. A study of rivastigmine with slow-dose escalation showed improved cognitive function, along with reduced behavioral problems and visual hallucinations in PDD without notable side effects *(98)*. A randomized, double-blind, placebo-controlled trial of rivastigmine in DLB demonstrated statistically and clinically significant behavioral effects *(99)*; however, there are no published studies of double-blind, placebo-controlled studies in PDD. The effect of memantine in PDD remains to be seen.

Trials of piracetam, phosphatidylserine, and olanzapine have not demonstrated improved cognitive performance *(100–102)*. Selegiline and tocopherol in the Deprenyl and tocopherol antioxidant therapy of Parkinsonism (DATATOP) trial did not significantly delay progression to dementia *(103)*.

9.3. Cognitive Effects of Surgical Treatment

The advent of surgical treatment for PD has raised new questions about patients with dementia or cognitive impairment. Surgical lesioning of the internal globus pallidus is related to improved motor control *(104)*. Surgical experience has provided additional evidence for the existence of distinct frontosubcortical circuits within the basal ganglia. A series of 26 patients were studied after lesioning of the globus pallidus. Lesions in the anteromedial region were associated with increased cognitive impairment. In the posterolateral region improvement in category-cued fluency and the Paced Auditory Serial Addition Test were noted. However, performance on other neuropsychological tests was inconclusive *(105)*.

More recently, implanted deep-brain stimulators (DBS) of the subthalamic nucleus have provided variable, reversible means of controlling motor symptoms *(106,107)*. Patients can then function on lower doses of levodopa and dopamine agonists with concomitant reduction in cognitive side effects of these drugs.

Limited data exist on the cognitive effects of chronic DBS itself. Up to 6 months after implantation of DBS 62 consecutive patients were assessed with a neuropsychological battery assessing 25 cognitive variables. Under stimulation, patients' performance improved on parts A and B of the Trail Making test, but deteriorated on literal and total verbal fluency *(107)*. In another series, patients were followed for up to 12 months after surgery. At 3 to 6 months, patients demonstrated significant declines in working memory, speed of mental processing, bimanual motor speed and coordination, set switching, phonemic fluency, consolidation of verbal material, and encoding of visuospatial material—never returning to baseline performance. The effects were more pronounced in patients older than 69 years *(108)*.

Motor circuits may be preserved at the expense of circuits subserving cognitive tasks. Seven patients suffering from PD with DBS "on" demonstrated improved motor symptoms but impaired letter fluency; the reverse was true in the "off" state *(109)*.

Future investigations may focus on possible cognitive benefit of "off" periods for DBS.

10. PROGNOSIS

Dementia in PD is associated with poor outcomes. Hip fractures occur more frequently (OR for men 3.4, 95% CI 2.5–4.8; OR for women 2.5, 95% CI 2.1–3.1 [*110*]). Dementia is a risk factor for nursing home placement *(10)*, and caregivers of demented patients with PD report increased distress *(111)*. A cross-sectional study of elderly people in southwestern France found the prevalence of dementia in PD to be 16.7% among people living at home when compared with 33.3% for those living in institutions. MMSE scores were lower for institutionalized PD patients than for community dwellers *(4)*.

Early epidemiological studies showed the low prevalence relative to incidence, which implies shortened life span for demented patients. Subsequent longitudinal studies confirmed that patients with PDD have an increased risk of death in comparison with both nondemented patients with PD and normal age-matched controls *(12,23)*.

11. CONCLUSION

Dementia is a common feature of PD and is associated with institutionalization and increased mortality. The biological substrate is not well-understood, as there is significant overlap with DLB and AD. Patients with confusion, psychosis, depression, or apathy should be evaluated for dementia. Loss of levodopa responsiveness may be associated with dementia and, in any event, is a point when dopaminergic therapy should be reduced. Although they may provide significant motor improvement and concomitant improvement in quality of life, DBS or pallidotomy may affect cognition adversely.

REFERENCES

1. Parkinson J. An Essay on the Shaking Palsy. In: Wilkins RH and Brody I, eds. Neurological Classics. American Association of Neurological Surgeons, Park Ridge, IL, 1997.
2. Martin WE, Loewenson RB, Resch JA, Baker AB. Parkinson's disease. Clinical analysis of 100 patients. Neurology 1973;23:783–790.
3. Mayeux R, Chen J, Mirabello E, et al. An estimate of the incidence of dementia in idiopathic Parkinson's disease. Neurology 1990;40:1513–1517.
4. Tison F, Dartigues JF, Auriacombe S, et al. Dementia in Parkinson's disease: a population-based study in ambulatory and institutionalized individuals. Neurology 1995;45:705–708.
5. Marder K, Tang MX, Cote L, et al. The frequency and associated risk factors for dementia in patients with Parkinson's disease. Arch Neurol 1995;52:695–701.
6. Levy G, Schupf N, Tang MX, et al. Combined effect of age and severity on the risk of dementia in Parkinson's disease. Ann Neurol 2002;51:722–729.
7. Aarsland D, Andersen K, Larsen JP, et al. Risk of dementia in Parkinson's disease: a community-based, prospective study. Neurology 2001;56:730–736.
8. Jacobs DM, Marder K, Cote LJ, et al. Neuropsychological characteristics of preclinical dementia in Parkinson's disease. Neurology 1995;45:1691–1696.
9. Levy G, Jacobs DM, Tang MX, et al. Memory and executive function impairment predict dementia in Parkinson's disease. Mov Disord 2002;17:1221–1226.
10. Aarsland D, Larsen JP, Tandberg E, Laake K. Predictors of nursing home placement in Parkinson's disease: a population-based, prospective study. J Am Geriatr Soc 2000;48:938–942.
11. Levy G, Tang MX, Louis ED, et al. The association of incident dementia with mortality in PD. Neurology 2002;59:1708–1713.
12. Louis ED, Marder K, Cote L, et al. Mortality from Parkinson disease. Arch Neurol 1997;54:260–264.
13. Brown RG, Marsden CD. How common is dementia in Parkinson's disease? Lancet 1984;2:1262–1265.
14. Cummings JL. The dementias of Parkinson's disease: prevalence, characteristics, neurobiology, and comparison with dementia of the Alzheimer type. Eur Neurol 1988;28(Suppl 1):15–23.

15. Marder K, Mayeux R. The epidemiology of dementia in patients with Parkinson's disease. Adv Exp Med Biol 1991;295:439–445.
16. American Psychiatric Association. Diagnostic and Statistical Manual of Mental Disorders, Revised 3rd ed. American Psychiatric Press, Washington, DC, 1987.
17. Mayeux R, Denaro J, Hemenegildo N, et al. A population-based investigation of Parkinson's disease with and without dementia. Relationship to age and gender. Arch Neurol 1992;49:492–497.
18. Ebmeier KP, Calder SA, Crawford JR, et al. Dementia in idiopathic Parkinson's disease: prevalence and relationship with symptoms and signs of Parkinsonism. Psychol Med 1991;21:69–76.
19. Aarsland D, Tandberg E, Larsen JP, Cummings JL. Frequency of dementia in Parkinson Disease. Arch Neurol 1996;53:538–542.
20. Biggins CA, Boyd JL, Harrop FM, et al. A controlled, longitudinal study of dementia in Parkinson's disease. J Neurol Neurosurg Psychiatry 1992;55:566–571.
21. Mahieux F, Fenelon G, Flahault A, et al. Neuropsychological prediction of dementia in Parkinson's disease. J Neurol Neurosurg Psychiatry 1998;64:178–183.
22. Hughes TA, Ross HF, Musa S, et al. A 10-year study of the incidence of and factors predicting dementia in Parkinson's disease. Neurology 2000;54:1596–1602.
23. Marder K, Leung D, Tang M, et al. Are demented patients with Parkinson's disease accurately reflected in prevalence surveys? A survival analysis. Neurology 1991;41:1240–1243.
24. Levin BE, Katzen HL, Klein B, Llabre ML. Cognitive decline affects subject attrition in longitudinal research. J Clin Exp Neuropsychol 2000;22:580–586.
25. Hughes AJ, Daniel SE, Kilford L, Lees AJ. Accuracy of clinical diagnosis of idiopathic Parkinson's disease: a clinicopathological study of 100 cases. J Neurol Neurosurg Psychiatry 1992;55:181–184.
26. Rinne JO, Rummukainen J, Paljarvi L, Rinne UK. Dementia in Parkinson's disease is related to neuronal loss in the medial substantia nigra. Ann Neurol 1989;26:47–50.
27. Zweig RM, Cardillo JE, Cohen M, et al. The locus ceruleus and dementia in Parkinson's disease. Neurology 1993;43:986–991.
28. Whitehouse PJ, Hedreen JC, White CL, III, Price DL. Basal forebrain neurons in the dementia of Parkinson disease. Ann Neurol 1983;13:243–248.
29. Gaspar P, Gray F. Dementia in idiopathic Parkinson's disease. A neuropathological study of 32 cases. Acta Neuropathol 1984;64:43–52.
30. Zarow C, Lyness SA, Mortimer JA, Chui HC. Neuronal loss is greater in the locus coeruleus than nucleus basalis and substantia nigra in Alzheimer and Parkinson diseases. Arch Neurol 2003;60:337–341.
31. Harding AJ and Halliday GM. Cortical Lewy body pathology in the diagnosis of dementia. Acta Neuropathol 2001;102:355–363.
32. Hughes AJ, Daniel SE, Blankson S, Lees AJ. A clinicopathologic study of 100 cases of Parkinson's disease. Arch Neurol 1993;50:140–148.
33. Jellinger KA. Morphological substrates of dementia in parkinsonism. A critical update. J Neural Transm Suppl 1997;51:57–82.
34. Renkawek K, Bosman GJ, de Jong WW. Expression of small heat-shock protein hsp 27 in reactive gliosis in Alzheimer disease and other types of dementia. Acta Neuropathol 1994;87:511–519.
35. Renkawek K, Bosman GJ, Gaestel M. Increased expression of heat-shock protein 27 kDa in Alzheimer disease: a preliminary study. Neuroreport 1993;5:14–16.
36. Renkawek K, Stege GJ, Bosman GJ. Dementia, gliosis and expression of the small heat shock proteins hsp27 and alpha B-crystallin in Parkinson's disease. Neuroreport 1999;10:2273–2276.
37. Renkawek K, Voorter CE, Bosman GJ, et al. Expression of alpha B-crystallin in Alzheimer's disease. Acta Neuropathol 1994;87:155–160.
38. Tagliavini F, Pilleri G, Bouras C, Constantinidis J. The basal nucleus of Meynert in idiopathic Parkinson's disease. Acta Neurol Scand 1984;70:20–28.
39. Nakano I, Hirano A. Parkinson's disease: neuron loss in the nucleus basalis without concomitant Alzheimer's disease. Ann Neurol 1984;15:415–418.
40. Hurtig HI, Trojanowski JQ, Galvin J, et al. Alpha-synuclein cortical Lewy bodies correlate with dementia in Parkinson's disease. Neurology 2000;54:1916–1921.
41. Mattila PM, Roytta M, Torikka H, et al. Cortical Lewy bodies and Alzheimer-type changes in patients with Parkinson's disease. Acta Neuropathol 1998;95:576–582.
42. McKeith IG, Galasko D, Kosaka K, et al. Consensus guidelines for the clinical and pathologic diagnosis of dementia with Lewy bodies (DLB): report of the consortium on DLB international workshop. Neurology 1996;47:1113–1124.
43. Apaydin H, Ahlskog JE, Parisi JE, et al. Parkinson disease neuropathology. Later-developing dementia and loss of the levodopa response. Arch Neurol 2002;59:102–112.
44. Ebmeier KP, Calder SA, Crawford JR, et al. Clinical features predicting dementia in idiopathic Parkinson's disease: a follow-up study. Neurology 1990;40:1222–1224.

45. Stern Y, Marder K, Tang MX, Mayeux R. Antecedent clinical features associated with dementia in Parkinson's disease. Neurology 1993;43:1690–1692.
46. Mindham RHS. The place of dementia in Parkinson's disease: a methodologic saga. Adv Neurol 1999;80:403–408.
47. Aarsland D, Andersen K, Larsen JP, et al. Prevalence and characteristics of dementia in Parkinson disease: an 8-year prospective study. Arch Neurol 2003;60:387–392.
48. Mayeux R, Denaro J, Hemenegildo N, et al. A population-based investigation of Parkinson's disease with and without dementia. Relationship to age and gender. Arch Neurol 1992;49:492–497.
49. Marder K, Flood P, Cote L, Mayeux R. A pilot study of risk factors for dementia in Parkinson's disease. Mov Disord 1990;5:156–161.
50. Breteler MM, de Groot RR, van Romunde LK, Hofman A. Risk of dementia in patients with Parkinson's disease, epilepsy, and severe head trauma: a register-based follow-up study. Am J Epidemiol 1995;142:1300–1305.
51. Glatt SL, Hubble JP, Lyons K, et al. Risk factors for dementia in Parkinson's disease: effect of education. Neuroepidemiology 1996;15:20–25.
52. Diamond SG, Markham CH, Hoehn MM, et al. An examination of male-female differences in progression and mortality of Parkinson's disease. Neurology 1990;40:763–766.
53. Levy G, Tang MX, Cote LJ, et al. Do risk factors for Alzheimer's disease predict dementia in Parkinson's disease? An exploratory study. Mov Disord 2002;17:250–257.
54. Marder K, Tang MX, Alfaro B, et al. Postmenopausal estrogen use and Parkinson's disease with and without dementia. Neurology 1998;50:1141–1143.
55. Marder K, Tang MX, Alfaro B, et al. Risk of Alzheimer's disease in relatives of Parkinson's disease patients with and without dementia. Neurology 1999;52:719–724.
56. Levy G, Louis ED, Mejia-Santana H, et al. Lack of familial aggregation of Parkinson disease and Alzheimer disease. Arch Neurol 2004;61:1033–1039.
57. Marder K, Maestre G, Cote L, et al. The apolipoprotein epsilon 4 allele in Parkinson's disease with and without dementia. Neurology 1994;44:1330–1331.
58. Koller WC, Glatt SL, Hubble JP, et al. Apolipoprotein E genotypes in Parkinson's disease with and without dementia. Ann Neurol 1995;37:242–245.
59. Whitehead AS, Bertrandy S, Finnan F, et al. Frequency of the apolipoprotein E epsilon 4 allele in a case-control study of early onset Parkinson's disease. J Neurol Neurosurg Psychiatry 1996;61:347–351.
60. Inzelberg R, Chapman J, Treves TA, et al. Apolipoprotein E4 in Parkinson disease and dementia: new data and meta-analysis of published studies. Alz Dis Assoc Disord 1998;12:45–48.
61. Parsian A, Racette B, Goldsmith LJ, Perlmutter JS. Parkinson's disease and apolipoprotein E: possible association with dementia but not age at onset. Genomics 2002;79:458–461.
62. Huang X, Chen PC, Kaufer DI, et al. APOE's role in dementia in Parkinson's disease: a meta-analysis. Neurology 2004;62(Suppl 5):(Abstract)A206.
63. Ramakrishnan R, Zareparsi S, Gancher S, et al. Risk factors for Parkinson's dementia: age, male gender, and apolipoprotein e2. Neurology 2001;56(Suppl 3):(Abstract) A113.
64. Harhangi BS, de Rijk MC, van Duijn CM, et al. APOE and the risk of PD with or without dementia in a population-based study. Neurology 2000;54:1272–1276.
65. Farrer M, Kachergus J, Forno L, et al. Comparison of kindreds with parkinsonism and alpha-synuclein multiplications. Ann Neurol 2004;55:174–179.
66. Zarranz JJ, Alegre J, Gomez-Esteban, JC, et al. The new mutation, E46K, of alpha-synuclein causes Parkinson and Lewy body dementia. Ann Neurol 2004;55:164–173.
67. Nussbaum RL, Ellis CE. Alzheimer's disease and Parkinson's disease. N Engl J Med 2003;348:1356–1364.
68. Ezquerra M, Pastor P, Valldeoriola F, et al. Identification of a novel polymorphism in the promoter region of the tau gene highly associated to progressive supranuclear palsy in humans. Neurosci Let 1999;19;275:183–186.
69. Pastor P, Ezquerra M, Tolosa E, et al. Further extension of the H1 haplotype associated with progressive supranuclear palsy. Mov Disord 2002;17:550–556.
70. Verpillat P, Camuzat A, Hannequin D, et al. Association between the extended tau haplotype and frontotemporal dementia. Arch Neurol 2002;59:935–939.
71. Farrer M, Skipper L, Berg M, et al. The tau H1 haplotype is associated with Parkinson's disease in the Norwegian population. Neurosci Let 2002;322:83–86.
72. Isoe-Wada K, Maeda M, Yong J, et al. Positive association between an estrogen receptor gene polymorphism and Parkinson's disease with dementia. Eur J Neurol 1999;6:431–435.
73. Mattila KM, Rinne JO, Roytta M, et al. Lack of association between an estrogen receptor 1 gene polymorphism and Parkinson's disease with dementia. Acta Neurol Scand 2002;106:128–130.
74. Hubble JP, Kurth JH, Glatt SL, et al. Gene-toxin interaction as a putative risk factor for Parkinson's disease with dementia. Neuroepidemiology 1998;17:96–104.
75. Hamilton M. A rating scale for depression. J Neurol Neurosurg Psychiatry 1960;23:56–62.

76. Starkstein SE, Bolduc PL, Mayberg HS, et al. Cognitive impairments and depression in Parkinson's disease: a followup study. J Neurol Neurosurg Psychiatry 1990;53:597–602.
77. Elizan TS, Sroka H, Maker H, et al. Dementia in idiopathic Parkinson's disease. Variables associated with its occurrence in 203 patients. J Neural Transm 1986;65:285–302.
78. Pluck GC, Brown RG. Apathy in Parkinson's disease. J Neurol Neurosurg Psychiatry 2002;73:636–642.
79. American Psychiatric Association. Diagnostic and Statistical Manual of Mental Disorders, 4th ed. American Psychiatric Association, Washington, DC, 1994.
80. Ballard CG, Aarsland D, McKeith I, et al. Fluctuations in attention: PD dementia vs. DLB with Parkinsonism. Neurology 2002;59:1714–1720.
81. Stern Y, Tang MX, Jacobs DM, et al. Prospective comparative study of the evolution of probable Alzheimer's disease and Parkinson's disease dementia. J Int Neuropsychol Soc 1998;4:279–284.
82. Pillon B, Dubois B, Ploska A, Agid Y. Severity and specificity of cognitive impairment in Alzheimer's, Huntington's, and Parkinson's diseases and progressive supranuclear palsy. Neurology 1991;41:634–643.
83. Helkala EL, Laulumaa V, Soininen H, Riekkinen PJ. Recall and recognition memory in patients with Alzheimer's and Parkinson's diseases. Ann Neurol 1988;24:214–217.
84. Stern Y, Langston JW. Intellectual changes in patients with MPTP-induced Parkinsonism. Neurology 1985;35:1506–1509.
85. Malapani C, Pillon B, Dubois B, Agid Y. Impaired simultaneous cognitive task performance in Parkinson's disease: a dopamine-related dysfunction. Neurology 1994;44:319–326.
86. Mayeux R, Stern Y, Cote L, Williams JB. Altered serotonin metabolism in depressed patients with Parkinson's disease. Neurology 1984;34:642–646.
87. Mayeux R, Stern Y, Sano M, Cote L. The relationship of serotonin to depression in Parkinson's disease. Mov Disord 1988;3:237–244.
88. Sano M, Stern Y, Williams J, et al. Coexisting dementia and depression in Parkinson's disease. Arch Neurol 1989;46:1284–1286.
89. Pillon B, Dubois B, Agid Y. Testing cognition may contribute to the diagnosis of movement disorders. Neurology 1996;46:329–334.
90. Spampinato U, Habert MO, Mas JL, et al. (99mTc)-HM-PAO SPECT and cognitive impairment in Parkinson's disease: a comparison with dementia of the Alzheimer type. J Neurol Neurosurg Psychiatry 1991;54:787–792.
91. Sawada H, Udaka F, Kameyama M, et al. SPECT findings in Parkinson's disease associated with dementia. J Neurol Neurosurg Psychiatry 1992;55:960–963.
92. Pizzolato G, Dam M, Borsato N, et al. [99mTc]-HM-PAO SPECT in Parkinson's disease. J Cereb Blood Flow Metab 1988;8:S101–S108.
93. Summerfield C, Gomez-Anson B, Tolosa E, et al. Dementia in Parkinson disease: a proton magnetic resonance spectroscopy study. Arch Neurol 2002;59:1415–1420.
94. Hu MT, Taylor-Robinson SD, Chaudhuri KR, et al. Cortical dysfunction in non-demented Parkinson's disease patients: a combined (31)P-MRS and (18)FDG-PET study. Brain 2000;123:340–352.
95. Ito K, Nagano-Saito A, Kato T, et al. Striatal and extrastriatal dysfunction in Parkinson's disease with dementia: a 6-[18F]fluoro-L-dopa PET study. [Erratum appears in Brain 2002;125:2144.] Brain 2002;125:1358–1365.
96. Aarsland D, Laake K, Larsen JP, Janvin C. Donepezil for cognitive impairment in Parkinson's disease: a randomised controlled study. [Erratum appears in J Neurol Neurosurg Psychiatry 2002;73:354.] J Neurol Neurosurg Psychiatry 2002;72:708–712.
97. Werber EA, Rabey JM. The beneficial effect of cholinesterase inhibitors on patients suffering from Parkinson's disease and dementia. J Neural Transm 2001;108:1319–1325.
98. Bullock R, Cameron A. Rivastigmine for the treatment of dementia and visual hallucinations associated with Parkinson's disease: a case series. Curr Med Res Opin 2002;18:258–264.
99. McKeith I, Del Ser T, Spano P, et al. Efficacy of rivastigmine in dementia with Lewy bodies: a randomized, double-blind, placebo-controlled international study. Lancet 2000;356:2031–2036.
100. Sano M, Stern Y, Marder K, Mayeux R. A controlled trial of piracetam in intellectually impaired patients with Parkinson's disease. Mov Disord 1990;5:230–234.
101. Funfgeld EW, Baggen M, Nedwidek P, et al. Double-blind study with phosphatidylserine (PS) in parkinsonian patients with senile dementia of Alzheimer's type (SDAT). Prog Clin Biol Res 1989;317:1235–46.
102. Marsh L, Lyketsos C, Reich SG. Olanzapine for the treatment of psychosis in patients with Parkinson's disease and dementia. Psychosomatics 2001;42:477–481.
103. Kieburtz K, McDermott M, Como P, et al. The effect of deprenyl and tocopherol on cognitive performance in early untreated Parkinson's disease. Neurology 1994;44:1756–1759.
104. Vitek JL, Bakay RA, Freeman A, et al. Randomized trial of pallidotomy versus medical therapy for Parkinson's disease. Ann Neurol 2003;53:558–569.
105. Lombardi WJ, Gross RE, Trepanier LL, et al. Relationship of lesion location to cognitive outcome following microelectrode-guided pallidotomy for Parkinson's disease: support for the existence of cognitive circuits in the human pallidum. Brain 2000;123:746–758.

106. Limousin P, Pollak P, Benazzouz A, et al. Effect of parkinsonian signs and symptoms of bilateral subthalamic nucleus stimulation. Lancet 1995;345:91–95.
107. Ardouin C, Pillon B, Peiffer E, et al. Bilateral subthalamic or pallidal stimulation for Parkinson's disease affects neither memory nor executive functions: a consecutive series of 62 patients. Ann Neurol 1999;46:217–223.
108. Saint-Cyr JA, Trepanier LL, Kumar R, et al. Neuropsychological consequences of chronic bilateral stimulation of the subthalamic nucleus in Parkinson's disease. Brain 2000;123:2091–2108.
109. Ceballos-Baumann A. Deep brain stimulation of the subthalamic nucleus in Parkinson's disease affects a fronto-temporal network associated with verbal fluency: a PET study. Neurology 2003;50(Supp 1):(Abstract) A125.
110. Pressley JC, Louis ED, Tang MX, et al. The impact of comorbid disease and injuries on resource use and expenditures in Parkinsonism. Neurology 2003;60:87–93.
111. Aarsland D, Larsen JP, Karlsen K, et al. Mental symptoms in Parkinson's disease are important contributors to caregiver distress. Int J Geriatr Psychiatry 1999;14:866–874.

5
Psychosis

Eric S. Molho and Stewart A. Factor

SUMMARY

There has been a growing recognition that psychosis, its impact on the treatment of motor symptoms, and its interaction with cognitive dysfunction, represent a major unmet need in the treatment of advanced Parkinson's disease (PD). Psychosis in PD is predominantly, although perhaps not exclusively, medication-induced. All anti-Parkinsonian drugs in current use, not just levodopa, are capable of producing drug-induced psychosis in patients with PD. Cognitive impairment and depression are strong predictors of risk for the development of hallucinations with PD. Hallucinations and psychosis can occur at any time in the course of PD, but they are most commonly seen as a late complication in susceptible individuals. Visual hallucinations are the most common feature of drug-induced psychosis in PD, although other types of hallucinations have also been reported. Insight that the images are not real may be retained. The mechanisms responsible for producing drug-induced psychosis in PD are poorly understood, and treatment can be approached in a stepwise manner. A triggering factor, such as infection, should be excluded. If one is not discovered, step-by-step tapering of anti-Parkinson medication should then be undertaken. If increased motor disability prevents adequate dosage reduction, quetiapine is a reasonable first-choice antipsychotic agent to employ.

Key Words: Drug-induced psychosis; dopaminergic mechanisms; hallucinosis; illusions; clozapine; quetiapine.

1. INTRODUCTION

With the development of levodopa therapy for Parkinson's disease (PD) in the late 1960s came great optimism that dopamine replacement therapy might provide a cure or, at least, a lasting reversal of symptoms. However, it was soon realized that levodopa therapy, despite being dramatically effective in controlling symptoms, was not a cure, and there were numerous long-term troublesome complications associated with its use. Among these problems were several drug-induced psychiatric states. The state that may be considered the most prominent and disabling is drug-induced psychosis (DIP; *1*). Studies have demonstrated that hallucinations in PD are a major risk factor for increased caregiver stress and strain *(2)*, as well as nursing home placement that is often permanent *(3)*. It has also been established that the occurrence of hallucinations and DIP, in general, heralds an alarmingly high mortality, particularly in the nursing home setting *(4,5)*. Recently, psychosis in PD has received increased attention because of the clearly demonstrated efficacy of clozapine (CLZ) in treating this problem *(6,7)* and the availability of other alternative "atypical" antipsychotic medications, each of which has been proposed as a safe and effective alternative to CLZ.

There has also been growing understanding that psychosis, its effect on the treatment of motor symptoms, and its relationship with cognitive dysfunction represent a significant need in the treatment of advanced PD.

From: *Current Clinical Neurology*
Parkinson's Disease and Nonmotor Dysfunction
Edited by: R. F. Pfeiffer and I. Bodis-Wollner © Humana Press Inc., Totowa, NJ

This report reviews the history, clinical features, and mechanisms of DIP in PD, analyzes recent literature concerning the treatment of DIP with atypical antipsychotic medications, and outlines an updated, practical approach to its treatment.

2. TERMINOLOGY AND HISTORY

In the past, the terms "levodopa psychosis," "dopaminomimetic psychosis," and "drug-induced psychosis" DIP have been used indiscriminately to describe several different psychiatric syndromes that occur in PD. Their broad application has hindered our understanding of the frequency, pathophysiology, and treatment of these disorders. It is now clear that there are several distinct psychiatric syndromes with psychotic features that occur in PD. Although Friedman *(8)* has suggested labeling these syndromes the levodopa psychoses, it is clear that levodopa is not the only drug with the capability of causing psychosis. There are also questions whether psychosis is purely a dopaminergic phenomenon; thus, the term "dopaminomimetic psychosis" may also be inaccurate. Finally, it remains uncertain that drugs are the only cause of psychosis in PD, although for the most part, psychosis does occur in treated patients. So the best term, and the one that will be used here, is DIP. For the sake of clarity, these syndromes are divided into two broad categories: those associated with a clear sensorium and those occurring on a background of confusion. Patients with a clear sensorium may suffer from delusions, hallucinations, or both. By *Diagnostic and Statistical Manual of Disorders* (DSM-III-R) criteria, these correspond to an organic delusional syndrome or an organic hallucinosis, respectively *(9)*. The organic confusional psychosis is seen in patients with a clouded sensorium and can vary in intensity from a mild confusional state to a frank delirium. These terms are no longer used in DSM-IV, but we feel they are still useful in the discussion of psychosis in PD. There seems to be general agreement that, despite that all these syndromes can be induced by dopaminergic medications, they are distinct in their epidemiology pathophysiology (including association with dementia), and response to treatment *(8,10–12)*. For clarification, the term DIP is used to refer to psychotic symptoms (hallucinations and delusions) occurring on the backdrop of a clear sensorium.

A historical review of psychosis in PD from the prelevodopa era indicates that not all psychotic symptoms are drug-related. Coexistent and premorbid psychiatric disease can occur, including schizophrenia *(8)*. There is also little question that psychiatric symptoms, such as psychosis, can be a prominent feature of secondary Parkinsonism, particularly the postencephalitic form *(13)*. The parkinsonian syndrome, Lewy body dementia (LBD; *14*) can also present with psychosis prior to any exposure to drugs. In all likelihood, those cases of PD with early prominent psychosis described in the 1960s and 70s were this disorder. However, the occurrence of hallucinations, delusions, and other psychotic symptoms as part of the natural history of PD is controversial, especially because a clear overlap between PD and LBD exists, leading to speculation that these are the same disease *(15,16)*.

In James Parkinson's original description of the disease, he concluded, "...by the absence of any injury to the senses and to the intellect, we are taught that the morbid state does not extend to the encephalon" *(17)*. This view of PD as a process that spares the intellect and psychological functioning was held for nearly a century. In 1903, Regis *(18)* categorized the mental disorders associated with Parkinsonism, specifically mentioning depression as an early phenomenon and hallucinations as symptoms associated with advanced disease. In 1922, 140 patients with PD were reviewed with an attempt to exclude postencephalitic Parkinsonism patients *(19)*. Depression was found in these patients and was thought to be reactive in nature, but no mention of psychotic symptoms was made. Another review in 1923 described several patients with "paralysis agitans" and prominent symptoms of psychosis *(20)*. Early features, such as sleep disturbance, withdrawal from social situations, and suspiciousness, were mentioned. Also discussed were more dramatic symptoms like paranoid delusions and even hallucinations that were "...generally limited to the organic sensations and tactile sense..." *(20)*. In 1950, Schwab et al. *(21)* described a number of psychiatric symptoms in "Parkinson's disease," including paroxysmal depression, paranoia, and schizoid reactions. However, it is clear from a review of the case histories in

Table 1
Frequency of Psychosis in PD: Summary of Recent Studies

Author/year	Patient population	Patient no.	% Psychosis[a]
Factor, 1990 *(33)*	Clinic	78	22%
Sanchez-Ramos, 1996 *(34)*	Clinic	214	26%
Barclay, 1997 *(35)*	Clinic	227	31%
Graham, 1997 *(36)*	Clinic	129	25%
Inzelberg, 1998 *(37)*	Clinic	121	37%
Aarsland, 1999 *(38)*	Population-based	235	25%
Fenelon, 2000 *(39)*	Clinic	216	46%[b]
Holroyd, 2001 *(40)*	Clinic	102	29%
Total		1322	30.8%

[a] Some studies included lifetime and recent occurrence. Lifetime numbers shown.
[b] Included minor symptoms.

this report that all the patients described had a history of encephalitis, oculogyric crisis, or both, and they likely had postencephalitic Parkinsonism rather than PD. Thus, it appears that psychosis may have occurred in PD prior to the levodopa era. However, it must have been rare, and some of these cases might have been secondary forms, especially postencephalitic Parkinsonism.

During the initial levodopa trials in the 1960s, it became apparent that various psychiatric syndromes were occurring with a much higher frequency than in untreated patients with PD. Unfortunately, it is difficult to determine the incidence with which these problems occurred because the early studies varied with regard to inclusion criteria, dosages of levodopa employed, and classification of the psychiatric side effects reported. Studies that included patients with postencephalitic Parkinsonism reported the incidence of psychiatric symptoms as high as 55% *(22)*. Most studies reporting a significant incidence of psychosis used levodopa dosages in excess of 4 g per day or did not specify the dosages used *(23–30)*. On the contrary, Cheifetz et al. *(31)* reported no incidence of psychosis in 34 patients treated with 4 g per day or less. In addition, some authors included patients with pre-existing psychiatric symptoms in their data, whereas others excluded these patients. When reporting side effects, confusional states were sometimes lumped with other forms of psychosis, but other studies attempted to be more specific in their definitions.

Despite these limitations, in 1971, Goodwin attempted to retrospectively review the psychiatric side effects that had occurred in 908 patients with PD treated in the early clinical trials using levodopa *(32)*. He found an average incidence of 20%, but the range was quite large (10–50%). Confusional states, including delirium, were the most common with an overall incidence of 4.4%. Psychosis, such as delusions and hallucinations, occurred with a frequency of 3.6%. These numbers are fairly low, but they only represent reports where the psychiatric side effects were clearly defined.

3. CURRENT EPIDEMIOLOGY AND RISK FACTORS

In the last 15 years, several studies have viewed the prevalence of hallucinations and psychosis in populations of patients with PD. Unlike older reviews on this topic, these studies reflect the modern era of PD treatment and the impact of the several adjunctive medications now available and in common use. Table 1 summarizes the results of eight publications since 1990, including 1322 patients *(33–40)*. The results are fairly consistent with the average overall incidence of psychotic symptoms being 30.8%. All these studies except one are based on movement disorder clinic populations, and they possibly overestimate the incidence of these problems because of selection bias. Fenelon et al. *(39)* found a particularly high incidence (46%), but they included so-called minor symptoms of psychosis like illusions and presence hallucinations. To avoid the problem of selection bias, Aarsland et al. *(38)*

performed the first extensive community-based survey of patients with PD and found that 15.8% had active symptoms of DIP at the time of the survey, and 9.8% specifically had hallucinations. When asked if the patient had ever had symptoms of DIP after the diagnosis of PD (lifetime prevalence), the reported frequency increased to 25%.

Recent reviews have also recognized that all of the anti-Parkinsonian drugs in current use, not just levodopa, are capable of causing DIP *(1,8,10,12)*. Individual reports on bromocriptine and pergolide have shown these agents to cause hallucinations, delusions, and confusional states with a frequency comparable to that of levodopa *(41–44)*. The latest available dopamine agonists, pramipexole and ropinirole, which are now in widespread use, have shown a similar tendency in advanced PD *(45)*. However, when pramipexole and ropinirole were compared to levodopa in studies of patients with early PD, the agonists were associated with a higher frequency of dip *(46,47)*. DIP has also been reported with experimental and less readily available dopamine agonists, e.g., cabergoline *(48)*, lisuride *(49)*, apomorphine *(50)*, lergotrile, and mesulergine *(51)*. Selegiline may be particularly prone to cause psychotic symptoms in susceptible individuals, especially when it is given concurrently with other anti-Parkinsonian medications *(52,53)*.

Nondopaminergic drugs are also known to cause psychosis in patients with PD. Propranolol, which is occasionally used in PD to treat tremors, has been reported to cause hallucinations *(54)*. Amantadine, an *N*-methyl-D-aspartate (NMDA) receptor antagonist, and anticholinergic drugs have also been associated with confusional and nonconfusional psychotic syndromes in patients with PD. When these drugs are given in isolation, the frequency of these problems is low *(55,56)*. Yet, when given in combination with dopaminergic medications, they are much more likely to cause an acute confusional psychosis *(10–12,57)*. The acute confusional syndromes seen with anticholinergic medications are more common in older or demented patients, and in some cases, result in a frank delirium *(12)*. Paradoxically, acute delirium has also been described with amantadine withdrawal in patients treated chronically with this agent *(58)*. It appears that this is particularly true if patients are demented and have been on doses of 300 mg or more per day.

The catechol-*O*-methyltransferase (COMT) inhibitors are a novel class of anti-Parkinsonian medication whose beneficial effect is achieved by increasing the bioavailability of concomitantly administered levodopa. Tolcapone was the first of these agents to be approved for use in PD. In clinical trials, tolcapone was shown to dramatically increase the duration of action and potency of levodopa, resulting in improvement of motor fluctuations *(59,60)*. Not surprisingly, patients treated with tolcapone also experienced an increase in dopaminergic side effects, including hallucinations. Sometimes dramatic reductions in the levodopa dosage were required to treat this complication of tolcapone treatment *(59,60)*. Clinical practice has confirmed that tolcapone must be used with caution in patients prone to cognitive side effects from levodopa. Some patients will experience DIP for the first time when beginning on this medication.

Entacapone, the second COMT inhibitor to become available, was approved for the adjunctive treatment of PD in 1999. In clinical trials, hallucinations and other dopaminergic side effects have been encountered with a frequency similar to tolcapone *(61)*, and it is clear from our personal experience with this medication that susceptible individuals have to be treated cautiously to avoid the onset or worsening of DIP.

Despite the fact that DIP is common, it has been clear since the early days of levodopa therapy that most patients do not experience this problem. Even in early reviews, the assertion was made that psychiatric side effects are much more likely to occur in patients with certain predisposing characteristics. Specifically, several authors mentioned dementia as a risk factor *(27,28,32,62)*. A confusional psychosis was believed to be particularly frequent in these patients. Other important risk factors mentioned in these early reviews were advanced age *(29)*, premorbid psychiatric illness *(27,31,32)*, and exposure to high daily doses of levodopa *(31)*.

Several recent publications have also analyzed the issue of risk factors for DIP. There has been consistent agreement that cognitive impairment *(34,35,38–40,63)* and depression *(34,35,38,40,63)* are strong predictors of risk for the development of hallucinations. More advanced age was found to be a risk in some studies *(34,38,63)*, but not others *(35,64)*. Similarly, duration or severity of PD was associated with the presence of DIP in some reports *(35,39,40,63)*, although not all *(34,40,64)*. Interestingly, none of these recent studies found a correlation between levodopa dose and DIP. However, there has been growing interest in disorders of sleep, not only as a risk factor for hallucinations *(34,39,63,65)*, but also as a clue to the pathophysiology of hallucinations in PD *(66)*. Visual loss has also been linked to hallucinations in patients with PD *(39,40,67)*. Combined with the fact that visual hallucinations occurring in the visually impaired, known as the Charles Bonnet syndrome *(68)*, clinically resemble those in patients with PD, these reports have fostered speculation that visual impairment may contribute to the pathophysiology of DIP *(39,63)*.

Although hallucinations can occur at any time in the course of illness, they are most commonly seen as a late complication of PD in susceptible individuals. In fact, Goetz et al. *(69)* have suggested that early-onset hallucinations (within 3 months of starting levodopa therapy) are not typical of idiopathic PD. Rather, the occurrence of hallucinations early in the course of levodopa treatment suggests the presence of premorbid psychiatric illness or an atypical Parkinsonian syndrome, such as LBD or Alzheimer's disease, with extrapyramidal signs.

Several attempts have been made to evaluate the occurrence of genetic risk factors for hallucinations as well. A recent study analyzing dopamine transporter gene polymorphisms found that a particular variant allele was more frequent in levodopa-treated patients with PD who were experiencing dyskinesia and psychosis *(70)*. However, the authors warned that this was a preliminary finding, and they could not exclude the possibility that other determinants like ethnicity might account for the differences observed. Another group looked at cholecystokinin (CCK) promoter polymorphisms. They found a trend toward more frequent representation of CCK-T in combination with the CCKAR-C polymorphism in hallucinators, but the differences when compared to nonhallucinators were not significant *(71)*.

4. CLINICAL FEATURES

The clinical features of DIP in PD are well-defined and have been described in numerous publications. Visual hallucinations are the most common symptoms *(10)* with recent estimates approximating 30% in treated individuals (*see* Table 1). Hallucinations can be defined as spontaneously fabricated perceptions occurring when awake (perceptions without stimulus). In PD, hallucinations usually occur on a background of a clear sensorium. However, a concomitant confusional state is not uncommon in older or demented patients *(10,11)*. Usually, hallucinations are fully formed, nonthreatening images of people, animals, or inanimate objects and tend to be recurrent, stereotyped, and reflect past experience for each patient *(10,11)*. For most, the imagined figures seem familiar and friendly, such as family members or friends who have died; whereas in others, they appear to be innocuous strangers or foggy shadows seen in dim light. Some patients will see adults sitting around their home as if they belong there. Others describe children wandering around the house. Another common scenario occurs when patients peer through a window and see children playing outside in the yard or men working (so-called kinetic scenes). One of our patients reported seeing a parade passing in front of her home on several occasions. Visions of animals are also common. Cats, dogs, and other benign furry creatures are typical, but small bugs and reptiles might also be seen. Occasionally, there will be an erotic overtone to the visions *(34)*, and about 28% of the time, the hallucinations will have a threatening or frightening quality *(56)*. Although the literature indicates that they are mostly nocturnal, they can, in fact, occur at any time. The hallucinations are typically brief, lasting minutes, with variable frequency. They may be in color or black and white, and figures may be miniature in size.

Oddly, many patients will claim to realize the fabricated nature of these images and yet describe them to family members and physicians in such neutral terms that to seem no more extraordinary than a visit from a neighbor. Others will insist they are real, and in these, the hallucinations will impact their behavior. In response to their hallucinations, one patient of ours was setting rat traps, whereas another was spraying bug spray to ward off imagined insects. The afflicted patients will often argue with their spouse about the real nature of the hallucinations. In most patients, these hallucinations are fleeting and may disappear if they look directly at the image, move toward it, blink their eyes, or try to touch it *(34)*. In most cases, visions of people are silent and relatively passive. Those without insight sometimes become frustrated because the hallucination (person) does not respond to their queries. A term commonly used to describe the experience of hallucinations with retained insight is "hallucinosis."

Two other forms of visual hallucinations have been well-described. "Passage hallucination" is seen transiently out of the corner of the eye. When the patient looks in that direction, it is usually gone. Another form is "presence hallucination" (extracampine), in which the patient usually has a sense of someone standing behind them or nearby. They don't actually see anyone, but they describe it as if they had *(34,39,72)*.

Pure auditory hallucinations are rare in PD, but a secondary auditory component has been reported in up to 40% of patients with visual hallucinations *(36,39)*. They are usually unrelated to the visual hallucinations despite occurring at the same time. In a recent review, auditory hallucinations accompanied visions in 8% of patients *(37)* and were described as human voices that were "nonimperative, nonparanoid, and often incomprehensible," like the background of voices at a party. In our own experience, we have had two patients who, in addition to benign visual hallucinations, also reported hearing music periodically, unconnected to their other hallucinations. Both claimed that the music was of a particular style, but could not identify a specific tune. One of these patients heard the music along with muffled voices that seemed to emanate from the air-conditioning ducts in her house. She actually attempted to record the sounds and play them back for her husband, who could not hear them. Music was heard by 14% of patients in prior studies *(37,39)*. Other noises can also be heard.

Other types of hallucinations also have been reported. Tactile and olfactory hallucinations occur, but these are extremely rare. Friedman et al. reviewed the data collected on 160 patients in two separate controlled clinical trials evaluating the treatment of DIP in PD *(73)*. In one study, 9% of patients and 22% of patients in the other, reported olfactory hallucinations. In these studies, 21% and 24% of patients, respectively, reported tactile hallucinations. Those with tactile hallucinations often appear to be taking something out of their hand and putting it down. This occurs more frequently in patients with dementia. In a recent report, a patient was described as "…feeling as if her bowels and bladder extruded from the distal parts of her upper limbs" *(74)*. The authors interpreted this as a somatic hallucination of visceral origin (cenesthetic hallucination). We have also had a patient with advanced PD and dementia who was certain he had been shot in the stomach. He related to his wife (who thought his stomach looked normal) that he could see and feel the bloody wound with his hands and feel the pain in his abdomen.

True illusions, which are distortions or misperceptions of actual visual stimuli, can also occur in some patients, but are less common than true hallucinations *(56)*. Typically, patients will report seeing faces in patterned fabric, misinterpret a curtain blown by the wind as a person moving, or mistake crumbs on a tablecloth for small bugs. One of our patients has intermittently reported that other people's faces appear to be distorted in grotesque ways. Illusions often occur in patients who also experience visual hallucinations *(39)*.

Clearly, the hallucinations described here are quite different from the more common hallucinatory syndromes seen with mind-altering drugs. Absent are the flashing lights, elaborate shifting patterns, and bizarre distortions of time and space seen with illicit hallucinogenic drugs *(75)*. Synesthesias, such as seeing sounds as colors, also do not occur in PD.

Abnormal dreaming and sleep disturbances seem to be closely related to the presence of hallucinations and other drug-induced psychiatric phenomena in patients with PD. In fact, Nausieda et al. *(76)* showed that 98% of patients with psychiatric side effects from their medications also experienced sleep disturbance in the form of sleep fragmentation, excessive daytime sleepiness, altered dreams, or parasomnias like sleeptalking, sleepwalking, and nocturnal myoclonus. They also found that hallucinations occurred in 39% of patients with sleep disturbances and in only 4% of patients with normal sleep patterns. Indeed, it is not unusual for hallucinations to blend indistinguishably with dream phenomena that possess similar themes *(11)*.

Delusions are not as common as hallucinations in PD, but they usually constitute a more serious problem for the patient and physician, often leading to hospitalization and sometimes suicide attempts. Delusions are false beliefs that are based on incorrect inference, held despite evidence to the contrary, and not ordinarily accepted by other members of one's culture *(9)*. In PD, delusions are usually paranoid in nature and most often occur on a background of a clear sensorium without other elements of a thought disorder, as are present in schizophrenia *(11)*. Delusions can occur as a side effect of any of the currently used antiparkinsonian medications *(10)*, including the COMT inhibitors, tolcapone, and entacapone (personal observation, Molho and Factor).

Klawans *(11)* indicated that about 3% of patients treated with levodopa for 2 or more years would experience this type of organic delusional syndrome. Friedman et al. *(73)* found that the most common delusional themes reported by patients with DIP participating in a clinical treatment trial involved stealing, spousal infidelity, abandonment, and the conviction that their spouse was an imposter or that they were not in their real home. In our own experience, delusions of spousal infidelity and elaborate conspiracies on the part of family members and even physicians are particularly common forms of delusions. Other examples mentioned in the literature include fears of being injured, poisoned, filmed, and even delusions of grandeur. Delusional misidentification syndromes are also well-described. Beliefs that family members or friends have been replaced by identical-appearing impostors (Capgras phenomenon) or that a familiar person is appearing in the guise of a stranger (Fregoli syndrome) have also been reported *(77)*. One of our patients, who was an artist, thought his paintings were being stolen and replaced by reproductions.

Another interesting delusional syndrome rarely described in PD is Cotards syndrome *(78)*. It is a fixed and unshakable belief that the person does not exist. Another interpretation is that the person thinks they are dead. One such case was described by Jenkins and Groh in 1970 *(29)*. This patient became psychotic and had the delusion that her husband was dead. "It was pointed out to her that she had been speaking to him, thereupon she developed the delusion that she herself was dead." We have seen a similar case. The patient was admitted by an ambulance to the hospital because she was immobile. She had stopped taking her PD medications, and when asked why, she claimed that she was dead and no longer had need for them. Her syndrome reversed with quetiapine therapy and medications were reinstituted.

Literature indicates quite clearly that the psychosis of PD is very different from that of schizophrenia. Verbal commands and ego-dystonic critical commentaries are not usually seen. In the study by Holroyd of 102 patients suffering from PD with DIP, no one had a schizophrenic-like syndrome *(40)*. However, it does occasionally occur, and we have seen two such cases. Both individuals had advanced PD. One heard voices telling her that she would be punished by having her PD medications withdrawn. This was very frightening to her because her "off" times were characterized by severe immobility. The other was hearing the voice of God commanding her to stop all medications or she would be punished. Neither patient had typical visual hallucinations, was demented, or had a history of premorbid psychotic disease, but one patient was hospitalized. Both were treated successfully with atypical antipsychotics.

5. MECHANISMS OF PSYCHOSIS

The mechanisms responsible for producing DIP in PD are poorly understood. In some patients, PD medications precipitate acute psychiatric symptoms by unmasking a premorbid psychiatric state. This has been shown to occur in schizophrenics *(79)* and patients with manic-depressive illness *(32)* who were exposed to levodopa. However, for the majority of patients with PD, there is no premorbid psychiatric disorder. Thus, other characteristics peculiar to patients with PD, PD medications, or both, must be important.

5.1. Pharmacological Mechanisms

5.1.1. Dopaminergic Mechanisms

It has been known for many years that drugs structurally similar to dopamine, e.g., lysergic acid diethylamide, mescaline, and amphetamines, can cause elaborate hallucinations and other psychotic symptoms in otherwise healthy individuals *(79)*. The discovery that levodopa could also precipitate psychiatric symptoms in animals and humans, coupled with the dramatic efficacy of dopamine receptor blockers (neuroleptics) in treating endogenous psychosis, has formed the basis for the dopamine theory of psychosis *(79)*. Clinical evidence that supports this hypothesis includes the *de novo* dose-related appearance of hallucinations in patients with PD who were treated with levodopa, the reliable disappearance of these symptoms with dose reduction, and the efficacy of traditional neuroleptics in treating this problem.

More recent theories have been based on the altered dopamine receptor physiology associated with PD and the varied effects of dopaminergic drugs on different dopamine-mediated systems in the brain. It is well-known that dysfunction of the nigrostriatal dopamine system and resulting insufficiency of dopamine at the receptor sites of otherwise normal striatal neurons is responsible for the motor symptoms of PD. This process also results in denervation hypersensitivity of striatal dopamine receptors. The early appearance of psychotic symptoms in patients treated with dopaminergic medications has been attributed to the stimulation of these hypersensitive receptors *(56)*.

To explain the late appearance of psychosis in PD, Klawans et al. *(80)* introduced the concept of levodopa-induced dopamine receptor hypersensitivity. In animal models, they showed that chronic stimulation of dopamine receptors can cause stereotyped behavior to appear with subthreshold doses and a shorter latency than in animals not chronically exposed to dopaminergic stimulation. Thus, chronic exposure to dopamine agonists causes hypersensitivity of dopamine receptors rather than the expected result, downregulation. In applying this model to levodopa-induced psychosis, Moskovitz et al. *(56)* proposed that two populations of dopamine sensitive neurons exist in the striatum and limbic cortex: dopamine-facilitated and -inhibited neuronal populations. Dopamine-inhibited neurons predominate in the striatum and exhibit downregulation and hyposensitivity when exposed to chronic dopaminergic stimulation. In contrast, dopamine-facilitated neurons respond to chronic stimulation by becoming hypersensitive. Moskovitz and colleagues suggested that this dopamine-facilitated neuronal population might predominate in the limbic cortex and therefore, be responsible for the psychotic symptoms indicated with chronic levodopa treatment.

Although the literature supporting the central role of dopamine in DIP is compelling, Goetz et al. have performed an experiment that casts some doubt on this concept *(81)*. They gave five nondemented patients with PD who were experiencing daily visual hallucinations high-dose intravenous infusions of levodopa, utilizing both steady and pulse infusion paradigms. None of the patients experienced hallucinations in response to the infusions, but some did experience an increase in dyskinesia. The investigators concluded that "visual hallucinations do not relate simply to high levels of levodopa or to sudden changes in plasma levels" *(81)*.

5.1.2. Serotonergic Mechanisms

Dysfunction of central serotonergic pathways has also been explored as a cause of DIP. Postmortem studies have demonstrated that patients with this complication have lower brainstem levels of serotonin (5-HT) *(76)*. In addition, acute administration of levodopa reduces brain serotonin levels by several possible mechanisms, including interfering with the transport of L-tryptophan across the gut and blood-brain barrier, inhibiting tryptophan hydroxylase, and replacing serotonin in presynaptic storage sites, leading to increased dopamine formation *(32,76)*. In animals, levodopa causes a decrease in 5HT levels but an increase in 5-hydroxyinduleacetic acid (5HIAA), suggesting an increase in release and turnover of serotonin that, in turn, brings forth increased receptor stimulation *(82)*. Dysfunction of serotonergic systems is also suggested by the frequent association of DIP with sleep disturbances and altered dreaming, both of which are thought to have a serotonergic basis *(34,65,76)*. Comella et al. *(83)* compared patients who had PD with and without hallucinations using polysomnography and found that hallucinators had reduced sleep efficiency, total rapid eye movement (REM) sleep, and the percentage of REM sleep. In another recent study, 24-hour ambulatory polysomnography was performed on 20 patients with PD experiencing visual hallucinations *(66)* and demonstrated a close temporal link between 33% of the hallucinations and the occurrence of non-REM sleep during the day or REM sleep patterns at night. These findings suggest that serotonergic neural mechanisms involved in generating sleep and dream phenomena may have a role in the occurrence of DIP in PD. The serotonin hypothesis is further strengthened by the discovery that ondansetron, a selective 5HT3 receptor antagonist, markedly improved psychotic symptoms in patients with PD *(82)*.

5.1.3. Cholinergic Mechanisms

Cholinergic pathways have also been implicated. Older studies *(84)* suggested this possibility because of the occurrence of hallucinations as an adverse event to anticholinergic drugs, because anticholinergic drug therapy was found to be a risk factor for the occurrence of psychosis, and because cholinergic deficiency was described in the brains of such patients. The recent finding that cholinesterase inhibitors provide relief of psychosis in PD also supports this possibility *(85)*.

5.2. Visual Mechanisms

Recent studies have suggested that hallucinations that occur in PD are similar to those of the Charles Bonnett syndrome *(39)*. This syndrome, first described in 1769, consists of fully formed hallucinations in patients who are blind from macular degeneration or other causes. Hallucinations occur in 21% of blind patients *(67)*, likely as a consequence of denervation hypersensitivity of the visual cortex *(68)*. Patients with PD may be prone to this phenomenon because they develop retinal dysfunction with abnormalities of contrast sensitivity and may also have several age-related visual problems, such as macular degeneration. Fenelon et al. found that ocular pathology in PD was an independent risk factor for hallucinations *(39)*. However, it remains uncertain whether such a link exists, because others did not confirm these results *(34,40)*. The most common hallucinations associated with the Charles Bonnett syndrome are simple evoked flashes and repetitive geometric patterns (tesselopsia); people or animals are seen less frequently *(68)*. Thus, it seems probable that there is no consistent relationship.

5.3. Neuroanatomy of Hallucinations

Although results have varied, there has been some success recently in elucidating the functional neuroanatomy of hallucinations in Parkinsonian disorders. Harding et al. *(86)* systematically reviewed the clinical features and neuropathological findings in 63 patients with LBD or PD with dementia. They found a striking association between the density of Lewy bodies in the temporal lobe and the presence of hallucinations in patients with LBD. The density of Lewy bodies was particularly high in the amygdala and the parahippocampus. Of course, these regions are also important for dementia, and the overlap is obvious. Harding and colleagues looked specifically at LBD, a disorder of dementia and Parkinsonism. The fact that psychosis is so much a part of this disorder raises the question of what the relationship is between dementia and its associated pathology, as well as the occurrence of hallucinations. Dementia is the most robust risk factor for the onset of hallucinations in PD, and hallucinations represent a possible risk factor for dementia *(5,34)*. Dementia may indeed be a necessary comorbidity because it may promote misinterpretation of visual stimuli. In LBD, hallucinations often occur in patients not on medication, but otherwise, the hallucinations are similar in both diseases. It has even been proposed that PD and LBD actually are the same disease with only the time sequence of dementia and Parkinsonism being different *(15,16)*.

Other brain regions may play an important role in the onset of hallucinations in PD. In one report, visual hallucinations were reliably induced by deep-brain stimulation of the subthalamic nucleus (STN-DBS) in a postsurgical patient with PD off of medications *(87)*, suggesting a role of the STN.

There is increasing evidence that altered occipital lobe function may also be important. Using functional magnetic resonance imaging (MRI), Goetz et al. *(88)* found that patients who had PD with chronic hallucinations respond to visual stimuli with prominent cingulate cortex activation and loss of the expected visual cortex activation seen in normal individuals. Decreased occipital activity has been demonstrated in positron emission tomography (PET) studies of PD dementia and LBD *(89,90)* and in an MRI spectroscopy study that showed a diminished *N*-acetylaspartate peak in PD dementia *(91)*. On the contrary, one study with functional MRI (fMRI) suggested that different regions are abnormal depending on the type of hallucinations. For instance, facial hallucinations were associated with temporal lobe abnormalities, whereas objects and kinetic scenes were associated with occipital lobe changes *(92)*. Because these are early findings, it is unclear which of the anatomical regions implicated by these studies is most important. Whether it is necessary that dysfunction be present in one or more of these areas for hallucinations to occur in PD is also unknown.

6. TREATMENT OF PSYCHOSIS

6.1. General Considerations

Some patients with psychotic symptoms secondary to dopaminergic medications do not require antipsychotic therapy. Those patients with hallucinosis on the background of a clear sensorium may not need or want therapeutic intervention, especially when the hallucinations are intermittent, brief, nonthreatening, and when the patient has preserved insight. In fact, some patients actually claim to gain pleasure from the symptoms. Yet, these patients should be watched carefully because escalation of psychotic symptoms may occur without provocation.

In patients with a sudden onset of psychotic symptoms, it is important to investigate for triggering events, such as urinary and pulmonary infections, metabolic disturbances, cerebrovascular events, or traumatic brain injury. Treatment of these underlying conditions is paramount and, if initiated immediately, will usually be sufficient. Postoperative psychosis is another condition that may not require specific therapy. In one study *(93)*, psychosis occurred in up to 60% of patients with PD who had surgical intervention. Our own experience with this situation suggests that once patients are allowed to increase activity and, more often, when they are discharged home, the psychosis will improve spontaneously. Other possible causes of postoperative psychosis include anesthetics, pain medications, altered environment, metabolic encephalopathy, or infection.

If the patient with PD has DIP and requires intervention, the first step is to decrease PD medications—this remains standard practice. Research indicates that reducing medications can be helpful and is usually well-tolerated. Marsden and Fahn *(94)* suggested decreasing and then removing adjunctive medications first before reducing levodopa. If psychosis persists as medications are individually stripped away, the patient will eventually experience intolerable worsening of motor symptoms. At this point, the addition of antipsychotic medication is usually considered.

In the 1970s and early 80s, some physicians utilized the "drug holiday" to treat patients who had with various late-stage complications, including psychosis. Medications were typically withdrawn for 5–14 days, and this invariably led to significant physical disability. Many patients became bedridden, unable to move or even swallow. As Friedman noted *(95)*, this was "not a holiday in the usual sense." It is now well-recognized that there are major drawbacks to the "drug holiday." First, it requires long-term hospitalization, which is costly. More importantly, patients have the terrifying experience of becoming completely immobile. Nursing care must be meticulous to prevent complications that may include decubitus ulcers, compression neuropathies, contractures, aspiration pneumonia, deep-venous thrombosis, pulmonary embolism and depression *(95)*. Additionally, the sudden cessation of dopaminergic medications can lead to a potentially lethal syndrome similar to the neuroleptic malignant syndrome *(95)*. Considering the gravity of these complications, a "drug holiday" should not be promoted as a routine therapeutic measure and, in fact, has been abandoned in many major medical centers.

In the not too distant past, drug therapy for DIP also included standard neuroleptics, particularly low-potency agents. Marsden and Fahn *(94)* indicated that, although the use of these agents was "illogical," the addition of small-dose thioridazine could allow a compromise between the relative disability imposed by psychosis or immobility. However, it is clear that in most cases, conventional neuroleptics (e.g., thioridazine) cause marked exacerbation of PD symptoms and dramatically increase disability *(96)*. Added to the risk of worsening PD disability, patients with PD, who are typically elderly, are consequently also at greater risk for the development of tardive dyskinesia and other tardive syndromes, as well as neuroleptic malignant syndrome. As a result, there is now a clear consensus that these drugs should be simply avoided in patients with PD.

6.2. Clozapine

CLZ is a unique drug that remains the treatment of choice for DIP in patients with PD. CLZ is considered to be an "atypical" antipsychotic because it does not cause catalepsy in laboratory animals (i.e., increase in muscle tone and postural abnormalities, *97*) and is associated with minimal risk of drug-induced Parkinsonism, dystonia, and akathisia *(96,97)*. It is this unique ability—to be able to effectively treat psychosis without causing Parkinsonism—that led to the initial attempts to use this drug in PD a decade ago. Since then, its safety and efficacy in patients who have PD with DIP has been demonstrated in numerous open-label studies *(98)*. This accumulated experience with CLZ has been remarkably uniform and has shown that CLZ can be used in small, well-tolerated doses to rapidly reverse the symptoms of psychosis.

In 1999, the results of two multicenter 4-week, double-blind, placebo-controlled trials were published and confirmed the results reported in previous open-label trials. The first was a North American trial organized by the Parkinson Study Group *(6,7)*. In this study, 30 patients with DIP were treated with CLZ, and 30 were randomized to placebo. CLZ was started at a very low dose of 6.25 mg at bedtime and increased as needed according to a standardized schedule to a maximum dose of 50 mg. Psychotic symptoms were measured with: (1) a seven-point clinical global impression scale; (2) the Brief Psychiatric Rating Scale (BPRS); (3) a modified form of the BPRS to remove four items thought to be more reflective of Parkinsonism than psychosis; and (4) the Survey Assessment of Positive Symptoms. The motor subscale of the Unified PD Rating Scale (UPDRS) was used to assess the worsening of Parkinsonism. Psychotic symptoms were significantly improved in the CLZ group when compared to placebo at a mean dose of 27 mg per day without decline of motor function. The double-blind study was followed by a 3-month open-label extension that confirmed this benefit *(7)*. A second double-blind, placebo-controlled study was organized by the French Parkinson Study Group *(99)*. They used similar methodology and reported very similar results. To date, CLZ remains the only drug proven with controlled trials to improve DIP without worsening motor symptoms, which is why it remains the gold standard to which other agents are compared.

Sedation is the most common side effect of CLZ, but its occurrence can be used to therapeutic advantage. Frequently, patients with DIP also have sleep disruption and some degree of reversal in their normal sleep–wake cycle. These patients often spend nights awake, agitated, hallucinating, and engaged in paranoid behaviors, such as looking through their house for intruders. Consequently, they will be sleepy and more disoriented the next day. Caregivers also become sleep-deprived, emotionally stressed, and physically exhausted. When CLZ therapy is started as a bedtime dose, the most dramatic initial benefit usually is restored restful sleep and normalization of the sleep–wake cycle. This is result is greatly appreciated by all involved and is also generally a sign that the CLZ dose is at, or very near, an effective antipsychotic dose. Dosing should begin at 6.25 mg at bedtime and increase every few days by 6.25 to 12.5 mg. Most patients will obtain these benefits with 50 mg at bedtime or less. Occasionally, acutely psychotic patients will need to be given doses as high as 150 to 200 mg per day until their symptoms are under control. Then, a smaller maintenance dose can be used to prevent recurrence. Some patients on a single bedtime dose will experience breakthrough symptoms during the day in the late afternoon or early evening. In this situation, a small additional daytime dose (usually ≤12.5 mg) is typically sufficient. If sedation is a problem in the morning, then the bedtime dose can be reduced or moved 1 to 2 hours earlier in the evening.

Once psychotic symptoms are adequately controlled and the patient is sleeping through the night, it is usually possible to carefully increase antiparkinsonian medication doses to improve motor functioning. Small increases in daytime levodopa doses are possible, but it is best to keep nighttime doses to the absolute minimum. Adjunctive medication (e.g., dopamine agonists, selegiline, or COMT inhibitors) will usually have been dramatically reduced in dose or eliminated prior to starting CLZ. These medications need to be used with caution in patients who require antipsychotic therapy; in patients with significant dementia, they should be avoided.

The adverse effect of most concern with CLZ is agranulocytosis (Agran). In 1975, the occurrence of eight deaths from septicemia out of 16 patients who developed Agran in Europe *(96,100)* delayed the marketing of this drug in the United States. The estimated risk of Agran in patients with schizophrenia treated with CLZ is 1 to 2% *(101),* which is higher than standard psychotropic medications. This figure is about the same in PD *(7),* indicating that this adverse effect is idiosyncratic and not dose-related. An apparent prodrome of 29 days, characterized by a gradual decrease in white blood cell (WBC) count, has been observed *(101).* However, precipitous drops in the WBC count from the normal range can also occur.

Current guidelines in the United States require weekly monitoring of the WBC count for the first 6 months of CLZ therapy and every other week monitoring thereafter. It is recommended that therapy should be interrupted if the WBC count drops to less than 3000 per mm^3 or the absolute neutrophil count drops to less than 1500/mm^3. Permanent discontinuation is recommended if the WBC is less than 2000/mm^3, or the neutrophil count becomes less than 1000 per mm^3. Also, patients with a baseline WBC of less than 3500 per mm^3, a neutrophil count of less than 1500 per mm^3, or a history of immune deficiency should not be treated.

Apparently, these guidelines have been effective in reducing the risk of Agran. Honigfeld et al. *(102)* reviewed the incidence of Agran in 99,502 patients treated with CLZ according to these guidelines between 1990 and 1994. They reported that 382 cases of Agran (0.38%) and 12 deaths had occurred; this was dramatically reduced from the 995 cases of Agran and 149 deaths that would have been predicted based on the preguideline incidence of 1 to 2%.

Other hematological side effects that may occur with CLZ include mild asymptomatic eosinophilia, chronic leukocytosis possibly associated with a low-grade fever, and lymphopenia (<600 lymphocytes/mm^3), which is usually asymptomatic or may be associated with diarrhea and fever *(97).* The etiology of these problems is unknown *(103).* One other adverse event of concern is neuroleptic malignant syndrome. Although CLZ causes few extrapyramidal side effects, neuroleptic malignant syndrome has been reported on rare occasions. One case was described in a patient on CLZ and carbamazepine therapy, the other in a patient taking CLZ in combination with lithium *(104).*

CLZ causes several other adverse effects of concern in patients with PD. Sialorrhea and delirium follow sedation in frequency *(8,97).* They appear to be dose-related adverse events and are often dose-limiting. CLZ-induced orthostatic hypotension can also cause difficulty for patients with PD because many already suffer from orthostatic hypotension owing to either PD medications or autonomic dysfunction. Seizures are of concern in schizophrenics, occurring in up to 4% of these patients *(97,105,106)* and related to electroencephalogram (EEG) changes that have been well-described. Both seizures and EEG changes are dose-related phenomena, which probably explains why no seizures have been reported thus far with the low doses used in PD. The incidence of seizures is less than 1% at doses under 300 mg per day, 2.7% at daily doses of 300 to 600 mg, and 4.4% at doses greater than 600 mg per day *(105).*

Serious, but fortunately rare, medical complications associated with CLZ use include venous thromboembolism *(107),* myocarditis *(108,109),* and possibly sudden death *(110).* The treating physician must be vigilant for these effects. There have also been several publications that reported poor blood sugar control in diabetics and increased risk of new-onset type 2 diabetes in patients treated with

Table 2
Summary of Distinguishing Characteristics of Atypical Antipsychotics

Characteristics	CLZ	RSP	OLZ	QTP	ZIP	ARI
Fails to induce catalepsy or antagonize amphetamine stereotypies	+	–	–	+	–	–
Inc. 5HT/D-2 binding	+	+	+	+	+	+
No prolactin elevation	+	–	+/–	+	–	+
Mesolimbic selectivity	+	–	+	+	?	–
Loose D-2 binding	+	–	–	+	–	–[a]
Improves negative symptoms	+	+	+	+	+	+
Decreased EPS	+	–	+	+	+	+
Not associated with TD	+	–	+/–	+	?	?

EPS, extrapyramidal side effects; TD, tardive dyskinesia; CLZ, clozapine; RSP, risperidone; OLZ, olanzapine; QTP, quetiapine; ZIP, ziprasidone; ARI, aripiprazole; ?, no reliable data available.

[a] Has partial dopamine agonist effects as well as antagonist effects.

CLZ *(111,112)*. These reports involved schizophrenics treated with high doses. The same increases in blood glucose were not seen in one study of patients with PD who were treated with much lower doses *(113)*. Olanzapine and other neuroleptic medications have been implicated as well, but this may not be a class effect *(114,115)*.

The main obstacle to long-term success with CLZ therapy in PD is the progression of underlying disease, particularly dementia. Greene et al. *(116)* found that of four patients with marked dementia treated with CLZ, only one improved, and the rest experienced adverse events. In a long-term trial, Factor et al. *(117)* showed that as dementia progressed (illustrated by a decrease in minimental status score), psychosis began to reemerge, and adverse effects became more of a dose-limiting problem. It is believed that nondemented patients can tolerate long-term therapy well. However, the efficacy and tolerance will decline in those with significant dementia.

6.3. Other Atypical Antipsychotics

Safe and effective alternatives for the treatment of DIP in PD have been sought because of the small, but significant, risk of Agran associated with CLZ and the need for mandatory blood monitoring. Five additional antipsychotic medications are now available that have an atypical pharmacological profile and do not carry the risk of Agran. Three have been utilized in the treatment of PD: risperidone (RSP), olanzapine (OLZ), and quetiapine (QTP). It is their atypical pharmacology that makes these drugs potential alternatives for patients with PD. But, what is the definition of 'atypical?' It has not been clearly defined pharmacologically. CLZ remains to be the prototype of this class of drugs and that to which all others are compared. CLZ is distinguished from typical antipsychotic drugs by its strong antipsychotic effect coupled with freedom from extrapyramidal syndromes. In essence, that is the clinical definition of atypical and the goal in developing new atypical agents, but what are the pharmacological properties that differentiate this drug?

The features most often discussed to define the atypical classification of drugs based on the unique pharmacology of CLZ are listed in Table 2, along with information as to how all currently available atypical agents fulfill these standards *(118)*. It should be noted from this table that, although RSP and OLZ share some features considered to define atypicality, it is QTP that is the most similar to CLZ in these respects. However, at this point, there does not appear to be a single pharmacological trait that strictly defines this class of agents.

A recent and compelling theory of the neurophysiological basis of atypicality has been derived from studies reviewing the way in which CLZ interacts with dopamine receptors. In vitro experiments

Table 3
Summary of Open-Label Reports With Risperidone in the Treatment of Psychosis in PD

Author/reference year	No. of patients	Dosage[a]	No. of psychosis improved	No. of PD worsened
Meco, 1994 *(122)*	6	0.67 mg/day	6	0
Ford, 1994 *(123)*	6	1.5 mg/day	6	6
Rich, 1995 *(124)*	6	0.5–4 mg/day	4	5
Allen, 1995 *(126)*	3	0.5–1 mg/day	3	0
McKeith, 1995 *(127)*	3	1 mg/day	0	3
Meco, 1997 *(125)*	10	0.73 mg/day	9	3
Workman, 1997 *(128)*	9	1.9 mg/day	8	0 (est)
Leopold, 2000 *(129)*	39	1.1 mg/day	33	6
Mohr, 2000 *(130)*	17	0.5–3 mg/day	16	0[b]

[a] Dosage is given as a mean or a range.
[b] Of 17 patients, 10 reported "hypokinesia" as an adverse event and 1 withdrew owing to worsening of gait.
est, estimated number based on available information in the publication.

using cloned human dopamine D2 receptors have shown that CLZ and QTP are loosely bound and easily displaced from these receptors *(119)*. All other antipsychotic drugs tested with this method, including RSP, OLZ, and traditional neuroleptics, show prolonged and tighter binding to D2 receptors (*see* Table 2). A second study utilizing in vivo PET scanning in 12 patients treated with QTP *(120)* demonstrated only transient high-dopamine D2 receptor occupancy. Based on these results, it has been speculated that the atypical clinical and pharmacological features seen most prominently in CLZ and QTP are because of this loose binding and fast dissociation from D2 receptors. In addition, it is thought that loose binding allows for a more physiological response to surges in endogenous dopamine, thus preventing the usual neuroleptic side effects like drug-induced Parkinsonism *(121)*. This feature may also contribute to mesolimbic selectivity and could be the reason for a faster relapse of psychosis in schizophrenia when the drugs are discontinued. If loose binding does define atypical behavior, then it might predict which agents will be safer and most useful in PD. Based on the limited clinical data available now, it appears to.

6.3.1. Risperidone

A summary of open-label studies published on the treatment of DIP in PD with RSP is shown in Table 3 *(122–130)*. The first report of its effect on PD psychosis was an open-label trial in only six patients reported in 1994, the same year it was approved for use in schizophrenia *(122)*. The results were promising, as all patients demonstrated improvement in psychosis with total elimination of symptoms in three. No change in the UPDRS scores or levodopa dose was reported. Two subsequent publications reported contrasting results *(123,124)*; both studies also involved six patients. Investigators found that RSP had effective antipsychotic properties in PD, but Parkinsonism worsened in 11 of 12 patients, even at low doses. Some patients became more confused. Meco et al. followed up their initial report with longer-term experience *(125)*. This time, 7 out of 10 subjects stopped using the drug within 1 year, despite improved psychosis in 9. Three patients had worsening of motor features, two of whom dropped out of the study. There also have been two reports regarding the use of RSP to treat psychosis in LBD. A total of six patients were treated; three experienced severe worsening of motor symptoms *(126,127)*.

Based on these reports and clinical experience, most PD specialists are in agreement that RSP is not appropriate to use in the setting of PD. However, three recently published papers have surprisingly detailed positive experiences. Unfortunately, each report has limitations that make the results difficult to interpret. Workman et al. *(128)* reported that 9 demented, agitated, and psychotic patients with PD in a psychiatric hospital did well on RSP when followed for a mean of 37 days. Unfortunately, as three

Table 4
Summary of Open-Label Reports With Olanzapine in the Treatment of PD With Psychosis

Author/reference year	No. of patients	Dosage[a]	No. of psychosis improved	No. of PD worsened
Wolters, 1996 *(132)*	15	6.5 mg/day	15 (est)	0
Jimenez, 1998 *(133)*	2	5 mg/day	1	2
Friedman, 1998 *(134)*	19	N/A	7	10
Friedman, 1998 *(135)*	12	4.4 mg/day	12	7
Weiner, 1998 *(137)*	21	5 mg/day	13	9
Graham, 1998 *(138)*	5	5 mg/day	5	4
Molho, 1999 *(136)*	12	6.3 mg/day	9	10
Stover, 1999 *(139)*	22	N/A	12	8

[a] Dosage is given as a mean or a range.
est, estimated number based on available information in the publication; N/A, data not available.

patients had been on typical neuroleptics at entry of the study, and the patients did not have their motor exams rated formally, the authors' conclusion that RSP did not worsen extrapyramidal symptoms can be questioned. In another report, Leopold *(129)* treated 39 Parkinsonian patients (32 PD, 6 LBD) with a mean RSP dose of 1.1 mg per day. Significant improvement in psychosis was seen in 23 patients and modest improvement in 10. Only 16 patients completed the 6-month trial, and in these cases, no worsening was seen in the UPDRS motor scores at 3 or 6 months. However, of the other 23 patients, 6 were clinically diagnosed as LBD and experienced severe worsening of motor function. No information regarding the motor exam was provided for the remaining 17 patients in the study. In the most recent report, Mohr et al. *(130)* treated 17 patients with 0.5 to 2 mg of RSP per day over 12 weeks and found a substantial improvement in psychotic symptoms with no statistical worsening in the UPDRS motor subscale. However, because 10 of the 17 patients reported hypokinesia as an adverse event, the authors' conclusion that RSP does not adversely affect the symptoms of PD is suspect.

In the only double-blind trial published on the use RSP in PD, Ellis et al. compared RSP to CLZ in 10 patients with PD and DIP *(131)*. Both medications improved psychosis, but RSP worsened motor features, whereas motor function actually improved on CLZ. Although these changes did not reach statistical significance, the authors advised caution when using RSP in this setting. Our conclusion is that RSP is not well-suited for use in PD.

6.3.2. *Olanzapine*

The next atypical antipsychotic medication that became available for use in patients with PD was OLZ, which was approved for use in schizophrenia in 1996. A summary of published open-label studies on the use of OLZ in PD is shown in Table 4 *(132–139)*. As with RSP, the initial report of OLZ for DIP in PD was very encouraging. Wolters et al. *(132)* found that OLZ was effective in 15 nondemented patients with PD. No decline of motor functioning was reported in this open-label prospective study. Unfortunately, the subsequent literature concerning the use of OLZ in this setting has, once again, been less impressive. Several open-label studies have found that disabling motor deterioration can be seen in some patients with PD *(133–135,137–139)*. Our own experience with OLZ has also been disappointing. In a retrospective analysis of 12 patients we had treated with OLZ, symptoms of psychosis were improved in 9 patients (75%), but 9 patients (75%) also experienced significant motor deterioration *(136)*. Only 1 of the original 12 subjects was still using OLZ successfully after 1 year, but even that patient stopped the drug shortly thereafter because of symptom worsening and recurrence of psychosis.

The reason for the disparity between the initial favorable results and subsequent studies is unclear, but it may relate to the differences in patient population and the method of dose titration used in these studies. Wolters et al. *(140)* suggested that the poor results reported in subsequent studies were related

Table 5
Summary of Open-Label Reports With Quetiapine in the Treatment of Patients Suffering From PD With Psychosis

Author/reference year	No. of patients	Dosage[a]	No. of psychosis improved	No. of PD worsened
Evatt, 1996 *(145)*	10	50 mg/day	10 (est)	0
Parsa, 1998 *(144)*	2	200, 400 mg/day	2	1
Juncos, 1998 *(146)*	15	70 mg/day	15 (est)	0
Juncos, 1999 *(147)*	40	25–800 mg/day	40 (est)	8 (est)
Samanta, 1998 *(149)*	10	37.5 mg/day	6	7
Fernandez, 1999 *(150)*	35	40.6 mg/day	25	0
Friedman, 1999 *(151)*	15	62.5 mg/day	12	4
Targum, 2000 *(148)*	11	25–300 mg/day	6	0
Reddy, 2002 *(152)*	43	54 mg/day	35	5
Fernandez, 2003 *(153)*	106	60 mg/day	87	34

[a] Dosage is given as a mean or a range.
est, estimated number based on available information in the publication.

to the inclusion of patients with atypical Parkinsonian syndromes and dementia. Additionally, the starting dose of OLZ in Wolters' report was 1 mg per day, which is less than half the initial dose of 2.5 to 5.0 mg per day used in subsequent studies (the lowest dose currently available in the United States is a 2.5-mg tablet).

Fortunately, the recent publication of three well-designed double-blind trials using OLZ to treat DIP seems to have resolved some of this confusion. In the first trial, Goetz et al. *(141)* compared OLZ to CLZ in a blinded fashion. A total of 15 patients were randomized to one of the two drugs. Motor function was measured with the UPDRS at baseline and weekly thereafter. After 15 patients had completed the study (the study was powered for 28), an independent interim safety analysis was performed, and safety-stopping rules were invoked because of significant worsening of Parkinsonism in the OLZ group, where six of seven patients withdrew. In the CLZ group, there was actually a small improvement in UPDRS scores with no dropouts. The poor results in the OLZ group occurred despite the fact that patients with dementia were excluded. CLZ was also more effective in improving psychosis. In the second trial, Ondo et al. *(142)* compared OLZ to placebo in 30 patients with PD and DIP. Psychosis did not significantly improve in the OLZ-treated patients when compared with placebo. Also, there was significant worsening of motor function in the active treatment group. Gait deterioration and increased bradykinesia accounted for this effect. Most recently, the results of two large multicenter randomized, placebo-controlled trials of OLZ in DIP were published together and reported results that were strikingly similar to the previous placebo-controlled trial *(143)*. A total of 160 patients were randomized between the two trials, one from the United States and the other from Europe. Once again, there was no significant improvement in psychosis in the OLZ group when compared with placebo. Motor worsening on OLZ was also indicated in both studies on several different measures of PD functioning; these differences did reach significance. Therefore, it would seem that OLZ is not well-suited for use in PD.

6.3.3. *Quetiapine*

The most promising atypical antipsychotic medication introduced as an alternative to CLZ for PD is QTP, which was approved for use in schizophrenia in 1998. A summary of published open-label studies is shown in Table 5 *(144–153)* Thus far, there have been several open-label studies in which QTP appears to be effective in treating DIP in PD at doses of 50 to 400 mg per day with mild impact on motor features. Unfortunately, no confirmatory double-blind studies have been completed as yet.

In one of the larger studies, Fernandez et al. *(150)* reported the results of an open trial of QTP in 35 patients with PD. In the study, 24 were neuroleptic-naive, 3 patients switched to QTP from OLZ and 8 patients switched to QTP from CLZ. Of the neuroleptic-naive patients, 20 had marked improvement or complete amelioration of psychosis at 4 weeks that was maintained through 8 weeks. Ten patients had baseline and week-4 BPRS measures, and significant improvement was observed. There was no worsening of Parkinsonism. Of the 11 switched to QTP, only 5 made the transition easily. In the other six patients, increased erratic behavior, confusion, and hallucinations were observed. These patients had to be switched back to their prior therapeutic agent. The authors concluded that the drug was a good antipsychotic agent for PD, but transition from another antipsychotic may be difficult. In a follow-up study *(151)*, 15 patients were switched more gradually from CLZ to QTP over an 8-week period. Patients tolerated this slower change more easily; 12 made the transition successfully and stayed on QTP. Motor features did not decrease except for transiently increased tremor in four patients.

Fernandez et al. have also provided long-term data regarding 106 of their patients with PD who were treated with QTP in the clinic *(153)*. The mean duration of therapy was 15 months, and the average QTP dose was 60 mg per day. Psychosis partially or completely remitted in 82%, whereas 18% did not improve. Some degree of motor worsening was seen in 32% of patients, but only 9% discontinued QTP because of this problem. The presence of dementia was associated with increased likelihood of motor decline as well as nonresponse relating to psychosis.

In our own evaluation *(152)*, 43 consecutive patients suffering from PD with DIP (mean duration 13 months) were treated with QTP at a mean dose of 54 mg per day for a mean duration of 10 months. Results showed 81% (35 patients) had improvement of psychotic symptoms, but it was not complete in all (23 complete amelioration and 12 partial). Five patients (12.5%) experienced mild worsening of motor symptoms, and two stopped therapy as a result. Twenty patients were demented; the rest were not. There was no difference in antipsychotic effect between the demented and nondemented groups, but mild worsening of motor symptoms was seen in the demented group as measured by UPDRS. All five of the patients with definite decline had some degree of dementia. None of the nondemented patients experienced worsening of motor symptoms. Levodopa dosage did not change. After the study was complete, 80% of patients chose to continue QTP.

Although some worsening of motor symptoms has been seen with QTP, judging from this preliminary literature and our own experience, it seems unlikely that this will constitute a significant clinical problem, as was the case with RSP and OLZ. However, QTP appears to be less potent than CLZ in relieving psychosis. The dose may need to be pushed aggressively into the range normally used to treat schizophrenia (≥400 mg/day) in some patients. Even then, some patients with DIP may not respond to QTP. We have also seen the occasional patient in our practice who has experienced a paradoxical worsening of agitation and psychosis when QTP was added at the usual starting dose of 25 mg at bedtime. Increasing the dose only exacerbated the problem in these rare patients. Generally, based on open-label experience, QTP seems well-suited for PD and has been often utilized in practice. However, results need to be confirmed in double-blind studies.

6.3.4. Aripiprazole and Ziprasidone

The two newest atypical antipsychotic medications available are aripiprazole and ziprasidone. No published results exist regarding the use of these medications for DIP in PD. Ziprasidone has dopamine receptor-binding characteristics similar to those of RSP and other typical antipsychotics and therefore may have a similar impact on PD *(119)*. Studies with aripiprazole are in progress.

6.4. Non-Neuroleptic Therapies

6.4.1. Ondansetron

Approaches to the treatment of DIP, other than atypical antipsychotic medications, have been used with some success. Ondansetron is one of these agents. It is a serotonin (5HT3) receptor antagonist that was approved by the Food and Drug Administration in 1991 for chemotherapy-induced emesis.

This drug has been utilized successfully in the treatment of schizophrenia *(154)* and only rarely has caused dystonia or akathisia *(155)*. It does not have significant dopamine receptor-blocking properties and, presumably as a result of this, there have been no clear cases of ondansetron-induced Parkinsonism. These features make this drug an appropriate candidate for use in PD and have led to early trials in this setting. Zoldan et al. *(82)* treated 16 patients suffering from PD with psychosis with ondansetron (12–24 mg/day) in an open-label fashion. All but one patient experienced moderate to marked improvement in psychiatric symptoms; the drug was well-tolerated. Yet, in one additional study, these optimistic findings were not fully reproduced *(156)*. Further studies of this interesting drug are clearly needed. However, a major obstacle to more widespread testing and use of this medication is its extremely high cost.

6.4.2. Cholinesterase Inhibitors

The cholinesterase inhibitors are another class of medication that has been investigated for potential efficacy in treating cognitive and psychiatric symptoms in PD. Donepezil, rivastigmine, and galantamine have all been shown to be beneficial in mild-to-moderate Alzheimer's disease in large double-blind, placebo-controlled trials *(157–159)*. The rationale for using these agents in parkinsonian disorders is based on the finding that more severe cholinergic deficits are seen in the neocortex of patients with LBD than in Alzheimer's disease *(160)*. These agents might also be better tolerated in PD than antipsychotic medications because they do not block dopamine receptors. Alternatively, a theoretical concern has been that these agents might worsen motor features of Parkinsonism by increasing cholinergic tone and upsetting the balance between acetylcholine and dopamine in the brain.

The results of preliminary studies have been encouraging, but they are far from definitive. McKeith et al. *(85)* reported improvements in delusions and hallucinations using rivastigmine in a double-blind placebo-controlled trial involving 120 patients with LBD. Patients were treated with up to 12 mg per day of rivastigmine for 20 weeks. Improvements were noted in subscores of the neuropsychiatric inventory scale. In PD specifically, two open-label trials examining psychotic symptoms have documented similar improvements in psychiatric symptoms in a small number of patients *(161,162)*. Significant reduction of motor symptoms was not seen in any of these studies. Donepezil was used to treat DIP in another small open-label study *(163)*. Six patients with PD were treated with donepezil (10 mg daily) for 6 weeks; 5 of the 6 patients experienced "clinically significant" improvement in symptoms of psychosis. No worsening of motor symptoms was observed. Clearly, larger well-designed trials are needed to fully assess the utility and safety of these medications in this setting.

6.5. Electroconvulsive Therapy

It has been suggested that electroconvulsive therapy (ECT) may be useful in the treatment of DIP *(8,164)*. Hurwitz et al. *(164)* treated two patients with PD suffering from chronic nonconfusional psychosis with bilateral ECT (one received six treatments and the other received three). It not only cleared the psychosis but also allowed for the use of higher doses of dopaminergic medications. At 5-month follow-up, one patient had still experienced no recurrence of psychosis; the others had experienced only occasional visual illusions 6 months after treatment. Likely, patients with confusional states will not achieve the same benefit and, in fact, confusion is considered to be a contraindication for ECT *(8,165)*. There also seems to be interest in using ECT to treat patients with PD because of its ability to improve motor symptoms *(166–168)*. This improvement may be the result of ECT-induced enhancement of dopamine transmission *(169)*. It is difficult to explain the antipsychotic effect of ECT on the background of increased responsiveness of dopamine receptors. Hurwitz et al. *(164)* suggest that improvement in psychosis may be owing to an effect via nondopaminergic mechanisms.

ECT-induced improvement of motor features of PD is most likely transient *(166,167)*. The antidepressant effects of ECT are also temporary, and patients should be treated with antidepressant agents for long-term maintenance. Generally, the temporary nature of its benefits does not support ECT as a logical choice to be a primary agent in the treatment of DIP in PD. The adverse effects of memory loss and delirium are also of concern. However, in those situations where CLZ does not improve psychosis, or when significant side effects occur at dose levels that are otherwise ineffective, ECT can be used as an adjunct, then low-dose CLZ may help maintain the benefit *(170)*.

6.6. Treatment Summary

The treatment of DIP in PD can be approached in a stepwise fashion. First, it is necessary to search for and treat any triggering factors (e.g., infection) that may have precipitated decompensation in an otherwise stable patient. If no such triggers are present, and the symptoms are mild, a modest reduction in antiparkinsonian medication dose will usually be sufficient. In more severely affected patients, the next step is to reduce or stop adjunctive medications. This should be done one drug at a time in order of decreasing risk-to-benefit ratio. If psychosis continues, an attempt should be made to decrease the dose of levodopa. If there is an increase in disability at any point, then an antipsychotic medication will be required.

CLZ is the only antipsychotic medication that has been proven in controlled clinical trials to effectively control DIP without worsening Parkinsonism. However, based on promising preliminary data, our own experience, and ease of use, we feel that QTP is a reasonable alternative as a first-choice agent. It is usually started with a bedtime dose, then daytime doses are added if necessary. If QTP is ineffective, or if side effects prevent further dose increases, we recommend CLZ as the antipsychotic of second choice. We have had patients treated with up to 400 mg per day of QTP without benefit, then respond to as little as 6.25 mg of CLZ. It is important to remember that patients with PD are particularly prone to sedation with these medications, and therapy should be initiated with a low dose and increased in small increments. Frequent communication between the physician and patient's caretakers is paramount during this difficult period. Once DIP is controlled, a smaller maintenance dose is usually possible, and a careful optimization of antiparkinsonian medications can be attempted.

In the rare patient who does not respond to either of these medications, a trial of one of the newer agents may be justified, but the patient should be carefully monitored for worsening of Parkinsonism. RSP, OLZ, and typical antipsychotics are not appropriate choices for treating DIP in PD and should be avoided. Occasional patients will not respond to the measures previously mentioned; thus, more drastic reductions in levodopa will be necessary. This consequence will usually be associated with severe worsening of Parkinsonism and should be done in a hospital setting under the supervision of a movement disorder specialist. Finally, in nondemented patients, a course of ECT can be used as a last resort.

7. LONG-TERM OUTCOMES

With the onset of hallucinations, it has been suggested that the prognosis of PD declines significantly. Several studies have examined the long-term outcome of patients who have DIP in an attempt to confirm this notion. Also, the question of whether treatment with atypical antipsychotics alters the outcome of hallucinating patients has been addressed in a limited way. Two studies examined the outcomes of patients prior to the availability of atypical agents. The first attempt was by Sweet et al. in 1976, who looked at the outcome of 18 patients with PD who were followed for about 6 years *(171)*. Five (27%) were placed in nursing homes, five (27%) died, six (33%) were incapacitated but living at home, and only two (11%) were home and semi-independent. However, there was a problem with patient selection, because these patients were a subset of 100 patients, and they had a mixture of dementia, agitation, delirium, mania, hallucinations, and other mental symptoms. Two studies by Goetz et al. have been the most frequently quoted reports on the subject. In 1993, they performed a case-control study to specifically examine the most frequent reason for nursing home placement in PD *(3)*. They studied 11 patients who had been placed and compared them to 22 who were still living at home. Hallucinations were significantly more common in patients placed in a nursing home. Motor impairment and dementia did not differentiate between the two groups, indicating that hallucinations were an independent cause of nursing home placement. This study was succeeded by a 2-year follow-up study to examine outcome; it was discovered that 100% of the nursing home patients had died with a mean duration of survival of 15.6 months *(4)*. The investigators also found that nursing home placement in these patients was permanent. These studies focused on hallucinations in relation to nursing home placement and likely involved the most severely affected cases.

Two studies have subsequently examined outcome after the availability of atypical antipsychotics. In the first, Juncos et al. examined the long-term outcome of 27 patients with PD treated with either QTP or CLZ for hallucinations *(172)*. Over the 36-month observation period, 50% were placed in nursing homes. The mortality of patients in nursing homes was 62% when compared with 52% in those still living at home. Finally, Factor et al. *(5)* examined 59 patients who were originally enrolled in a double-blind placebo-controlled clinical trial that examined CLZ therapy for DIP in PD. Long-term outcome data were collected for a mean of 22 months following enrollment. The patients were more typical of those seen in practice, living at home for the most part, requiring antipsychotic therapy, and receiving clozapine. Over the follow-up period, many switched to other agents or came off antipsychotics completely. The participants in this study were not the most severely affected patients with DIP, because enrollment included those who could withstand 1 month of placebo therapy. At baseline, 12% were living in a nursing home, 95% had hallucinations, and 60% had paranoia. On follow-up, 25% were dead, nursing home placement occurred in 42%, psychosis was persistent in 69%, and dementia was diagnosed in 68%. Of those in a nursing home, 28% had died over the 2-year period, including two of the seven patients in a nursing home at baseline. Of those with persistent psychosis, 97% had hallucinations, and 27% had paranoia. Comparison of the studies completed prior to and after the availability of atypical agents is limited, but data suggest that these agents have a positive effect on long-term outcome. The death rate in nursing home patients is clearly diminished, suggesting an improvement in survival. In addition, the study by Factor et al. *(5)* demonstrated a significant decrease in the percentage of patients with paranoia, a complex symptom associated with increased nursing home placement. It is interesting to note that the persistence (or lack) of psychosis at follow-up did not have an impact on the final outcome of these patients. A similar percentage of psychotic and nonpsychotic patients died, were placed in a nursing facility, were treated with antipsychotics, and became demented. This may suggest that the hallucinations themselves are not necessarily associated with a poor outcome, but they may be indicators of the development of a high-risk stage of the disease.

Factor et al. *(5)* also examined possible risk factors (from baseline data) that might predict poor outcome in patients with PD in addition to DIP. There were no predictors for death. Older age and the presence of paranoia were risk factors for nursing home placement, whereas older age, older age of onset, and lower baseline minimental status exam scores conferred greater risk for developing dementia. On the other hand, younger age of onset and longer duration of disease are risk factors for persistent psychosis.

In combination, the data indicate that older patients tend to end up in nursing homes with paranoia or develop dementia with poor survival, where younger onset patients tend to continue to have hallucinations and remain in the community. The goal should be to alter the outcome of patients suffering from PD with DIP, and the examination of predictors for the individual outcome measures might lead to improved treatment approaches. This was the first study to determine modifiable risk factors that could lead to such an alteration. Some possibilities come to mind. For instance, nursing home placement was associated with paranoid psychosis in addition to the visual hallucinations usually seen. The occurrence of this problem should lead to more vigorous antipsychotic treatment, perhaps using higher doses than typically prescribed or in those with a clear sensorium, ECT if the drugs are not effective. Better control of paranoia may catalyze the prevention or delay of placement and, in turn, longer survival. Patients with onset of psychosis at an older age are not only more likely to be placed in a nursing home, but are also more likely to develop dementia, particularly those patients with a decreased minimental status exam score. That background should signal an earlier intervention for cognitive difficulties, possibly with a cholinesterase inhibitor. The approach might be to use an atypical antipsychotic and cholinesterase inhibitor concurrently from the beginning. Finally, younger patients with long-term disease are more likely to have persistent psychosis. This scenario should encourage more aggressive dosing with antipsychotic drugs, perhaps using higher doses than those routinely used. These strategies will have to be tested, but they represent a starting point toward the improvement in prognosis of this patient population.

REFERENCES

1. Fischer P, Danielczyk W, Simanyi M, Streifler MB. Dopaminergic psychosis in advanced Parkinson's disease. Adv Neurol 1990;53:391–397.
2. Carter JH, Archbold PG, Stewart BJ. Family caregiving. In: Factor SA, Weiner WJ, eds. Parkinson's Disease: Diagnosis and Clinical Management. Demos Medical Publishing, New York, 2002, pp. 627–637.
3. Goetz CG, Stebbins GT. Risk factors for nursing home placement in advanced Parkinson's disease. Neurology 1993;43:2227–2229.
4. Goetz CG, Stebbins GT. Mortality and hallucinations in nursing home patients with advanced Parkinson's disease. Neurology 1995;45:669–671.
5. Factor SA, Feustel PJ, Friedman JH, et al. Longitudinal outcome of Parkinson's disease patients with psychosis. Neurology 2003;60:1756–1761.
6. The Parkinson Study Group. Low-dose clozapine for the treatment of drug-induced psychosis in Parkinson's disease. N Engl J Med 1999;340:757–763.
7. Factor SA, Friedman JH, Lannon MC, et al. and the Parkinson Study Group. Clozapine for the treatment of drug-induced psychosis in Parkinson's disease: results of the 12 week open label extension in the PSYCLOPS trial. Mov Disord 2001;16:135–139.
8. Friedman JH. The management of the levodopa psychoses. Clin Neuropharmacol 1991;14:283–295.
9. American Psychiatric Association. Diagnostic and Statistical Manual of Mental Disorders, 3rd Ed. Revised. American Psychiatric Association, Washington, DC, 1987.
10. Cummings JL. Behavioral complications of drug treatment of Parkinson's disease. J Am Geriatr Soc 1991;33:708–716.
11. Klawans HL. Levodopa-induced psychosis. Psychiatric Ann 1978;8:447–451.
12. Mayeux R. PD: a review of cognitive and psychiatric disorders. Neuropsychiatry Neuropsychol Behav Neurol 1990;3:3–14.
13. Hoehn MM, Yahr MD. Parkinsonism: onset, progression and mortality. Neurology 1967;17:427–442.
14. McKeith IG, Galasko D, Kosaka K, et al. Consensus guidelines for the clinical and pathological diagnosis of dementia with Lewy bodies (DLB): report of the consortium on DLB international workshop. Neurology 1996;47:1113–1124.
15. Hurtig HI, Trojanowski JQ, Galvin J, et al. Alpha-synuclein cortical Lewy bodies correlate with dementia in Parkinson's disease. Neurology 2000;54:1916–1921.
16. Apaydin H, Ahlskog JE, Parisi JE, et al. Parkinson's disease neuropathology: later-developing dementia and loss of the levodopa response. Arch Neurol 2002;59:102–112.
17. Parkinson J. An Essay on the Shaking Palsy. Neely and Jones, Sherwood, London, 1817.
18. Regis E. Precis de Psychiatrie. Gaston Doiz, Paris, 1906.
19. Patrick HT, Levy DM. PD: a clinical study of one hundred and forty-six cases. Arch Neurol Psychiatry 1922;7:711–720.
20. Jackson JA, Free GBM, Pike HV. The psychic manifestations in paralysis agitans. Arch Neurol Psychiatry 1923;10:680–684.
21. Schwab RS, Fabing HD, Prichard JS. Psychiatric symptoms and syndromes in Parkinson's disease. Am J Psychiatry 1950;107:901–907.
22. Calne DB, Stern GM, Laurence DR, et al. L-dopa in post-encephalitic Parkinsonism. Lancet 1969;1:744–746.
23. Celesia GG, Barr AN. Psychosis and other psychiatric manifestations of levodopa therapy. Arch Neurol 1970;23:193–200.
24. Yahr MD, Duvoisin RC, Schear MJ, et al. Treatment of Parkinsonism with levodopa. Arch Neurol 1969;21:343–354.
25. Cotzias GC, Papavasilou PS, Gellene R. Modification of Parkinsonism: chronic treatment with L-dopa. N Engl J Med 1969;280:337–345.
26. McDowell F, Lee JE, Swift T, et al. Treatment of Parkinson's syndrome with L-dihydroxyphenyl-alanine (levodopa). Ann Intern Med 1970;72:29–35.
27. Damasio AR, Lobo-Antunes J, Macedo C. Psychiatric aspects in Parkinsonism treated with L-dopa. J Neurol Neurosurg Psychiatry 1971;34:502–507.
28. Mawdsley C. Treatment of Parkinsonism with laevo-dopa. Brit Med J 1970;1:331–337.
29. Jenkins RB, Groh RH. Mental symptoms in parkinsonian patients with L-dopa. Lancet 1970;2:177–180.
30. Celesia GG, Wanamaker WM. Psychiatric disturbances in Parkinson's disease. Dis Nerv Syst 1972;33:577–583.
31. Cheifetz DI, Garron DC, Leavitt F, et al. Emotional disturbance accompanying the treatment of Parkinsonism with L-dopa. Clin Pharmacol Ther 1970;12:56–61.
32. Goodwin FK. Psychiatric side effects of levodopa in man. JAMA 1971;218:1915–1920.

33. Factor SA, McAlarney T, Sanchez-Ramos JR, Weiner WJ. Sleep disorders and sleep effect in Parkinson's disease. Mov Disord 1990;5:280–285.
34. Sanchez-Ramos JR, Ortoll R, Paulson GW. Visual hallucinations associated with Parkinson's disease. Arch Neurol 1996;53:1265–1268.
35. Barclay CL, Hildebrand K, Gray P, et al. Risk factor for the development of psychosis in Parkinson's disease [abstract]. Mov Disord 1997;12(Suppl 1):108.
36. Graham JM, Grunewald RA, Sagar HJ. Hallucinosis in idiopathic Parkinson's disease. J Neurol Neurosurg Psychiatry 1997;63:434–440.
37. Inzelberg R, Kipervasser S, Korczyn AD. Auditory hallucinations in Parkinson's disease. J Neurol Neurosurg Psychiatry 1998;64:533–535.
38. Aarsland D, Larsen JP, Cummings JL, Laake K. Prevalence and clinical correlates of psychotic symptoms in Parkinson's disease. Arch Neurol 1999;56:595–601.
39. Fenelon G, Mahieux F, Huon R, Ziegler M. Hallucinations in Parkinson's disease: prevalence, phenomenology and risk factors. Brain 2000;123:733–745.
40. Holroyd S, Currie L, Wooten GF. Prospective study of hallucinations and delusions in Parkinson's disease. J Neurol Neurosurg Psychiatry 2001;70:734–738.
41. Lipper S. Psychosis in patients on bromocriptine and levodopa with carbidopa. Lancet 1976;2:571–572.
42. White AC, Murphy TJC. Hallucinations caused by bromocriptine. Br J Psychiatry 1977;130:104.
43. Kurlan R, Miller C, Levy R, et al. Long-term experience with pergolide therapy of advanced Parkinsonism. Neurology 1985;35:738–742.
44. Stern Y, Mayeux R, Ilson J, et al. Pergolide therapy for Parkinson's disease: neurobehavioral changes. Neurology 1984;34:201–204.
45. Factor SA. Dopamine agonists. Med Clin North Am 1999;83:415–443.
46. Parkinson Study Group. Pramipexole vs levodopa as initial treatment for Parkinson's disease: a randomized controlled trial. JAMA 2000;284;1931–1938.
47. Rascol O, Brooks DJ, Korczyn AD, et al. A five-year study of the incidence of dyskinesia in patients with early Parkinson's disease who were treated with ropinirole or levodopa. N Engl J Med 2000;342:1484–1491.
48. Hutton JJ, Morris JL, Brewer MA. Controlled study of the antiparkinsonian activity and tolerability of cabergoline. Neurology 1993;43:613–616.
49. Rinne UK. Lisuride, a dopamine agonist in the treatment of early Parkinson's disease. Neurology 1989;39:336–339.
50. Frankel JP, Lees AJ, Kempster PA, Stern GM. Subcutaneous apomorphine in the treatment of Parkinson's disease. J Neurol Neurosurg Psychiatry 1990;53:96–101.
51. Lieberman AN, Goldstein M, Gopinathan G, Neophytides A. D-1 and D-2 agonists in Parkinson's disease. Can J Neurol Sci 1987;14:466–473.
52. Boyson SJ. Psychiatric effects of selegiline. Arch Neurol 1991;48(Letter):902.
53. Venezia P, Mohr E, Grimes D. Deprenyl in Parkinson's disease: mechanisms, neuroprotective effect, indications and adverse effects. Can J Neurol Sci 1992;19:142–146.
54. Fleminger R. Visual hallucinations and illusions with propranolol. Brit Med J 1978;1:1182.
55. Weiner WJ, Bergen D. Prevention and management of the side effects of levodopa. In: Klawans HL, ed. Clinical Neuropharmacology, vol. 2. Raven Press, New York, 1977, pp. 1–23.
56. Moskovitz C, Moses H, Klawans HL. Levodopa-induced psychosis: a kindling phenomenon. Am J Psychiatry 1978;135:669–675.
57. Schwab RS, England AC, Poskanzer DC, Young RR. Amantadine in the treatment of Parkinson's disease. JAMA 1969;208:1168–1170.
58. Factor SA, Molho ES, Brown DL. Acute delirium after withdrawal of amantadine in Parkinson's disease. Neurology 1998;50:1456–1458.
59. Adler CH, Singer C, O'Brien C, et al. Randomized, placebo-controlled study of tolcapone in patients with fluctuating Parkinson's disease treated with levodopa-carbidopa. Arch Neurol 1998;55:1089–1095.
60. Rajput AH, Martin W, Saint-Hilaire MH, et al. Tolcapone improves motor function in parkinsonian patients with the "wearing-off" phenomenon: a double-blind, placebo-controlled, multicenter trial. Neurology 1997;49:1066–1071.
61. Parkinson Study Group. Entacapone improves motor fluctuations in levodopa-treated Parkinson's disease patients. Ann Neurol 1997;42:747–755.
62. Sacks OW, Kohl MS, Messeloff CR, Schwartz WF. Effects of levodopa in parkinsonian patients with dementia. Neurology 1972;22:516–519.
63. Barnes J, David AS. Visual hallucinations in Parkinson's disease: a review and phenomenological survey. J Neurol Neurosurg Psychiatry 2001;70:727–733.
64. Goetz CG, Leurgans S, Pappert EJ, et al. Prospective longitudinal assessment of hallucinations in Parkinson's disease. Neurology 2001;57:2078–2082.
65. Pappert EJ, Goetz CG, Niederman FG, et al. Hallucinations, sleep fragmentation, and altered dream phenomena in Parkinson's disease. Mov Disord 1999;14:117–121.

66. Manni R, Pacchetti C, Terzaghi M, et al. Hallucinations and sleep-wake cycle in PD: a 24-hour continuous polysomnographic study. Neurology 2002;59:1979–1981.
67. Lepore FE. Visual loss as a causative factor in visual hallucinations associated with Parkinson's disease. Arch Neurol 1997;54:799.
68. Burke W. The neural basis of Charles Bonnet hallucinations: a hypothesis. J Neurol Neurosurg Psychiatry 2002;73:535–541.
69. Goetz CG, Vogel C, Tanner CM, Stebbins GT. Early dopaminergic drug-induced hallucinations in Parkinsonian patients. Neurology 1998;51:811–814.
70. Kaiser R, Hofer A, Grapengiesser A, et al. L-Dopa-induced adverse effects in PD and dopamine transporter gene polymorphism. Neurology 2003;60:1750–1755.
71. Goldman JG, Goetz CG, Berry-Kravis E, et al. Genetic polymorphisms in Parkinson's disease patients with and without hallucinations: an analysis of the cholecystokinin (CCK) system. Neurology 2003;60(Suppl 1):A282.
72. Chan D, Rosser MN. "-but who is that on the other side of you?" Extracampine hallucinations revisited. Lancet 2002;360:2064–2066.
73. Friedman JH, Messing S, Oakes D, et al. and the Parkinson Study Group. A descriptive and comparative analysis of psychotic symptoms in three placebo-controlled, double-blinded trials of atypical antipsychotic drugs in the treatment of drug-induced psychosis in Parkinson's disease [abstract]. Mov Disord 2002;17:1105.
74. Jimenez-Jimenez FJ, Orti-Pareja M, Gasalla T, et al. Cenesthetic hallucinations in a patient with Parkinson's disease. J Neurol Neurosurg Psychiatry 1997;63:120.
75. Kluver H. Neurobiology of normal and abnormal perception. In: Hoch P, Zubin J, eds. Psychopathology of Perceptions. Grune & Stratton, New York, NY, 1965.
76. Nausieda PA, Weiner WJ, Kaplan LR, et al. Sleep disruption in the course of chronic levodopa therapy: an early feature of the levodopa psychosis. Clin Neuropharmacol 1982;5:183–194.
77. Roane DM, Rogers JD, Robinson JH, Feinberg TE. Delusional misidentification in association with Parkinsonism. J Neuropsychiatry Clin NeuroSci 1998;10:194–198.
78. Pearn J, Gardner-Thorpe C. Jules Cotard (1840–1889): His life and the unique syndrome which bears his name. Neurology 2002;58:1400–1403.
79. Yaryura-Tobias JA, Diamond B, Merlis S. Psychiatric manifestations of levodopa. Dis Nerv System 1970;31:60–63.
80. Klawans HL, Goetz CG, Nausieda PA, Weiner WJ. Levodopa-induced dopamine receptor hypersensitivity. Ann Neurol 1977;2:125–129.
81. Goetz CG, Pappert EJ, Blasucci LM, et al. Intravenous levodopa in hallucinating Parkinson's disease patients: high-dose challenge does not precipitate hallucinations. Neurology 1998;50:515–517
82. Zoldan J, Friedberg G, Livneh M, Melamed E. Psychosis in advanced Parkinson's disease: treatment with ondansetron, a 5-HT3 receptor antagonist. Neurology 1995;45:1305–1308.
83. Comella CL, Tanner CM, Ristanovic RK. Polysomnographic sleep measures in Parkinson's disease patients with treatment-induced hallucination. Ann Neurol 1993;34:710–714.
84. Tanner CM, Vogel C, Goetz CG, Klawans HL. Hallucinations in Parkinson's Disease: a population study. Ann Neurol 1983;14(Abstract):136.
85. McKeith I, Del Ser T, Spano P, et al. Efficacy of rivastigmine in dementia with Lewy bodies: a randomized, double-blind, placebo-controlled international study. Lancet 2000;356:2031–2036.
86. Harding AJ, Broe GA, Halliday GM. Visual hallucinations in Lewy body disease relate to Lewy bodies in the temporal lobe. Brain 2002;125:391–403.
87. Diederich NJ, Alesch F, Goetz CG. Visual hallucinations induced by deep brain stimulation in Parkinson's disease. Clin Neuropharmacol 2000;23:287–289.
88. Goetz CG, Medina D, Carrillo M, et al. Functional neuroimaging in Parkinson's disease patients with hallucinations. Neurology 2002;58(Suppl 3):A201.
89. Albin RL, Minoshima S, D'Amato CJ, et al. Fluoro-deoxyglucose positron emission tomography in diffuse Lewy body disease. Neurology 1996;47:462–466.
90. Vanderborght T, Minoshima S, Giordani B, et al. Cerebral metabolic differences in Parkinson's and Alzheimer's diseases matched for dementia severity. J Nucl Med 1997;38:797–802.
91. Summerfield C, Gomez-Anson B, Tolosa E, et al. Dementia in Parkinson's disease: a proton magnetic resonance spectroscopy study. Arch Neurol 2002;59:1415–1420.
92. Santhouse AM, Howard RJ, Ffytche DH. Visual hallucinatory syndromes and the anatomy of the visual brain. Brain 2000;123:2055–2064.
93. Golden WE, Lavender RC, Metzer WS. Acute postoperative confusion and hallucinations in Parkinson's disease. Ann Int Med 1989;111:218–222.
94. Marsden CD, Fahn S. Problems in PD. In: Marsden CD, and Fahn S, eds. Movement Disorders. Butterworth Scientific, London, 1981, pp. 1–7.
95. Friedman JH, "Drug Holidays" in the treatment of Parkinson's disease: a brief review. Arch Intern Med 1985;145:913–915.
96. Friedman JH, Lannon MC. Clozapine in the treatment of psychosis in Parkinson's disease. Neurology 1989;39:1219–1221.

97. Baldesserini RJ, Frankenburg FR. Clozapine: a novel antipsychotic agent. N Engl J Med 1991;324:740–754.
98. Factor SA, Friedman JH. The emerging role of clozapine in the treatment of movement disorders. Mov Disord 1997;12:483–496.
99. French Clozapine Parkinson Study Group. Clozapine in drug-induced psychosis in Parkinson's disease. Lancet 1999;353:2041–2042.
100. Scholz E, Dichgans J. Treatment of drug-induced exogenous psychosis in Parkinsonism with clozapine and fluperlapine. Eur Arch Psychiatr Neurol Sci 1985;235:60–64.
101. Alvir JMJ, Lieberman JA, Safferman AZ, et al. Clozapine-induced agranulocytosis: incidence and risk factors in the United States. N Engl J Med 1993;329:162–167.
102. Honigfeld G, Arellano F, Sethi J, et al. Reducing clozapine-related morbidity and mortality: 5 years experience with the Clozaril National Registry. J Clin Psychiatry 1998;59(Suppl 3):3–9.
103. Gerson SL. Clozapine-deciphering the risks. N Engl J Med 1993;329:204–205.
104. Factor SA, Singer C. Neuroleptic malignant syndrome. In: Lang AE, and Weiner WJ, eds. Drug-induced Movement Disorders. Futura Publishing Co. Inc., Mount Kisco, NY, 1992, pp. 199–230.
105. Devinsky O, Honigfeld G, Patin J. Clozapine-related seizures. Neurology 1991;41:369–371.
106. Alphs LD, Meltzer HY, Bastani B, Ramirez LF. Side effects of clozapine and their management. Pharmacol Psychiatry 1991;24:46.
107. Hagg S, Spigset O, Soderstrom TG. Association of venous thromboembolism and clozapine. Lancet 2000;355:1155–1156.
108. Kilian JG, Kerr K, Lawrence C, Celermajer DS. Myocarditis and cardiomyopathy associated with clozapine. Lancet 1999;354:1841–1842.
109. La Grenade L, Graham D, Trontell A. Myocarditis and cardiomyopathy associated with clozapine use in the United States. N Engl J Med 2001;345(Letter):224.
110. Devarajan S, Kutcher SP, Dursun SM. Clozapine and sudden death. Lancet 2000;355(Letter):841.
111. Liebzeit KA, Markowitz JS, Caley CF. New Onset diabetes and atypical antipsychotics. Eur Neuropsychopharmacol 2001;11:25–32.
112. Henderson D, Cagliero E, Gray C, et al. Clozapine, diabetes mellitus, weight gain, and lipid abnormalities: a 5-year naturalistic study. Am J Psychiatry 2000;157:975–981.
113. Fernandez HH, Friedman JH, Factor SA, et al. New onset diabetes among parkinsonian patients on long-term clozapine use. Mov Disord 2002;17(Suppl 5):S47.
114. Gianfrancesco FD, Grogg AL, Mahmoud RA, et al. Differential effects of risperidone, olanzapine, clozapine, and conventional antipsychotics on type 2 diabetes: findings from a large health plan database. J Clin Psychiatry 2002;63:920–930.
115. Koro CE, Fedder DO, L'Italian GJ, et al. Assessment of independent effect of olanzapine and risperidone on risk of diabetes among patients with schizophrenia: population based nested case-control study. Brit Med J 2002;325:243–247.
116. Greene P, Cote L, Fahn S. Treatment of drug-induced psychosis in Parkinson's disease with clozapine. Adv Neurol 1993;60:703–706.
117. Factor SA, Brown D, Molho ES, Podskalny GD. Clozapine: a two year open trial in Parkinson's disease patients with psychosis. Neurology 1994;44:544–546.
118. Friedman JH, Factor SA. Atypical antipsychotics in the treatment of drug-induced psychosis in Parkinson's disease. Mov Disord 2000;15:201–211.
119. Seeman P, Tallerico T. Rapid release of antipsychotic drugs from dopamine D2 receptors: an explanation for low receptor occupancy and early clinical relapse upon withdrawal of clozapine or quetiapine. Am J Psychiatry 1999;156:876–884.
120. Kapur S, Seeman P. Does fast dissociation from the dopamine D2 receptor explain the action of atypical antipsychotics?: a new hypothesis. Am J Psychiatry 2001;158:360–369.
121. Kapur S, Zipursky R, Jones C, et al. A positron emission tomography study of quetiapine in schizophrenia: a preliminary finding of an antipsychotic effect with only transiently high dopamine D2 receptor occupancy. Arch Gen Psychiatry 2000;57:553–559.
122. Meco G, Alessandria A, Bonifati V, Giustini P. Risperidone for hallucinations in levodopa-treated Parkinson's disease patients. Lancet 1994;343:1370–1371.
123. Ford B, Lynch T, Greene P. Risperidone in Parkinson's disease. Lancet 1994;344:681.
124. Rich SS, Friedman JH, Ott BR. Risperidone versus clozapine in the treatment of psychosis in six patients with Parkinson's disease and other akinetic-rigid syndromes. J Clin Psychiatry 1995;56:556–559.
125. Meco G, Alessandria A, Giustini P, Bonifati V. Risperidone in levodopa-induced psychosis in advanced Parkinson's disease: an open-label, long-term study. Mov Disord 1997;12:610–611.
126. Allen RL, Walker Z, D'Ath PJ, Katona CL. Risperidone for psychotic and behavioral symptoms in Lewy body dementia. Lancet 1995;346:185.
127. McKeith IG, Ballard CG, Harrison RWS. Neuroleptic sensitivity to risperidone in Lewy body dementia. Lancet 1995;346:699.
128. Workman RJ Jr., Orengo CA, Bakey AA, et al. The use of risperidone for psychosis and agitation in demented patients with Parkinson's disease. J Neuropsychiatry Clin Neurosci 1997;9:594–597.
129. Leopold NA. Risperidone treatment of drug-related psychosis in patients with Parkinsonism. Mov Disord 2000;15:301–304.

130. Mohr E, Mendis T, Hildebrand IC, DeDeyn PP. Risperidone in the treatment of dopamine-induced psychosis in Parkinson's disease: An open pilot trial. Mov Disord 2000;15:1230–1237.
131. Ellis T, Cudkowicz ME, Sexton PM, Growdon JH. Clozapine and risperidone treatment of psychosis in Parkinson's disease. J Neuropsychiatry Clin Neurosci 2000;12:364–369.
132. Wolters EC, Jansen ENH, Tuynman-Qua HG, Bergmans PLM. Olanzapine in the treatment of dopaminomimetic psychosis in patients with Parkinson's disease. Neurology 1996;47:1085–1087.
133. Jimenez-Jimenez FJ, Tallon-Barranco A, Orti-Pareja M, et al. Olanzapine can worsen Parkinsonism. Neurology 1998;50:1183–1184.
134. Friedman JH. Olanzapine in the treatment of dopaminomimetic psychosis in patients with Parkinson's disease. Neurology 1998;50(Letter):1195–1196.
135. Friedman JH, Goldstein SM, Jacques C. Substituting clozapine for olanzapine in psychiatrically stable Parkinson's disease patients; Results of an open-label pilot trial. Clin Neuropharmacol 1998;21:285–288.
136. Molho ES, Factor SA. Worsening of motor features of Parkinson's disease with olanzapine. Mov Disord 1999;14:1014–1016.
137. Weiner WJ, Minagar A, Shulman LM. Olanzapine for the treatment of hallucinations/delusions in Parkinson's disease. Mov Disord 1998;13:862.
138. Graham JM, Sussman JD, Ford KS, Sagar HJ. Olanzapine in the treatment of hallucinosis in idiopathic Parkinson's disease: a cautionary note. J Neurol Neurosurg Psychiatry 1998;65:774–777.
139. Stover NP, Juncos JL. Olanzapine treatment of parkinsonian patients with psychosis. Neurology 1999;52(Suppl 2):A215.
140. Wolters EC, Jansen ENH, Tuynman-Qua HG, et al. Olanzapine in the treatment of dopaminomimetic psychosis in patients with Parkinson's disease. Neurology 1998;50(Letter):1196.
141. Goetz CG, Blasucci CM, Leurgans S, Pappert EJ. Olanzapine and clozapine: comparative effects on motor function in hallucinating Parkinson's disease patients. Neurology 2000;55:789–794.
142. Ondo WG, Levy JK, Vuong KD, Hunter C, Jankovic J. Olanzapine treatment for dopaminergic-induced hallucinations. Mov Disord 2002;17:1031–1035.
143. Breier A, Sutton VK, Feldman PD, et al. Olanzapine in the treatment of dopamimetic-induced psychosis in patients with Parkinson's disease. Biol Psychiatry 2002;52:438–445.
144. Parsa MA, Bastani B. Quetiapine (Seroquel) in the treatment of psychosis in patients with Parkinson's disease. J Neuropsychiatry Clin Neurosci 1998;10:1–4.
145. Evatt ML, Jewart D, Juncos JL. "Seroquel" (ICI 204,636) treatment of psychosis in Parkinsonism. Mov Disord 1996;11:595.
146. Juncos JL, Evatt ML, Jewert D. Long term effects of quetiapine fumarate in Parkinsonism complicated by psychosis. Neurology 1998;50(Suppl 4):A70–A71.
147. Juncos JL, Arvanitis L, Sweitzer D, et al. Quetiapine improves psychotic symptoms associated with Parkinson's disease. Neurology 1999;52(Suppl 2):A262.
148. Targum SD, Abbott JL. Efficacy of quetiapine in Parkinson's patients with psychosis. J Clin Psychopharmacol 2000;20:54–60.
149. Samanta J, Stacy M. Quetiapine in the treatment of hallucinations in advanced Parkinson's disease. Mov Disord 1998;13(Suppl 2):274.
150. Fernandez HH, Friedman JH, Jacques C, Rosenfeld M. Quetiapine for the treatment of drug-induced psychosis in Parkinson's Disease. Mov Disord 1999;14:484–487.
151. Friedman JH, Fernandez HH, Jacques C, Rosenfeld M. Quetiapine for the treatment of drug-induced psychosis in Parkinson's disease. Neurology 1999;52(Suppl 2):A215.
152. Reddy S, Factor SA, Molho ES, Feustel PJ. The effect of quetiapine on psychosis and motor function in parkinsonian patients with and without dementia. Mov Disord 2002;17:676–681.
153. Fernandez HH, Trieschmann ME, Burke MA, et al. Long-term outcome of quetiapine use for psychosis among parkinsonian patients. Mov Disord 2003;18:510–514.
154. White A, Corn TH, Feetham C, Faulconbridge C. Ondansetron in treatment of schizophrenia. Lancet 1991;337:1173.
155. Halperin JR, Murphy B. Extrapyramidal reaction to ondansetron. Cancer 1992;69:1275.
156. Eichhorn TE, Brunt E, Oertel WH. Ondansetron treatment of L-dopa-induced psychosis. Neurology 1996;47:1608–1609.
157. Rogers SL, Friedhoff LT, and the Donepezil Study Group. The efficacy and safety of donepezil in patients with Alzheimer's disease: results of a US multicenter, randomized, double-blind, placebo-controlled trial. Dementia 1996;7:293–303.
158. Rosler M, Anand R, Cicin-Sain A, et al. Efficacy and safety of rivastigmine in patients with Alzheimer's disease: international randomized controlled trial. Br Med J 1999;31:633–640.
159. Raskind MA, Peskind ER, Wessel T, Yuan W, and the Galantamine USA-1 Study Group. Galantamine in AD: a 6-month randomized, placebo-controlled trial with a 6-month extension. Neurology 2000;54:2261–2268.
160. Perry EK, Haroutunian V, Davis KL, et al. Neocortical cholinergic activities differentiate Lewy body dementia from classical Alzheimer's disease. Neuroreport 1994;5:747–749.
161. Reading PJ, Luce AK, McKeith IG. Rivastigmine in the treatment of parkinsonian psychosis and cognitive impairment: preliminary findings from an open trial. Mov Disord 2001;16:1171–1174.

162. Van Laar T, de Vries JJ, Leenders KL. Rivastigmine as anti-psychotic treatment in patients with Parkinson's disease. Parkinsonism Relat Disord 2001;7(Suppl 1):S73.
163. Bergman J, Lerner V. Successful use of donepezil for the treatment of psychotic symptoms in patients with Parkinson's disease. Clin Neuropharmacol 2002;25:107–110.
164. Hurwitz TA, Calne DB, Waterman K. Treatment of dopaminomimetic psychosis in Parkinson's disease with electroconvulsive therapy. Can J Neurol Sci 1988;15:32–34.
165. Brown GI. Parkinsonism depression and ECT. Am J Psychiatry 1975;132:1084.
166. Stern MB. Electroconvulsive therapy in untreated Parkinson's disease. Mov Disord 1991;6:265.
167. Douyon R, Serby M, Klutchko B, Rotrosen J. ECT and Parkinson's disease revisited: a "naturalistic" study. Am J Psychiatry 1989;146:1451–1455.
168. Abrams R. ECT for Parkinson's disease. Am J Psychiatry 1989;146:1391–1393.
169. Fochtmann L. A mechanism for the efficacy of ECT in Parkinson's disease. Convulsive Therapy 1988;4:321–327.
170. Factor SA, Molho ES, Brown DL. Combined clozapine and electroconvulsive therapy for the treatment of drug-induced psychosis in Parkinson's disease. J Neuropsychiatry Clin Neurosci 1995;7:304–307.
171. Sweet RD, McDowell FH, Feigenson JS, et al. Mental symptoms in Parkinson's disease during chronic treatment with levodopa. Neurology 1976;26:305–310.
172. Juncos JL, Jewart RD, Neparizde N, Hanfelt J. Long-term prognosis of hallucinating Parkinson's disease patients treated with quetiapine or clozapine. Neurology 2002;58(Abstract):A435.

6
Postsurgical Behavioral Changes

Laurie M. Rilling, John A. Lucas, and Ryan J. Uitti

SUMMARY

Evaluation of postsurgical behavioral changes in patients with Parkinson's disease (PD) is a complicated subject. Reasons for this complexity stem from the progressive nature of PD, its propensity to include neurobehavioral changes, and the variability in motor and nonmotor results that follow various types of surgical treatment. Studies of postsurgical behavioral changes also have not had the benefit of comparison with randomized, controlled, longitudinal follow-up of patients who have not had surgical treatment. Nevertheless, it appears that most modern-day lesioning and deep-brain stimulation (DBS) operations performed at experienced surgical centers are relatively safe from a cognitive perspective. Surgical interventions appear to involve minimal psychiatric morbidity in most instances. When neurocognitive declines are observed, they most often involve verbal fluency, regardless of the surgical technique and target. This decline in verbal fluency occurs more often after dominant hemisphere-sided operations and may persist for 1 year or more, independent of motor speech changes. Other selective changes have been observed in working memory, attention, and episodic memory, but only in a minority of studies and patients.

A small number of studies have reported severe cognitive and psychiatric complications, including both severe declines in memory and dementia. Although it is impossible to predict definitively which factors determine such declines, the following likely increase the risk for postoperative neurobehavioral morbidity: age (particularly > 70 years), bilateral or language-dominant hemisphere surgery (not necessarily ablative), lesion location in the anteromedial versus posterolateral aspect of the globus pallidus interna (GPi), pre-existing psychiatric disturbance, and preexisting dementia or marked frontal–subcortical syndrome. Lesion volume has not convincingly or consistently been identified as a correlate of cognitive outcome. Claims that DBS is neuropsychologically safer than ablative surgery are not adequately supported in the literature at this time. There is also no clear indication that certain targets (GPi versus subthalamic nucleus [STN]) are better from a cognitive standpoint. Future randomized, preferably blinded, studies are needed to compare interventions (target and treatment methods) directly in terms of their effects on neurobehavioral functioning.

Key Words: Parkinson's disease (PD); thalamotomy; pallidotomy; subthalamotomy; deep-brain stimulation; cognition,

1. INTRODUCTION

Over the past decade, surgical intervention has regained widespread acceptance as a safe and effective treatment for the disabling motor symptoms associated with idiopathic Parkinson's disease (PD). Surgical treatment, employing various lesioning methods, had been popular in the 1950s and 1960s but was largely supplanted by pharmacological therapy with levodopa in the late 1960s. More recent advances in the understanding of neuroanatomic structures and underlying pathophysiology, in combination with improved surgical, radiological, and stereotactical techniques, have led to more

From: *Current Clinical Neurology*
Parkinson's Disease and Nonmotor Dysfunction
Edited by: R. F. Pfeiffer and I. Bodis-Wollner © Humana Press Inc., Totowa, NJ

successful symptom relief and significant reductions in postoperative morbidity *(1,2)*. Nevertheless, early anecdotal reports of deleterious postoperative neurobehavioral changes highlighted the need for systematic investigation of potential contributing factors. Patient characteristics, type of surgical procedure, and target location have all been implicated to varying degrees; however, methodological limitations and procedural differences have presented challenges in the interpretation of existing studies and their clinical significance. The topic is further complicated when the variability in surgical treatment is considered, such as unilateral versus bilateral, single versus staged bilateral procedure, and dominant versus nondominant hemispheric surgery. The extent to which these and other factors influence neurobehavioral outcomes remains the focus of ongoing empirical investigations.

Behavioral changes in patients with PD are important determinants of quality of life and survival. As such, any deleterious or protective consequences secondary to surgical therapy for PD may have profound repercussions on the recommended therapy for this disorder. Unfortunately, the data currently available are limited in scope and duration with regard to follow-up. Furthermore, a prolonged follow-up series may be subject to study retention biases that could inappropriately influence apparent results. Given these potential shortcomings, the data presented here should be considered with caution.

This chapter presents a brief overview of the neuropathological and neurophysiological correlations of motor dysfunction in PD and the rationale for specific surgical targets. The overview is followed by a more comprehensive evaluation of the current literature examining neurobehavioral changes associated with ablation and deep-brain stimulation (DBS) at various target locations, including the thalamus, globus pallidus (GP), and subthalamic nucleus (STN). The neurobehavioral sequelae associated with intrastriatal transplantation are also addressed to a limited degree. Finally, implications for clinical practice are discussed and suggestions for future scientific investigations are provided.

2. NEUROPATHOLOGY OF PD AND SURGICAL TARGETS

Idiopathic PD is a neurodegenerative movement disorder characterized by symptomatic onset of resting tremor, rigidity, bradykinesia, and postural instability, typically in the sixth or seventh decade of life. The motor dysfunction associated with PD results from a disproportionate loss of dopaminergic cells in the substantia nigra (SN) pars compacta that begins perhaps a decade prior to symptoms. The subsequent disruption of normal excitatory and inhibitory influences within the basal ganglia, initially most dramatic in the dopaminergic neurons of the ventrolateral tier of the SN that innervate the posterior putamen, causes abnormal activity in associated thalamocortical circuits. Inputs from the basal ganglia originate in various cortical regions and project to the striatum, SN, GP, STN, and thalamus via a system of five parallel segregated cortico-striato-thalamo-cortical loops *(3)*. Within the direct pathway, the striatum receives excitatory input from cortical regions and projects inhibitory efferents to the globus pallidus interna (GPi)/SN pars reticulata (SNpr) complex. These structures, in turn, have an inhibitory influence on the thalamus, which ultimately projects excitatory efferents back to the cortex *(4)*. There is also an indirect pathway, in which inhibitory efferents project from the striatum to the globus pallidus externa and extend to the STN, which then projects excitatory efferents back to the GPi–SNpr complex *(5)*. The loss of dopamine within the direct pathway leads to a decrease in the normal inhibitory activity from the putamen to the GPi, resulting in an excessive inhibition of the thalamus and net decrease in cortical excitation. DeLong and colleagues *(6)* have proposed that this net inhibition of thalamocortical projections within the motor circuit may account for motor signs like bradykinesia in PD. With this model in mind, several neuroanatomical targets (thalamus, GPi, and STN) and surgical techniques (ablation, stimulation, and transplantation) have been explored in an attempt to alleviate the motor symptoms associated with PD (*see* ref. *7* for a more comprehensive review of the scientific basis for surgical targets).

3. NEUROBEHAVIORAL OUTCOME AND SURGICAL TARGETS

3.1. Thalamus

3.1.1. Surgical Lesioning of the Ventrolateral/Ventral Anterior Nuclei

3.1.1.1. Postoperative Changes in Cognition

In the prelevodopa era, the issue of cognitive morbidity following thalamotomy received little attention in the literature. When cognitive changes were observed postoperatively, these were often described in passing in very general terms or on a case-by-case basis. For example, in one of the earliest anecdotal reports, Spiegel and colleagues *(8)* briefly commented on postoperative changes in memory, orientation, and sense of time in several patients who underwent bilateral thalamotomy, but no formal cognitive measures were administered. The implementation of formal neurocognitive evaluation has undoubtedly aided in our understanding of the cognitive sequelae associated with thalamotomy; however, reliable estimates of cognitive morbidity in early thalamotomy studies are still difficult to ascertain because of the inconsistent use of assessment measures, inclusion of mixed diagnostic samples (*see* ref. *9*), multiple or combined lesion sites, as well as different lesioning techniques (*see* ref. *10*). However, there is some evidence that suggests preexisting cognitive impairment and bilateral lesioning increased the risk for cognitive decline following thalamotomy. For example, formal cognitive assessment of 11 patients pre- and postunilateral thalamotomy revealed significant cognitive decline in three patients who were considered cognitively impaired prior to surgery *(11)*. In a sample of eight unilateral and three bilateral operates, formal testing revealed a greater incidence of postoperative cognitive impairment in patients who received bilateral compared to unilateral thalamic lesions *(12)*. Based on his review of figures reported in some of the early studies, Burchiel *(13)* estimated that 39% of thalamotomy patients demonstrated declines in speech, language, and/or memory, with declines being more common among bilateral than unilateral operates (60% versus 31%). Although it is likely that preoperative cognitive impairment and bilateral lesioning have an additive effect in terms of cognitive morbidity, this was not examined systematically in early thalamotomy studies.

A detailed review of early thalamotomy studies that employed objective neuropsychological evaluation is provided by Wilkinson and Tröster *(14)*. Generally, early studies found that verbal memory declined after unilateral left and bilateral thalamotomy *(10,15–22)*, but not after unilateral right *(17,18,20,22)*. Findings for visual memory were less consistent. Riklan et al. *(23)*, Shapiro et al. *(15)*, as well as Vilkki and Laitinen *(24,25)*, observed no changes in visual memory, whereas others reported declines following unilateral left *(26)* or both unilateral left and right thalamotomy *(27)*. Improvement in visual memory after right thalamotomy has also been reported *(22)*. Most deficits appeared soon after surgery and resolved in less than 18 months *(28–30)*, yet Perret and Siegfried *(27)* observed memory deficits up to 18 months postoperatively. VanBuren et al. *(31)* also reported that of 78 unilateral operants, 4 patients who underwent left thalamotomy had significant memory problems postoperatively and were unable to live independently up to 7 years after surgery.

In addition to changes in memory, several studies reported changes in global intellectual functioning (i.e., verbal and/or performance IQ) after unilateral thalamotomy with declines being more common after left thalamic lesions *(18,27,32,33)*. In a study comparing surgical targets, unilateral left thalamotomy was associated with slightly greater decline in verbal IQ than pallidotomy *(17)*. However, the majority of postoperative declines in IQ were mild and highly transient in nature, and there are several studies in which no significant change in IQ was observed *(16,28)*. Transient declines in attention have also been noted after left and bilateral thalamotomy *(31,34)*.

Numerous early studies examined language and speech. In a controlled study (using a nonsurgical PD control group), declines in letter and category fluency were observed following left and bilateral thalamotomy, but these resolved within 5 months *(34,35)*. Reductions in verbal fluency were also reported by Perret and Siegfried *(27)*, Vilkki and Laitinen *(24)*, and are indeed concluded by Riklan and Cooper *(36)* to best describe the early consequences of left thalamotomy. Although not as common, dysnomia has been observed after unilateral left, not right thalamotomy *(37,38)*.

In one of the few studies that included postmortem data, Samra and colleagues *(39)* reported lesion size was unrelated to postoperative changes on formal measures of speech and language in 27 patients who had undergone thalamotomy. Unlike speech changes, language disturbances were typically transient and related to lesion laterality with declines more commonly occurring after left thalamotomy. Quaglieri and Celesia *(40)* found that when compared to a nonsurgical PD group, patients who were 8-years postthalamotomy performed more poorly on measures of speech but not language.

The few contemporary studies that exist suggest that modern thalamotomy may be safer than its earlier counterpart. In the largest reported series of unilateral thalamotomy patients (28 right and 25 left), formal neuropsychological measures showed little change 3 months after surgery and, in fact, reported mild improvement on a verbal memory (dichotic listening) and a "visual closure" task *(41)*. A smaller sample of 13 patients showed no deficits on a limited neuropsychological test battery 4 weeks after unilateral thalamotomy *(42)*, but another study reported side effects (including dysphasia) in 8% of thalamotomy patients *(43)*. Not unexpectedly, γ knife thalamotomy initially appears to involve few cognitive side effects (1.5–2% complication rate; *44*), but formal, detailed, and long-term neuropsychological data have not been reported.

3.1.1.2. Postoperative Changes in Mood, Behavior, and Quality of Life

There is little consensus among the few detailed studies of psychiatric complications following thalamotomy available in the current literature. For example, Angelini and colleagues *(45,46)* observed several cases of significant depression following surgery. In contrast, several investigators have reported reduction in depressive and obsessive symptomatology postoperatively *(30,47)*. Although Narabayashi and colleagues *(48)* found no postoperative changes among eight thalamotomy patients using a modified Minnesota Multiphasic Personality Inventory (MMPI), decreases in depression and social isolation were seen in a slightly larger sample of 13 unilateral (6 left and 7 right) thalamotomy patients *(42)*. Persistent neuropsychiatric changes, including "childlike" behavior, decreased motivation, catatonic features, and hallucinations, have been observed following bilateral thalamotomy *(49)*. Okun et al. *(50)* described a case of pseudobulbar laughter following unilateral right gamma knife thalamotomy, but symptoms were successfully managed with medication *(51)*. In the only published study to employ formal measures of quality of life (QOL) pre- and postthalamotomy, significant improvements in social stigma and physical discomfort were observed in a sample of 33 unilateral thalamotomy patients at 3 to 6 months after surgery *(52)*. The absence of significant postoperative improvement on other indices of QOL may reflect a selection bias toward patients with less severe tremor-predominant disease that may only negatively impact specific aspects of daily functioning.

3.1.2. Ventral Intermediate Nucleus–Deep-Brain Stimulation

3.1.2.1. Postoperative Changes in Cognition

Several published studies have reported no change in the overall level of cognitive functioning following ventral intermediate nucleus (Vim)–DBS for PD *(53–55)*. Contrary to thalamotomy, thalamic stimulation does not seem to be associated with declines in verbal fluency or memory in patients with PD. In fact, improvements (possibly practice effects) on tasks of problems solving, verbal fluency, naming, and delayed recall were observed up to 12 months *(54–56)*. These studies examined combined samples of patients with left and right sided surgery, and material-specific cognitive changes have yet to be delineated. This will be important to study in the future, given the evidence from thalamotomy studies that left-sided surgical intervention carries a greater risk of cognitive morbidity than right-sided surgery.

The interpretation of cognitive changes following Vim–DBS surgery is even more challenging than postablation changes. In addition to medication and practice effects, neurocognitive changes observed on formal assessment measures may reflect a microthalamotomy effect. Preliminary evidence also suggests that stimulation parameters (unipolar versus bipolar; amplitude, frequency, and pulse width) may play a role in cognitive outcome *(57)*. Indeed, studies employing intraoperative stimulation *(20,58–60)* found lower frequencies (60 Hz) more predictive of memory impairment following thalamotomy than higher frequencies (200 Hz), the latter of which are typically utilized in chronic Vim–DBS. Tröster et al. *(61)* examined the combined effect of medications and stimulation on postoperative cognitive functioning in a single patient with PD under four different conditions: with or without stimulation and "on" or "off" medications. Although a decrement in verbal fluency was observed postoperatively, this improved with stimulation in both medication conditions, suggesting that stimulation alone may alleviate potential cognitive sequelae associated with the microthalamotomy effect.

3.1.2.2. Postoperative Changes in Mood, Behavior, and Quality of Life

Despite the increasingly common use of Vim–DBS as a treatment for tremor in patients with PD, few studies have included formal measures of mood, behavior, or QOL. Preliminary evidence suggests that Vim–DBS may lead to fewer reported symptoms of depression and anxiety within 1 week *(54)* and up to 12 months *(56)* postsurgery. Improvement in mood state at the 12-month mark has also been noted after Vim–DBS in patients with essential tremor (ET) *(62)*. However, no detectable change in depressive symptomatology was evident at 3 months following surgery in a sample of patients who demonstrated significantly improved motor functioning *(63)*. The relationship between Vim-DBS and QOL remains unclear. Straits-Tröster et al. *(63)* failed to detect changes in QOL at 3 months after Vim-DBS surgery, likely because of the use of a generic QOL measure and small-sample size. Indeed, Woods et al. *(56)* employed a disease-specific measure of QOL and found that a similar sample of patients ($n = 6$) reported significant improvements in QOL that were maintained at 12 months following unilateral Vim–DBS surgery. Nevertheless, improvements in several aspects of QOL that failed to reach significance highlight the need for investigation of QOL in patients with PD following Vim-DBS using disease-specific measures in larger samples.

3.2. Globus Pallidus

3.2.1. Surgical Lesioning-GPi

3.2.1.1. Changes in Cognition

As with early thalamotomy studies, few formal neuropsychological measures were consistently employed in early studies of pallidotomy. In one study that utilized objective measures of cognition, a mixed sample of pallidotomy and thalamotomy patients who underwent either unilateral or bilateral procedures showed no significant change in IQ. However, pallidotomy was associated with responses on projective personality measures, suggesting possible "frontal" dysfunction *(64)*. Svennilson and colleagues reported that among 78 unilateral pallidotomy cases, 4 developed postoperative dementia and 11 developed "a significant memory impairment" *(65)*.

The majority of modern studies show that unilateral pallidotomy does not result in significant cognitive morbidity. Although lateral-specific deficits are observed after surgery, these tend to be mild, transient, and of little clinical significance. In a recent meta-analysis, Alkhani and Lozano *(66)* estimated that transient memory deficits occur in 1.3% of cases after either unilateral or bilateral pallidotomy, whereas persistent memory deficits are indicated in less than 1% of cases. However, these results may underestimate the prevalence of memory impairment after surgery because not all studies included in the analysis had shown whether memory deficits occurred, and it is doubtful that formal neuropsychological assessment was employed by all studies.

The most commonly reported postoperative cognitive change involves a decline in verbal fluency after left pallidotomy *(67–82)*; but such declines are not evident when unilateral right pallidotomy patients are included in analyses *(83–85)*. Verbal fluency changes are likely unrelated to changes in medication because the decrements are observed in both the "on" and "off " states *(86)*. Indeed, some evidence suggests they may be related to changes in underlying executive mechanisms, such as ability to efficiently switch between phonemic or semantic clusters or categories *(67,87)*. Age appears to be a predictor of postoperative verbal fluency decline, where older patients are at greater risk *(78,88)*. Yet, preoperative severity of motor impairment is not a reliable predictor *(80)*. Mini-Mental-Status Examination (MMSE) scores are also not predictive of verbal fluency decline *(80)*. This likely reflects the insensitivity of the MMSE to cognitive dysfunction in PD and the restricted range of MMSE scores represented in the study sample. In one study, 8 of 11 patients with PD who did not respond with significant motor improvement following unilateral pallidotomy demonstrated preoperative "frontal behavioral syndromes" that were undetected by the MMSE *(89)*. Given that nonresponders were more likely than responders to have this frontal behavioral syndrome prior to surgery, this behavioral profile might serve as a relative contraindication to pallidotomy.

Some studies report lesion location as an important determinant of postoperative cognitive deficits. Anteromedial lesions have been associated with greater impairment than posterolateral lesions *(90,91)*; however, some studies have failed to find a relationship between lesion location and cognitive outcome on select measures *(88,92)*. The implementation of standardized procedures across sites and the use of stimulation-confirmed target locations might have restricted the range of values regarding lesion location such that a relationship may be undetectable.

Several studies have reported more wide ranging cognitive deficits after pallidotomy *(67,93)* or select deficits in domains aside from verbal fluency. Specifically, postoperative deficits have been observed in verbal and nonverbal memory *(42,67,68,70,80,94–96)*, working memory and attention *(67,70,76,97)*, and executive functions, such as categories achieved *(68,79)* or perseverative responses on a card-sorting task *(75,79)*. Some studies have reported mild improvements in verbal memory *(67,70,79)* or aspects of nonverbal memory *(70)* following right pallidotomy. Alterman et al. *(98)* reported progressive dementia in 5 of 60 unilateral pallidotomy cases, and only 1 of these 5 patients showed evidence of possible dementia prior to surgery.

Bilateral pallidotomy is assumed to involve greater risk for cognitive dysfunction than unilateral pallidotomy, but findings are inconsistent and based on small samples. Iacono et al. *(99)* reported that average Wechsler Memory Scale-Revised Index scores improved in 10 bilateral pallidotomy patients; yet, actual scores were not presented, and it is difficult to determine the role of possible practice effects. Therefore, the results are of questionable clinical significance. Scott et al. *(73)* found no significant adverse cognitive effects among eight bilaterally operated patients, other than verbal fluency declines that were also observed in unilateral operates. However, other studies have reported, at least anecdotally, profound deficits after bilateral pallidotomy. Svennilson et al. *(65)* found that all three of their bilaterally operated patients had significant memory deficits and dementia after surgery. Ghika et al. *(100)* reported either profound overall changes (likely reflecting dementia) or marked executive or memory impairments in two of four patients after bilateral pallidotomy. Trépanier et al. *(81)* reported global cognitive decline after the second operation in two of three bilateral pallidotomy patients who had atypical cognitive profiles before surgery. Among 8 of 12 patients with clinical follow-up, 4 had poorer speech and 1 had worse memory after staged bilateral surgery *(82)*. Gálvez-Jiménez et al. *(101)* noted that no overt cognitive changes were observed among four patients undergoing GPi-DBS after contralateral pallidotomy, but detailed data was not reported.

3.2.1.2. Changes in Mood, Behavior, and Quality of Life

Numerous studies mention psychiatric outcomes following pallidotomy only anecdotally. Bezerra and colleagues *(102)* reported persistent depression in 5 of 41 patients after unilateral pallidotomy. However, several studies using formal measures of mood have reported either improvements in depressive symptomatology *(56,63,69,70,72,80,82,103)*, or no significant change in mood state *(71,73,78,81,84,104,105)*. Junqué et al. *(106)* reported improvement in scores on a measure of obsessive-compulsive behavior. In contrast, Trépanier et al. *(67,81)* found that, up to 41% of patients' caregivers observed frontal lobe behavioral changes, including lack of insight, lability, impulsivity, poor social judgment, and environmental dependency after their family member underwent unilateral pallidotomy. Ghika et al. *(100)* also reported profound personality/behavioral changes and depression in two of four bilateral pallidotomy patients who demonstrated postoperative cognitive dysfunction, as well as another patient who developed obsessive-compulsive features. In a study that employed an objective personality measure (i.e., MMPI), patients reported fewer somatic symptoms and better energy after unilateral pallidotomy *(42)*. However, it is difficult to determine whether this reflects a surgical effect versus a placebo effect, the latter of which may also have a physiological basis.

Studies utilizing formal measures of QOL generally indicate improvements in a wide range of aspects of QOL after unilateral pallidotomy *(63,73,103,104,107)*. The study by D'Antonio *(107)* is noteworthy because it includes a nonsurgical control group. In this study, patients in the surgical group (combined unilateral pallidotomy, bilateral pallidotomy, and pallidotomy plus thalamotomy group) reported improvements in QOL at 4-months postsurgery, whereas the medically treated wait-list control group did not. Unfortunately, the conclusion is weakened by sizeable subject attrition (about 33%). The studies by D'Antonio et al. *(107)* and Martinez-Martin et al. *(103)* both suggest that improvement in QOL is related to improvement in motor function in the "off " state, and Tröster et al. *(109)* have found that physical aspects of QOL are related to residual motor disability after pallidotomy. Changes in QOL also relate to changes in anxiety *(103)*, depressive symptoms *(63)*, coping method, and social stressors and resources *(108)*. Older individuals tend to show less QOL improvement after pallidotomy *(109)*.

3.2.2. Deep-Brain Stimulation-GPi

3.2.2.1. Changes in Cognition

Preliminary studies of patients undergoing unilateral pallidal DBS have found no significant changes in the overall status of cognitive functioning 3-month postsurgery *(110–112)*. Declines in visuoconstructional ability and verbal fluency have been observed, but these changes were rarely of any clinical importance. Subsequent studies yielded similar findings. Vingerhoets et al. *(111)* also calculated an impairment index (the percentage of measures falling <1 standard deviation [SD] below the mean of normative samples) and noted that 6 of 20 patients showed a decrement (i.e., any magnitude increase in percentage of tests in the impaired range). These patients tended to be older and were taking higher medication dosages prior to surgery than patients who showed no change or improvement.

Safety of bilateral GPi-DBS has been addressed in only a few studies, but the majority of these suggest that the procedure is relatively safe from a cognitive standpoint. Ardouin et al. *(113)* found no significant changes in average test scores for up to 6 months after bilateral GPi-DBS in 13 cases. Similarly, Pillon et al. *(114)* found no cognitive morbidity using clinical tests in a similar group of patients at 12 months postoperatively. Ghika et al. *(115)* found no serious changes in neuropsychological test scores 3 months after contemporaneous bilateral GPi-DBS electrode implantation (n = 6). Staged bilateral GPi-DBS electrode implantation does not appear to pose any significant risk of cognitive decline *(116)*.

Only a single case study with magnetic resonance imaging-confirmed electrode location has reported significant executive dysfunction after bilateral GPi-DBS *(117)*. Importantly, this study indicates the role that stimulation played in this impairment. When the stimulators were turned off, the impairment was partially reversed. Relatively isolated cognitive impairments were reported by the Toronto group *(81)*. Among four patients, there was a significant decrease only in backward digit span. Verbal fluency testing was administered to only one patient, who demonstrated a decline on this task.

Whether unilateral GPi-DBS is cognitively safer than pallidotomy has not been adequately addressed, but studies by Merello et al. *(112)* and Fields et al. *(118)* suggest that the safety of these procedures from a cognitive perspective is comparable.

3.2.2.2. Changes in Mood, Behavior, and Quality of Life

Unilateral GPi-DBS does not appear to significantly impact depressive symptomatology; *(63,114,115,120)* yet, small but significant reductions in anxiety have been observed *(116)*. Relatively little data has been published regarding the occurrence of prominent neurobehavioral changes following GPi-DBS *(121)*. However, Miyawaki et al. *(122)* described a single patient who underwent bilateral-staged GPi-DBS surgery and developed manic episodes after his second (right GPi) surgery with both unilateral and bilateral stimulation. This patient was eventually able to benefit from bilateral GPi stimulation and without psychiatric sequelae after a reduction in his levodopa dosage, suggesting that interactions between stimulation and medication may have an important role in neurobehavioral morbidity in GPi-DBS.

Despite the lack of change in mood following GPi-DBS surgery, preliminary studies using formal assessment measures have found major postoperative improvements on generic measures of QOL. Vingerhoets et al. *(119)* reported a significant increase in physical, psychosocial, and overall functioning at 3 months postunilateral GPi-DBS with particular gains in ambulation, body care, movement, communication, sleep, rest, and eating. Grace et al. *(123)* observed similar improvements in physical and overall functioning in a smaller sample (n = 9) of patients with unilateral GPi-DBS. But studies with disease-specific QOL measures are absent from the current literature.

3.3. Subthalamic Nucleus

3.3.1. Surgical Lesioning

3.3.1.1. Changes in Cognition

Until recently, subthalamotomy (involving the STN proper) was avoided owing to fear of inducing hemiballism. Two centers that now perform these operations have published detailed neuropsychological findings. McCarter et al. *(124)* evaluated neuropsychological functioning in 12 patients undergoing procedures on the dorsolateral portion of the nucleus: two left subthalamic nucleotomy, three right subthalamic nucleotomy, three bilateral subthalamic nucleotomy, and four right subthalamic nucleotomy plus left subthalamic DBS. Evaluation was carried out 2 days before surgery and an average of 6 months after surgery. Poorer postoperative performance was observed on a complex auditory attention/working memory task, whereas statistically significant (albeit, probably not clinically significant) gains were observed in verbal IQ and immediate recall of stories. Thirty-three percent of bilateral subthalamic nucleotomy patients showed reliable decreases in phonemic verbal fluency, but no reliable change in fluency was observed in the other groups (unilateral nucleotomy or nucleotomy plus contralateral DBS). One third of the nucleotomy plus DBS group showed reliable decrements on several attention measures and on a list-learning task. None of the patients with right-sided unilateral surgery demonstrated reliable decrements on any cognitive measure, whereas the patients with left unilateral surgery tended to experience decrements in attention, facial recognition, word list recall, and an executive function task (i.e., a tower-building task). Although modern subthalamic nucleotomy likely does not lead to global deterioration in cognition, this study suggests that mild deficits in select domains may occur overall. The duration and clinical significance of these deficits remains unclear, but cognitive changes seem less likely after unilateral right-sided ablations. Clearly, additional research is needed before reliable practice parameters can be generated.

3.3.1.2. Changes in Mood, Behavior, and Quality of Life

Early subthalamotomy never gained widespread popularity, partly as a result of adverse neurobehavioral outcomes. Spiegel et al. *(8)* reported a 30% incidence of "psycho-organic syndrome" among 33 patients who underwent subthalamic ablation. In a sample of 58 patients, all 6 bilateral operates developed a lasting (of several years' duration) loss of initiative and spontaneity, and diminished interest in the environment *(125)*. After a second operation, one patient developed a "jovial, carefree attitude." Over one third of the patients manifested increased desire for food, and some actually became obese. Unlike Speigel and colleagues, who performed subthalamic ablations by lesioning Forel's Field H and interrupting pallidofugal fibers (known as campotomy), Mundinger and colleagues *(126)* placed the bulk of the subthalamotomy lesion in the zona incerta. Reporting on outcomes in 456 interventions for PD, they noted that only 32% of individuals were free of "speech symptoms" postoperatively. However, specific neurobehavioral morbidity data were not reported. No formal studies of psychiatric symptoms or QOL issues following STN ablation have been reported in the literature.

3.3.2. Deep-Brain Stimulation-STN

3.3.2.1. Changes in Cognition

In the largest patient series ($n = 49$) reported to date, Ardouin et al. *(113)* discovered few significant changes in cognition 3–6 months after bilateral STN-DBS. Similar to Vim-DBS, cognitive declines with bilateral STN stimulation were primarily observed on measures of verbal fluency, and these were maintained in a subgroup of patients evaluated at 12-months postsurgery *(114)*. Improvements were seen on tasks of basic attention and psychomotor speed at 6- and 12-month postsurgery, but performance on tasks of divided attention were mixed. Patients also demonstrated improvements on experimental measures of executive functioning/working memory 6 months following surgery. Other studies with smaller samples also reported only few significant cognitive changes *(127–130)*.

The effect of STN-DBS on working memory and executive functioning appears somewhat complicated, partly because of the potentially heterogeneous effects on the various aspects of frontal-subcortical systems. Studies with neurophysiological measures provide some evidence of this heterogeneous effect on frontal-executive functioning. For example, Gerschlager et al. *(131)* found improvement on a physiological index of "frontal" function during an executive-planning task with STN-DBS. Yet, other investigators *(132)* have reported no change in preoperative P300 abnormalities (thought to be a physiological marker of frontally mediated attentional dysfunction).

Two groups have described more wide-ranging adverse cognitive effects in small-patient series *(81,133,134)*. Saint-Cyr and colleagues *(81)* observed poorer performance on tasks of divided attention, verbal fluency, and memory for both visual and verbal material in a series of 11 patients at 3–6 months postbilateral STN-DBS surgery. These deficits were still evident at 12-month follow-up *(133)*. Although declines in several cognitive domains were observed at 12, but not 3–6 months, these changes likely reflect disease progression, subject selection bias, and/or attrition. Alegret and coworkers *(134)* reported similar declines in attention, verbal fluency, and memory, as well as visuospatial in a sample of 15 patients who were tested off medication, but the investigators interpreted these changes as clinically insignificant.

Cognitive outcomes after bilateral STN-DBS may vary within individual patients and across studies. Dujardin and colleagues *(135)* evaluated nine patients 3 months after bilateral STN-DBS surgery and found that, as a group, patients demonstrated relatively isolated cognitive declines in verbal memory and verbal fluency, as well as some improvement in basic attention and reaction time. However, when patients' performances were examined individually, approximately one-third of the patients had a more generalized pattern of cognitive declines (defined as a decline of one or more standard deviations on 20% of the tests administered). At 12-month follow-up, a subset of the original group demonstrated a similar global cognitive decline, but one patient considered globally impaired at 3 months had returned to baseline by 1-year follow-up. Morrison et al. *(136)*, the only investigators to publish neuropsychological findings pertaining to unilateral STN-DBS, reported few cognitive changes. Patients demonstrated reduction in lexical and semantic verbal fluency, but no definitive laterality effects related to fluency changes were observed. In contrast, poorer performance on tasks of divided or alternating attention was seen only in unilateral left operants. Although the sample is too small to reliably evaluate laterality effects of STN-DBS, it appears changes can occur after both left and right STN-DBS.

Risk factors for cognitive deterioration are difficult to identify, given the generally small sample sizes of studies. Nonetheless, more advanced age (>69 years; *81,133,136*), and preexisting cognitive deficits *(137)* may predispose patients to cognitive decline. Age also appears to be a factor in the occurrence of transient postoperative confusion *(138)*. The identification of reliable prognostic indicators of notable decline or impairment will be important, given the heterogeneity of cognitive outcomes among individual patients.

3.3.2.2. Changes in Mood, Behavior, and Quality of Life

Several studies have reported improvement in depressive symptomatology *(113,130,133)* on self-report questionnaires. Saint-Cyr et al. *(133)* reported increased "frontal" behavior changes on a care-

Table 1
Factors Potentially Influencing the Risk of Cognitive and Behavioral Morbidity Following Surgical Treatment of Parkinson's Disease

Increased Risk
Age more than 69 years at time of surgery
Bilateral surgery
Unilateral surgery involving the language-dominant hemisphere
Anteromedial lesions of the GPi
Psychiatric or behavioral disturbance
Dementia
Prominent "frontal" behavioral symptoms
No increased risk
Type of surgical intervention (ablative versus stimulation)
Surgical target (Vim, STN, GPi)
Lesion volume (if confined to intended target location)
Uncertain risk (insufficient data)
Stimulation parameters (amplitude, frequency, and pulse width)
Disease duration
Medication effects

GPi, globus pallidus interna; Vim, ventral intermediate nucleus; STN, subthalamic nucleus.

giver-rated personality scale in two of six patients older than 69 years. Although the most serious problems were rare, caregivers endorsed concerns regarding perseveration, impulsivity, diminished social judgment, diminished insight, lability, and lack of awareness in some patients. Isolated cases of pathological laughter, euphoria, and severe depression *(139–142)* have also been reported following STN-DBS. In fact, depression may be relatively common after STN-DBS. In the largest series of STN-DBS to date, Benabid et al. *(141)* observed significant depression in 16 of 137 patients. Volkmann and colleagues *(130)* also found that depression and anhedonia occurred more frequently in patients receiving STN as opposed to GPi-DBS.

Detailed QOL data have not been published for STN-DBS. Yet, Capus et al. *(143)* reported up to 50% improvement in QOL (on a disease-specific questionnaire) in seven patients at 14.5-months postsurgery.

4. TRANSPLANTATION

4.1. Adrenal Medullary Autografts

Intrastriatal implantation of autologous adrenal medullary tissue is no longer carried out because of lack of benefit. Although the few studies formally evaluating cognition did not indicate any significant morbidity *(144–146)*, significant psychiatric morbidity was reported *(147,148)*.

4.2. Fetal Mesencephalic Transplants

Intrastriatal grafting of fetal mesencephalic tissue can provide lasting motor benefit in some patients with clinical benefit predicted by 18-fluorodopa uptake (an index of graft viability; *149,150*), but studies differ in tissue preparation, site (unilateral versus bilateral; caudate and/or putamen), and number of implants. Observed neurobehavioral changes may reflect disease progression, medication, associated surgical lesion, or the sprouting of implanted tissue (*see* ref. *151*). Transient improvements (up to 2 years) in memory have been reported *(152)*, but cognitive (and speech) outcomes vary across individuals *(153–155)*. Although most individuals have not shown significant cognitive changes after surgery, some cognitive decline may occur in patients with preoperative deficits *(153,154)*.

Table 2
Suggested Measures to Evaluate Change in Neuropsychological Functioning, Mood, Behavior, and Quality of Life From Baseline to Postoperative Follow-Up at 3 Months and 1 Year

Domain	Assessment measure
Global cognitive screening	Mattis Dementia Rating Scale (DRS)
Information/psychomotor processing	Trailmaking Test, part A
Speed	WAIS-III Arithmetic
	WAIS-III Symbol Search
	Stroop Color-Word Test, Word Reading Trial
Attention/working memory	WAIS-III Digit Span
	WAIS-III Letter-Number Sequencing
	Stroop Color-Word Test, Interference Trial
	Trailmaking Test, part B
Frontal/executive functioning	Wisconsin Card Sorting Test (WCST)
	WAIS-III Matrix Reasoning
	WAIS-III Similarities
Language	Boston Naming Test
	COWAT Phonemic Fluency (FAS/CFL)
	Category Fluency
Verbal learning and memory	Hopkins Verbal Learning Test-Revised (HVLT-R)[a]
	WMS-R Logical Memory I & II
Visuospatial functioning	Benton Judgment of Line Orientation (JLO)
	WAIS-III Block Design
Mood, behavior, and quality of life	Geriatric Depression Scale (GDS)
	Profile of Mood States-Short Form (POMS-SF)[b]
	Frontal Systems Behavior Scale (FrSBe)
	Medical Outcomes Short Form-23 (MOS-SF-36)[b]
	Parkinson's Disease Quality of Life (PDQL) Scale

[a] HVLT-R is preferred for the availability of multiple alternate forms.
[b] Short forms are suggested owing to time constraints.
Note: WAIS-III, Wechsler Adult Intelligence Test-Third Edition; COWAT, Controlled Oral Word Association Test; WMS-R, Wechsler Memory Scale-Revised. All tests are described in Spreen and Strauss *(163),* with the exception of the WAIS-III *(164),* HVLT-R *(165)* FrSBe *(166),* MOS-SF-36 *(167),* and PDQL *(168).*

Psychiatric complications, such as depression, paranoia, and hallucinations, are more common with open *(156,157)* versus stereotactic procedures *(158).* Unfortunately, a recent report of a well-controlled study (using a "placebo" control group) did not describe neuropsychological or QOL outcomes, despite reports that such data were gathered *(159).*

Hagell and colleagues *(160)* investigated QOL using a generic rating scale and reported significant benefits in QOL after bilateral grafting, particularly in terms of patients' satisfaction with mobility, energy, and emotional well-being.

5. CONCLUSIONS AND RECOMMENDATIONS

Levodopa-era surgical interventions for PD appear relatively safe from a cognitive standpoint and may produce significant gains in QOL. When cognitive declines are observed, they typically involve verbal fluency, regardless of the surgical technique and target location. The decline in verbal fluency occurs more often after left-sided surgeries, and may persist for 1 year or more, independent of speech changes (i.e., dysarthria). These declines do not usually have sufficient clinical severity to impact QOL. Other cognitive changes have been observed with tasks of working memory, problem solving, attention, and memory, but findings vary across studies and likely reflect differences in methodology, sample characteristics, or disease progression.

To date, the lack of significant neurobehavioral morbidity demonstrated should not be interpreted as an indication that surgical intervention poses no risk for certain patients with PD. In fact, several studies have reported severe, but isolated, cases of cognitive and psychiatric decline, including memory deficits that eventually progress to dementia. The question remains then as to what factors present the most significant risk for decreased cognition. Unfortunately, studies are still too few in quantity and have too many methodological limitations at this early stage to identify the risk factors for neurobehavioral morbidity with accuracy. Nonetheless, some preliminary observations are warranted and summarized in Table 1. Randomized, preferably blinded, studies are still needed to compare interventions (target and treatment type) directly pertaining to their effects on neurobehavioral functioning and QOL. Examination of several other factors, including medication levels, disease duration, and stimulation parameters, will help to better characterize their potential effect on neurobehavioral outcome (*see* ref. *121*). Finally, carefully controlled studies that include a nonsurgical patient group are required to identify the conditions under which patients with PD may optimally benefit from these neurosurgical interventions. It will be of utmost importance that these studies include formal assessments measures of cognition, mood, and behavioral functioning, as well as a disease-specific measure of QOL. Table 2 presents measures that may be used to characterize neurobehavioral outcome following movement disorder surgery (*see also* ref. *162* for additional suggestions).

REFERENCES

1. Goetz CG, Diederich NJ. There is a renaissance of interest in pallidotomy for Parkinson's disease. Nature Med 1996;2:510–514.
2. Koller WC, Wilkenson S, Pahwa R, Miyawaki EK. Surgical treatment options in Parkinson's disease. Neurosurg Clin North Am 1998;9:295–306.
3. Alexander GE, Delong MR, Strick PL. Parallel organization of functionally segregated circuits linking basal ganglia and cortex. Ann Rev Neurosci 1986;9:357–381.
4. Wichman T, DeLong MR. Model of basal ganglia function and pathophysiology of movement disorders. Neurosurg Clin North Am 1998;9:223–236.
5. Alexander GE, Crutcher MD, DeLong MR. Basal ganglia-thalamocortical circuits: Parallel substrates for motor, oculomotor, "prefrontal" and "limbic" functions. Prog Brain Res 1990;85:119–146.
6. DeLong MR. Primate models of movement disorders of basal ganglia origin. Trends Neurosci 1990;13:281–285.
7. Uitti RJ, Adler CH, Wszolek ZK, Wharen RE. Surgical treatment of movement disorders. In: Gilman S, ed. MedLink Neurology. MedLink Corporation, San Diego, CA, (CDROM) Website available at: www.medlink.com last accessed March 28, 2003.
8. Spiegel E, Wycis H, Orchinik C, Freed H. Thalamic chronotaraxis. Arch Neurol Psychiatry 1955;73:469–471.
9. Almgren PE, Andersson AL, Kullberg G. Differences in verbally expressed cognition following left and right ventrolateral thalamotomy. Scand J Psychol 1969;10:243–249.
10. Levita E, Riklan M, Cooper IS. Verbal and perceptual functions after surgery of subcortical structures. Percept Mot Skills 1964;18:195–202.
11. Niebuhr Jr. H. Some psychological aspects of patients with Parkinson's disease before and after ventrolateral thalamotomy. In: Spiegel EA, Wycis HT, eds. Stereoencephalotomy. Part II Clinical and Physiological Applications, vol. 2, Grune and Stratton, New York, 1962, pp. 349–357.
12. Fünfgeld EW. Die psychischen Hirnfunktionen bei hirnatrophischen Zustandsbildern nach operativer Belastung (stereotaktische Hirnoperationen älterer Parkinsonpatienten). Acta. Neurochir (Wien) 1961;(Suppl)7:539–544.
13. Burchiel KJ. Thalamotomy for movement disorders. Neurosurg Clin North Am 1995;6:55–71.
14. Wilkinson SB, Tröster AI. Surgical interventions in neurodegenerative disease: impact on memory and cognition. In: Tröster AI, ed. Memory in Neurodegenerative Disease: Biological, Cognitive, and Clinical Perspectives. Cambridge University Press, Cambridge, UK, 1998, pp. 362–376.
15. Shapiro DY, Sadowsky DA, Henderson WG, Van Buren JM. An assessment of cognitive function in postthalamotomy Parkinson patients. Confin. Neurol 1973;35:144–166.
16. Asso D, Crown S, Russell JA, Logue V. Psychological aspects of the stereotactic treatment of Parkinsonism. Br J Psychiatry 1969;115:541–553.
17. McFie J. Psychological effects of stereotaxic operations for the relief of parkinsonian symptoms. J Ment Sci 1960; 106:1512–1517.

18. Riklan M, Diller L, Weiner H, Cooper IS. Psychological studies on effects of chemosurgery of the basal ganglia in Parkinsonism. I. Intellectual functioning. Arch Gen Psychiatry 1960;2:22–31.
19. Krayenbühl H, Wyss OAM, Yasargil MG. Bilateral thalamotomy and pallidotomy as treatment for bilateral Parkinsonism. J Neurosurg 1961;18:429–444.
20. Ojemann GA, Hoyenga KB, Ward Jr, AA. Prediction of short-term verbal memory disturbance after ventrolateral thalamotomy. J Neurosurg 1971;35:203–210.
21. Kocher U, Siegfried J, Perret E. Verbal and nonverbal learning ability of Parkinson patients before and after unilateral ventrolateral thalamotomy. Appl Neurophysiol 1982;45:311–316.
22. Krayenbühl H, Siegfried J, Kohenof M, Yasargil MG. Is there a dominant thalamus? Confin Neurol 1965;26:246–249.
23. Riklan M, Levita E, Cooper IS. Psychological effects of bilateral subcortical surgery for Parkinson's disease. J Nerv Ment Dis 1966;141:403–409.
24. Vilkki J, Laitinen LV. Differential effects of left and right ventrolateral thalamotomy on receptive and expressive verbal performances and face-matching. Neuropsychologia 1974;12:11–19.
25. Vilkki J, Laitinen LV. Effects of pulvinotomy and ventrolateral thalamotomy on some cognitive functions. Neuropsychologia 1976;14:67–78.
26. Jurko MF, Andy OJ. Psychological aspects of diencephalotomy. J Neurol Neurosurg Psychiatry 1964;27:516–521.
27. Perret E, Siegfried J. Memory and learning performance of Parkinson patients before and after thalamotomy. In: Gillingham FJ, Donaldson I. ML, eds. Third Symposium on Parkinson's Disease. E & S Livingstone Ltd., Edinburgh, UK, 1968, pp. 164–168.
28. Jurko MF, Andy OJ. Psychological changes correlated with thalamotomy site. J Neurol Neurosurg Psychiatry 1973;36:846–852.
29. Almgren PE, Andersson AL, Kullberg G. Long-term effects on verbally expressed cognition following left and right ventrolateral thalamotomy. Confin Neurol 1972;34:162–168.
30. Hays P, Krikler B, Walsh LS, Woolfson G. Psychological changes following surgical treatment of Parkinsonism. Am J Psychiatry 1966;123:657–663.
31. Van Buren JM, Li CL, Shapiro DY, et al. A qualitative and quantitative evaluation of parkinsonians three to six years following thalamotomy. Confin Neurol 1973;35:202–235.
32. Riklan M, Diller L, Weiner H. Psychological studies on the effects of chemosurgery of the basal ganglia in Parkinsonism. II. Aspects of personality. Arch Gen Psychiatry 1960;3:267–275.
33. Choppy M, Zimbacca N, Le Beau J. Psychological changes after selective frontal surgery (especially cingulotomy) and after stereotactic surgery of the basal ganglia. In: Laitinen LV, Livingston KE, eds. Surgical Approaches in Psychiatry. Medical and Technical Publishing, Lancaster, UK, 1973, pp. 175–181.
34. Riklan M, Levita E. Psychological studies of thalamic lesions in humans. J Nerv Ment Dis 1970;150:251–265.
35. Riklan M, Levita E, Zimmerman J, Cooper IS. Thalamic correlates of language and speech. J Neurol Sci 1969;8:307–328.
36. Riklan M, Cooper IS. Psychometric studies of verbal functions following thalamic lesions in humans. Brain Lang 1975;2:45–64.
37. Bell DS. Speech functions of the thalamus inferred from the effects of thalamotomy. Brain 1968;91:619–638.
38. Petrovici JN. Speech disturbances following stereotaxic surgery in ventrolateral thalamus. Neurosurg Rev 1980;3:189–195.
39. Samra K, Riklan M, Levita E, et al. Language and speech correlates of anatomically verified lesions in thalamic surgery for Parkinsonism. J Speech Hear Res 1969;12:510–540.
40. Quaglieri CE, Celesia GG. Effect of thalamotomy and levodopa therapy on the speech of Parkinson patients. Eur Neurol 1977;15:34–39.
41. Lund-Johansen M, Hugdahl K, Wester K. Cognitive function in patients with Parkinson's disease undergoing stereotaxic thalamotomy. J Neurol Neurosurg Psychiatry 1996;60:564–571.
42. Fukuda M, Kameyama S, Yoshino M, et al. Neuropsychological outcome following pallidotomy and thalamotomy for Parkinson's disease. Stereotact. Funct Neurosurg 2000;74:11–20.
43. Broggi G, Dones I, Ferroli P, et al. Surgery for movement disorders: complications and complication avoidance. Semin Neurosurg 2001;12:225–231.
44. Young RF. Gamma knife treatment for movement disorders. Semin Neurosurg 2001;12:233–243.
45. Angelini L, Bono R, Broggi G, et al. Psychological implications of stereotactic thalamotomies for cerebral palsy. Ital J Neurol Sci 1979;1:32–36.
46. Angelini L, Nardocci N, Bono R, Broggi G. Depression after stereotactic thalamotomy in patients with abnormal movements. Ital J Neurol Sci 1982;3:301–310.
47. Müller VC, Yasargil MG. Zur Psychiatrie der stereotaktischen Hirnoperationen bei extrapyramidalen Erkrankungen. Schweiz Arch Neurol Neurochirurgie Psychiatrie 1959;84:136–154.
48. Narabayashi H, Miyashita N, Hattori Y, et al. Posteroventral pallidotomy: its effect on motor symptoms and scores of MMPI test in patients with Parkinson's disease. Parkinsonism Relat Disord 1997;3:7–20.
49. Jurko MF, Andy OJ. Electrical and behavioral changes following thalamotomy. Surg Forum 1961;12:404–406.
50. Okun MS, Stover NP, Subramanian T, et al. Complications of gamma knife surgery for Parkinson's Disease. Arch Neurol 2001;58:1995–2002.

51. Okun MS, Heilman KM, Vitek JL. Treatment of pseudobulbar laughter after gamma knife thalamotomy. Mov Disord 2002;17:622–624.
52. Gray A, McNamara I, Aziz T, et al. Quality of life outcomes following surgical treatment of Parkinson's disease. Mov Disord 2002;17:68–75.
53. Blond S, Caparros-Lefebvre D, Parker F, et al. Control of tremor and involuntary movement disorders by chronic stereotactic stimulation of the ventral intermediate thalamic nucleus. J Neurosurg 1992;77:62–68.
54. Caparros-Lefebvre D, Blond S, Pécheux N, et al. Evaluation neuropsychologique avant et après stimulation thalamique chez 9 parkinsoniens. Rev Neurol 1992;148:117–122.
55. Tröster AI, Fields JA, Wilkinson SB, et al. Neuropsychological functioning before and after unilateral thalamic stimulating electrode implantation in Parkinson's disease [electronic manuscript]. Neurosurg Focus 1997;2:Article 9.
56. Woods SP, Fields JA, Lyons KE, et al. Neuropsychological and quality of life changes following unilateral thalamic deep brain stimulation in Parkinson's disease: A one-year follow-up. Acta Neurochir (Wein) 2001;143:1273–1278.
57. Tröster AI. Introduction to neurobehavioral issues in the neurosurgical treatment of movement disorders: basic issues thalamotomy, and nonablative treatments. Brain Cogn 2000;42:173–182.
58. Hugdahl K, Wester K. Lateralized thalamic stimulation: effects on verbal memory. Neuropsychiatry Neuropsychol. Behav Neurol 1997;10:155–161.
59. Wester K, Hugdahl K. Thalamotomy and thalamic stimulation: effects on cognition. Stereotact Funct Neurosurg 1997;69:80–85.
60. Hugdahl K, Wester K. Neurocognitive correlates of stereotactic thalamotomy and thalamic stimulation in Parkinsonian patients. Brain Cogn 2000;42:231–252.
61. Tröster AI, Wilkinson SB, Fields JA, et al. Chronic electrical stimulation of the left ventrointermediate (Vim) thalamic nucleus for the treatment of pharmacotherapy-resistant Parkinson's disease: a differential impact on access to semantic and episodic memory? Brain Cogn 1998;38:125–149.
62. Fields JA, Tröster AI, Woods SP, et al. Neuropsychological and quality of life outcomes 12 months after unilateral thalamic stimulation for essential tremor. J Neurol Neurosurg Psychiatry 2003;74:305–311.
63. Straits-Tröster K, Fields JA, Wilkinson SB, et al. Health-related quality of life in Parkinson's disease after pallidotomy and deep brain stimulation. Brain Cogn 2000;42:399–416.
64. Christensen AL, Juul-Jensen P, Malmros R, Harmsen A. Psychological evaluation of intelligence and personality in Parkinsonism before and after stereotaxic surgery. Acta Neurol Scand 1970;46:527–537.
65. Svennilson E, Torvik A, Lowe R, Leksell L. Treatment of Parkinsonism by stereotactic thermolesions in the pallidal region: a clinical evaluation of 83 cases. Acta Psych Neurol Scand 1960;35:358–377.
66. Alkhani A, Lozano AM. Pallidotomy for parkinson disease: a review of contemporary literature. J Neurosurg 2001;94:43–49.
67. Trépanier LL, Saint-Cyr JA, Lozano AM, Lang AE. Neuropsychological consequences of posteroventral pallidotomy for the treatment of Parkinson's disease. Neurology 1998;51:207–215.
68. Green J, Barnhart H. The impact of lesion laterality on neuropsychological change following posterior pallidotomy: A review of current findings. Brain Cogn 2000;42:379–398.
69. Schmand B, de Bie RM, Koning-Haanstra M, et al. Unilateral pallidotomy in PD: A controlled study of cognitive and behavioral effects. The Netherlands Pallidotomy Study (NEPAS) group. Neurology 2000;54:1058–1064.
70. Riordan HJ, Flashman LA, Roberts DW. Neurocognitive and psychosocial correlates of ventroposterolateral pallidotomy surgery in Parkinson's disease [electronic manuscript]. Neurosurg Focus 1997;2:Manuscript 7.
71. Cahn DA, Sullivan EV, Shear PK, et al. Neuropsychological and motor functioning after unilateral anatomically guided posterior ventral pallidotomy: Preoperative performance and three-month follow-up. Neuropsychiatry Neuropsychol Behav Neurol 1998;11:136–145.
72. Masterman D, DeSalles A, Baloh RW, et al. Motor, cognitive, and behavioral performance following unilateral ventroposterior pallidotomy for Parkinson disease. Arch Neurol 1998;55:1201–1208.
73. Scott R, Gregory R, Hines N, et al. Neuropsychological, neurological and functional outcome following pallidotomy for Parkinson's disease. A consecutive series of eight simultaneous bilateral and twelve unilateral procedures. Brain 1998;121:659–675.
74. Rilling LM, Filoteo JV, Roberts JW, Heilbrun MP. Neuropsychological Functioning in Patients with Parkinson's Disease Pre and Post Pallidotomy. Arch Clin Neuropsychology 1996;11(Abstract):442.
75. Tröster AI, Fields JA, Wilkinson SB, Koller WC. Neurobehavioral outcome of left and right pallidotomy for Parkinson's disease. Clin Neuropsychologist 1998;12(Abstract):268–269.
76. Yokoyama T, Imamura Y, Sugiyama K, et al. Prefrontal dysfunction following unilateral posteroventral pallidotomy in Parkinson's disease. J Neurosurg 1999;90:1005–1010.
77. Dewey Jr. RB, Giller CA, Broline SK, et al. Clinical outcome of unilateral stereotactic pallidotomy without microelectrode recording for intractable Parkinson's disease. Parkinsonism Relat Disord 2000;6:7–16.
78. Kubu CS, Grace GM, Parrent AG. Cognitive outcome following pallidotomy: the influence of side of surgery and age of patient at disease onset. J Neurosurg 2000;92:384–389.
79. Lacritz LH, Cullum CM, Frol AB, et al. Neuropsychological outcome following unilateral stereotactic pallidotomy in intractable Parkinson's disease. Brain Cogn 2000;42:364–378.

80. Rettig GM, York MK, Lai EC, et al. Neuropsychological outcome after unilateral pallidotomy for the treatment of Parkinson's disease. J Neurol Neurosurg Psychiatry 2000;69:326–336.
81. Trépanier LL, Kumar R, Lozano AM, et al. Neuropsychological outcome of GPi pallidotomy and GPi or STN deep brain stimulation in Parkinson's disease. Brain Cogn 2000;42:324–347.
82. Intemann PM, Masterman D, Subramanian I, et al. Staged bilateral pallidotomy for treatment of Parkinson disease. J Neurosurg 2001;94:437–444.
83. Soukup VM, Ingram F, Schiess MC, et al. Cognitive sequelae of unilateral posteroventral pallidotomy. Arch Neurol 1997;54:947–950.
84. Perrine K, Dogali M, Fazzini E, et al. Cognitive functioning after pallidotomy for refractory Parkinson's disease. J Neurol Neurosurg Psychiatry 1998;65:150–154.
85. Kuzis G, Sabe L, Tiberti C, et al. Neuropsychological effects of pallidotomy in patients with Parkinson's disease. J Neurol Neurosurg Psychiatry 2001;71(Letter):563.
86. Alegret M, Vendrell P, Junqué C, et al. Effects of unilateral posteroventral pallidotomy on 'on-off' cognitive fluctuations in Parkinson's disease. Neuropsychologia 2000;38:628–633.
87. Tröster AI, Fields JA, Hanisch C, Beatty WW. Clustering and switching on semantic verbal fluency in Parkinson's disease after unilateral, microelectrode-guided pallidotomy. J Int Neuropsychol Soc 1999;5(Abstract):273.
88. Obwegeser AA, Uitti RJ, Lucas JA, et al. Predictors of neuropsychological outcome in patients following microelectrode-guided pallidotomy for Parkinson's disease. J Neurosurg 2000;93:410–420.
89. Van Horn G, Hassenbusch SJ, Zouridakis G, et al. Pallidotomy: a comparison of responders and nonresponders. Neurosurgery 2001;48:263–273.
90. Lombardi WJ, Gross RE, Trépanier LL, et al. Relationship of lesion location to cognitive outcome following microelectrode-guided pallidotomy for Parkinson's disease: support for the existence of cognitive circuits in the human pallidum. Brain 2000;123:746–758.
91. Yokochi F, Okiyama R, Taniguchi M, et al. Relationship between lesion location and the outcome of pallidotomy for Parkinson's disease. J Neurol 2001;248:32–36.
92. Burns JM, Wilkinson S, Kieltyka J, et al. Analysis of pallidotomy lesion positions using three-dimensional reconstruction of pallidal lesions, the basal ganglia, and the optic tract. Neurosurgery 1997;41:1303–1316.
93. Shannon KM, Penn RD, Kroin JS, et al. Stereotactic pallidotomy for the treatment of Parkinson's disease. Efficacy and adverse effects at 6 months in 26 patients. Neurology 1998;50:434–438.
94. Crowe SF, O'Sullivan JD, Peppard RF, et al. Left posteroventral pallidotomy results in a deficit in verbal memory. Behav Neurol 1998;11:79–84.
95. Rettig GM, Lai EC, Krauss JK, et al. Neuropsychological evaluation of patients with Parkinson's disease before and after pallidal surgery. In: Krauss JK, Grossman RG, Jankovic J, eds. Pallidal Surgery for the Treatment of Parkinson's Disease and Movement Disorders. Lippincott-Raven, Philadelphia, PA, 1998, pp. 211–231.
96. Peppard RF, Crowe SF. Cognitive changes due to neurosurgical ablative and stimulating procedures in PD patients. In: Wolters EC, Scheltens P, Berendse HW, eds. Mental Dysfunction in Parkinson's Disease II, vol. 2. Academic Pharmaceutical Productions, Utrecht, The Netherlands, 1999, pp. 177–188.
97. Stebbins GT, Gabrieli JD, Shannon KM, et al. Impaired frontostriatal cognitive functioning following posteroventral pallidotomy in advanced Parkinson's disease. Brain Cogn 2000;42:348–363.
98. Alterman RL, Kelly P, Sterio D, et al. Selection criteria for unilateral posteroventral pallidotomy. Acta Neurochir Suppl 1997;68:18–23.
99. Iacono RP, Carlson JD, Kuniyoshi S, Mohamed A, Meltzer C, Yamada S. Contemporaneous bilateral pallidotomy [electronic manuscript]. Neurosurg Focus 1997;2:1–5.
100. Ghika J, Ghika-Schmid F, Fankhauser H, et al. Bilateral contemporaneous posteroventral pallidotomy for the treatment of Parkinson's disease: neuropsychological and neurological side effects. Report of four cases and review of the literature. J Neurosurg 1999;91:313–321.
101. Gálvez-Jiménez N, Lozano A, Tasker R, et al. Pallidal stimulation in Parkinson's disease patients with a prior unilateral pallidotomy. Can J Neurol Sci 1998;25:300–305.
102. Bezerra MLS, Martinez JVL, Nasser JA. Transient acute depression induced by high-frequency deep-brain stimulation [correspondence]. N Engl J Med 1999;341:1003–1004.
103. Martínez-Martín P, Valldeoriola F, Molinuevo JL, et al. Pallidotomy and quality of life in patients with Parkinson's disease: an early study. Mov Disord 2000;15:65–70.
104. Baron MS, Vitek JL, Bakay RA, et al. Treatment of advanced Parkinson's disease by posterior GPi pallidotomy: 1-year results of a pilot study. Ann Neurol 1996;40:355–366.
105. Uitti RJ, Wharen RE, Duffy JR, et al. Unilateral pallidotomy for Parkinson's disease: speech, motor, and neuropsychological outcome measurements. Parkinsonism Relat Disord 2000;6:133–143.
106. Junqué C, Alegret M, Nobbe FA, et al. Cognitive and behavioral changes after unilateral posteroventral pallidotomy: relationship with lesional data from MRI. Mov Disord 1999;14:780–789.
107. D'Antonio LL, Zimmerman GJ, Iacono RP. Changes in health related quality of life in patients with Parkinson's disease with and without posteroventral pallidotomy. Acta Neurochir 2000;142:759–767.

108. Hailey D, Harstall C. Posteroventral pallidotomy for Parkinson's disease: assessment and policy on a technology in transition. Health Policy 1998;43:55–64.
109. Tröster AI, Fields JA, Straits-Tröster KA, et al. Motoric and psychosocial correlates of quality of life in Parkinson's disease four months after unilateral pallidotomy. Neurology 1998;50(Abstract):A299.
110. Tröster AI, Fields JA, Wilkinson SB, et al. Unilateral pallidal stimulation for Parkinson's disease: neurobehavioral functioning before and 3 months after electrode implantation. Neurology 1997;49:1078–1083.
111. Vingerhoets G, van der Linden C, Lannoo E, et al. Cognitive outcome after unilateral pallidal stimulation in Parkinson's disease. J Neurol Neurosurg Psychiatry 1999;66:297–304.
112. Merello M, Nouzeilles MI, Kuzis G, et al. Unilateral radiofrequency lesion versus electrostimulation of posteroventral pallidum: a prospective randomized comparison. Mov Disord 1999;14:50–56.
113. Ardouin C, Pillon B, Peiffer E, et al. Bilateral subthalamic or pallidal stimulation for Parkinson's disease affects neither memory nor executive functions: a consecutive series of 62 patients. Ann Neurol 1999;46:217–223.
114. Pillon B, Ardouin C, Damier P, et al. Neuropsychological changes between "off" and "on" STN or GPi stimulation in Parkinson's disease. Neurology 2000;55:411–418.
115. Ghika J, Villemure JG, Fankhauser H, et al. Efficiency and safety of bilateral contemporaneous pallidal stimulation (deep brain stimulation) in levodopa-responsive patients with Parkinson's disease with severe motor fluctuations: a 2-year follow-up review. J Neurosurg 1998;89:713–718.
116. Fields JA, Tröster AI, Wilkinson SB, et al. Cognitive outcome following staged bilateral pallidal stimulation for the treatment of Parkinson's disease. Clin Neurol Neurosurg 1999;101:182–188.
117. Dujardin K, Krystkowiak P, Defebvre L, et al. A case of severe dysexecutive syndrome consecutive to chronic bilateral pallidal stimulation. Neuropsychologia 2000;38:1305–1315.
118. Fields JA, Tröster AI, Wilkinson SB, et al. Comparison of the cognitive safety of unilateral pallidal stimulation and pallidotomy. Neurology 1998;50(Abstract):A389.
119. Vingerhoets G, Lannoo E, van der Linden C, et al. Changes in quality of life following unilateral pallidal stimulation in Parkinson's disease. J Psychosom Res 1999;46:247–255.
120. Pahwa R, Lyons KE, Wilkinson SB, et al. Comparison of thalamotomy to deep brain stimulation of the thalamus in essential tremor. Mov Disord 2001;16:140–143.
121. Fields JA, Tröster AI. Cognitive outcomes after deep brain stimulation for Parkinson's disease: a review of initial studies and recommendations for future research. Brain Cogn 2000;42:268–293.
122. Miyawaki E, Perlmutter JS, Tröster AI, et al. The behavioral complications of pallidal stimulation: a case report. Brain Cogn 2000;42:417–434.
123. Grace J, Stout JC, Malloy PF. Assessing frontal lobe behavioral syndromes with the frontal lobe personality scale. Assessment 1999;6:269–284.
124. McCarter RJ, Walton NH, Rowan AF, et al. Cognitive functioning after subthalamic nucleotomy for refractory Parkinson's disease. J Neurol Neurosurg Psychiatry 2000;69:60–66.
125. Andy OJ, Jurko MF, Sias Jr FR. Subthalamotomy in treatment of parkinsonian tremor. J Neurosurg 1963;20:861–871.
126. Mundinger F. Results of 500 subthalamotomies in the region of the zona incerta. In: Gillingham FJ, Donaldson IML, eds. Third Symposium on Parkinson's Disease. E & S Livingstone Ltd., Edinburgh, UK, 1968, pp. 261–265.
127. Moro E, Scerrati M, Romito LM, et al. Chronic subthalamic nucleus stimulation reduces medication requirements in Parkinson's disease. Neurology 1999;53:85–90.
128. Lopiano L, Rizzone M, Bergamasco B, et al. Deep brain stimulation of the subthalamic nucleus: Clinical effectiveness and safety. Neurology 2001;56:552–554.
129. Lopiano L, Rizzone M, Perozzo P, et al. Deep brain stimulation of the subthalamic nucleus: selection of patients and clinical results. Neurol Sci 2001;22:67–68.
130. Volkmann J, Allert N, Voges J, et al. Safety and efficacy of pallidal or subthalamic nucleus stimulation in advanced PD. Neurology 2001;56:548–551.
131. Gerschlager W, Alesch F, Cunnington R, et al. Bilateral subthalamic nucleus stimulation improves frontal cortex function in Parkinson's disease. An electrophysiological study of the contingent negative variation. Brain 1999;122:2365–2373.
132. Gerschlager W, Bloem BR, Alesch F, et al. Bilateral subthalamic nucleus stimulation does not improve prolonged P300 latencies in Parkinson's disease. J Neurol 2001;248:285–289.
133. Saint-Cyr JA, Trépanier LL, Kumar R, et al. Neuropsychological consequences of chronic bilateral stimulation of the subthalamic nucleus in Parkinson's disease. Brain 2000;123:2091–2108.
134. Alegret M, Junqué C, Valldeoriola F, et al. Effects of bilateral subthalamic stimulation on cognitive function in Parkinson disease. Arch Neurol 2001;58:1223–1227.
135. Dujardin KLD, Krystkowiak P, Blond S, Destée A. Influence of chronic bilateral stimulation of the subthalamic nucleus on cognitive function in Parkinson's disease. J Neurol 2001;248:603–611.
136. Morrison CE, Borod JC, Brin MF, et al. A program for neuropsychological investigation of deep brain stimulation (PNIDBS) in movement disorder patients: Development, feasibility, and preliminary data. Neuropsychiatry Neuropsychol Behav Neurol 2000;13:204–219.

137. Hariz MI, Johansson F, Shamsgovara P, et al. Bilateral subthalamic nucleus stimulation in a parkinsonian patient with preoperative deficits in speech and cognition: Persistent improvement in mobility but increased dependency: a case study. Mov Disord 2000;15:136–139.
138. Benabid AI, Koudsié A, Benazzouz A, et al. Neurosurgical therapy in Parkinson's disease. In: Wolters EC, Scheltens P, Berendse HW, eds. Mental Dysfunction in Parkinson's Disease II, vol. 2. Academic Pharmaceutical Productions, Utrecht, The Netherlands, 1999, pp. 131–139.
139. Bejjani BP, Damier P, Arnulf I, et al. Transient acute depression induced by high-frequency deep-brain stimulation. N Engl J Med 1999;340:1476–1480.
140. Kumar R, Lozano AM, Sime E, et al. Comparative effects of unilateral and bilateral subthalamic nucleus deep brain stimulation. Neurology 1999;53:561–566.
141. Benabid AL, Koudsié A, Benazzouz A, et al. Deep brain stimulation of the corpus luysi (subthalamic nucleus) and other targets in Parkinson's disease. Extension to new indications such as dystonia and epilepsy. J Neurol 2001;248:37–47.
142. Houeto JL, Damier P, Bejjani PB, et al. Subthalamic stimulation in Parkinson disease: a multidisciplinary approach. Arch Neurol 2000;57:461–465.
143. Capus L, Melatini A, Zorzon M, et al. Chronic bilateral electrical stimulation of the subthalamic nucleus for the treatment of advanced Parkinson's disease. Neurol Sci 2001;22:57–58.
144. Ostrosky-Solis F, Quintanar L, Madrazo I, et al. Neuropsychological effects of brain autograft of adrenal medullary tissue for the treatment of Parkinson's disease. Neurology 1988;38:1442–1450.
145. Goetz CG, Tanner CM, Penn RD, et al. Adrenal medullary transplant to the striatum of patients with advanced Parkinson's disease: 1-year motor and psychomotor data. Neurology 1990;40:273–276.
146. Madrazo I, Franco-Bourland R, Aguilera M, et al. Autologous adrenal medullary, fetal mesencephalic, and fetal adrenal brain transplantation in Parkinson's disease: a longterm postoperative follow-up. J Neural Transplant Plast 1991;2:157–164.
147. Goetz CG, Stebbins GT, Klawans HL, et al. United Parkinson Foundation Neurotransplantation Registry on adrenal medullary transplants: Presurgical, and 1- and 2-year follow-up. Neurology 1991;41:1719–1722.
148. Stebbins GT, Tanner, CM. Behavioral effects of intrastriatal adrenal medullary surgery in Parkinson's disease. In: Huber SJ, Cummings JL, eds. Parkinson's Disease: Neurobehavioral Aspects. Oxford University Press, New York, 1992, pp. 328–345.
149. Rehncrona S. A critical review of the current status and possible developments in brain transplantation. In: Cohadon F, Dolenc VV, Lobo Antunes J, et al., eds. Advances and Technical Standards in Neurosurgery, vol. 23. Springer, Vienna, Austria, 1997, pp. 3–46.
150. Hagell P, Schrag A, Piccini P, et al. Sequential bilateral transplantation in Parkinson's disease: effects of the second graft. Brain 1999;122:1121–1132.
151. Diederich NJ, Goetz CG. Neuropsychological and behavioral aspects of transplants in Parkinson's disease and Huntington's disease. Brain Cogn 2000;42:294–306.
152. Sass KJ, Buchanan CP, Westerveld M, et al. General cognitive ability following unilateral and bilateral fetal ventral mesencephalic tissue transplantation for treatment of Parkinson's disease. Arch Neurol 1995;52:680–686.
153. Leroy A, Michelet D, Mahieux F, et al. Examen neuropsychologique de 5 patients parkinsoniens avant et après greffe neuronale. Rev Neurol 1996;152:158–164.
154. Thompson LL, Cullum CM, O'Neill S, Freed CR. Effects of fetal cell transplantation on cognitive and psychological functioning in Parkinson's disease. Arch Clin Neuropsychology 1997 (Abstract);12:416.
155. Baker KK, Ramig LO, Johnson AB, Freed CR. Preliminary voice and speech analysis following fetal dopamine transplants in 5 individuals with Parkinson disease. J Speech Lang Hear Res 1997;40:615–626.
156. Molina H, Quinones, Alvarez L, et al. Transplantation of human fetal mesencephalic tissue in caudate nucleus as treatment for Parkinson's disease: the Cuban experience. In: Lindvall I, Björklund A, Widner H, eds. Intracerebral Transplantation in Movement. Disorders: Experimental Basis and Clinical Experiences. Elsevier, Amsterdam, 1991, pp. 99–110.
157. Madrazo I, Franco-Bourland RE, Castrejon H, et al. Fetal striatal homotransplantations for Huntington's disease: first two case reports. Neurol Res 1995;17:312–315.
158. Price LH, Spencer DD, Marek KL, et al. Psychiatric status after human fetal mesencephalic tissue transplantation in Parkinson's disease. Biol Psychiatry 1995;38:498–505.
159. Freed CR, Greene PE, Breeze R. E, et al. Transplantation of embryonic dopamine neurons for severe Parkinson's disease. N Engl J Med 2001;344:710–719.
160. Hagell P, Crabb L, Pogarell O, et al. Health-related quality of life following bilateral intrastriatal transplantation in Parkinson's disease. Mov Disord 2000;15:224–229.
161. Schumacher M, Ellias SA, Palmer EP, et al. Transplantation of embryonic porcine mesencephalic tissue in patients with PD. Neurology 2000;54:1042–1050.
162. Saint-Cyr JA, Trépanier LL. Neuropsychological Assessment of Patients for Movement Disorder Surgery. Mov Disord 2000;15:771–783.
163. Spreen O, Strauss EA. Compendium of Neuropsychological Tests: Administration, Norms, and Commentary, 2nd ed. Oxford University Press, New York,1998.

164. Wechsler D. Wechsler Adult Intelligence Test, Third Edition (WAIS-III). Administration and Scoring Manual. The Psychology Corporation, San Antonio, TX, 1997.
165. Brandt J, Benedict RHB. Hopkins Verbal Learning Test-Revised (HVLT-R). Professional Manual. Psychological Assessment Resources, Inc, Lutz, FL, 2002.
166. Grace J, Malloy P. Frontal Systems Behavior Scale (FrSBe) Professional Manual. Psychological Assessment Resources, Inc., Lutz, FL, 2002.
167. Ware JE, Snow KK, Kosinski M, Gandek B. SF-36 Health Survey Manual and Interpretation Guide. The Health Institute, New England Medical Center, Boston, MA, 1993.
168. de Boer AG, Wijker W, Speelman JD, et al. Quality of life in patients with Parkinson's disease: Development of a questionnaire. J Neurol Neurosurg Psychiatry 1996;61:70–74.

II Autonomic Dysfunction in Parkinson's Disease

7
Dysphagia

Norman A. Leopold

SUMMARY

Dysphagia is an often unrecognized complication that occurs in a majority of patients with Parkinson's disease (PD). Although dysphagia is usually asymptomatic in PD, a detailed clinical and radiological examination of patients with symptomatic dysphagia typically identifies multiple abnormalities in each phase of ingestion. Dysphagia treatment options are discussed, but there is inconsistent benefit from medications and no documented evidence for paramedical modalities.

Key Words: Parkinson's disease; dysphagia; swallowing; ingestion; videofluoroscopy; dysphagia therapy.

"Whilst at meals the fork not being duly directed frequently fails to raise the morsel from the plate: Which, when seized, is with much difficulty conveyed to the mouth." "...so much are the actions of the muscles of the tongue, pharynx, &c. impeded by impaired action and perpetual agitation, that the food is with difficulty retained in the mouth until masticated; and then as difficultly swallowed." "...the saliva fails of being directed to the back part of the fauces, and hence is continually draining from the mouth, mixed with the particles of food, which he is no longer able to clear from the inside of the mouth." James Parkinson, 1817 (1).

1. INTRODUCTION

James Parkinson unambiguously portrayed advanced dysphagia in "The Shaking Palsy" *(1)*. Despite his obvious references to aspects of ingestion that precede or overlap swallow initiation, early investigators of deglutition in Parkinson's disease (PD) attributed dysphagia to disturbed esophageal swallowing, a conclusion supported both by the presence of Lewy bodies in the vagal dorsal motor nucleus *(2)* and esophageal myenteric plexus *(3)*, as well as numerous radiologic observations of esophageal dysmotility *(4–13)*. More recently, considerations of motoric features preceding esophageal transport have insinuated themselves into investigations of dysphagia in this disorder *(14–18)*. Analysis of this research identifies multiple abnormalities that support a role for the basal ganglia in directing bolus movement and also challenge some general views of the relationship between the swallow and dysphagia.

2. DEFINITION OF DYSPHAGIA

Dysphagia is commonly defined as disordered swallowing. However, the standard lingual, pharyngeal, and esophageal stages of swallowing inadequately incorporate other motor and cognitive behaviors that may impact swallow efficiency and safety. Therefore, dysphagia is most inclusively not just a disorder of the swallow, but of ingestion *(19)*, a complex motor cascade beginning prior to the swallow and ending when a bolus passes the lower esophageal sphincter.

From: *Current Clinical Neurology*
Parkinson's Disease and Nonmotor Dysfunction
Edited by: R. F. Pfeiffer and I. Bodis-Wollner © Humana Press Inc., Totowa, NJ

Table 1
Ingestion Questionnaire

1.	Do you have difficulty swallowing?
2.	Do you choke or gag on food?
3.	Do you choke or gag on liquids?
4.	Do you choke or gag on your own saliva?
5.	Do you have difficulty starting to swallow?
6.	Do you drool? If so, when?
7.	Do you have difficulty chewing?
8.	Do you have difficulty moving food about in your mouth?
9.	Does food feel like it gets stuck when you go to swallow? If so, where—mouth, throat, or chest?
10.	Do you have heartburn?
11.	Do you have reflux?
12.	Do you belch frequently?
13.	Do you get full at meals too quickly?
14.	Do you have a poor appetite?
15.	Do you have a fear of swallowing food or pills?
16.	Does your mouth feel too dry?
17.	Does it take too long to eat?

3. ANATOMIC CONSIDERATIONS

Reflexive deglutition begins *in utero (20,21)* and is likely driven solely by a medullary central pattern generator *(22)*. This functional center includes, but is not limited to, the nucleus solitarius, dorsal and ventral vagal nuclei, and intervening reticular-activating system *(23)*. Exposed by neuroanatomic-labeling techniques, additional polysynaptic connections that assist to control and coordinate complex oromotor behaviors extend throughout the brainstem from the hypoglossal nucleus to the substantia nigra zona reticulata *(24,25)*. With brain maturation, more suprasegmental innervation diminishes the primacy of the reflex swallow and merges it into the final phase of ingestion. Transcortical magnetic stimulation *(26,27)* and functional brain imaging (positron emission tomography and functional magnetic resonance imaging; *28,29*) have identified the cingulate, premotor, prefrontal, and primary motor and sensory cortices (insula, cerebellum, and the basal ganglia-thalamic-cortical circuitry) as active regions in nonreflexive swallowing *(29)*. Therefore, many integrated neuronal systems, including those known to be defective in PD, control both bulbar and automatic extremity and commanded movements. This extensive, functionally related circuitry provides robust evidence against the concept of hierarchical control of ingestion, but in favor of modular or distributed governance *(29)*.

4. PREVALENCE OF DYSPHAGIA IN PD

The exact prevalence of dysphagia in PD remains uncertain, but may range from about 50–100% *(16,30,31)*. Disparate results among studies relate partly to inconsistent criteria used to define dysphagia. In the first systematic investigation of dysphagia in PD, Eadie and Tyrer *(31)*, claimed that 47% of their cohort had "symptomatic" dysphagia. Edwards et al. *(32)*, used a more elaborate questionnaire and reinforced this conclusion. However, an additional 28% of both study cohorts had sialorrhea, a complaint often owing to an abnormality of swallow and not to dysautonomic salivary overproduction *(33,34)*.

The prevalence of dysphagia in PD increases if its definition encompasses those asymptomatic patients with radiological abnormalities of swallowing. Logemann and colleagues *(35)* found that 95% of studied patients with PD referred for dysphagia therapy had cineradiographic swallowing disturbances, but only 15–20% were clinically symptomatic. Other investigations of dysphagia in PD using varying inclusions criteria also highlight the disparity between symptomatic and radiological dysphagia *(14–17,32,36,37)*. These examples of diminished awareness of dysphagia in PD allow the conclusion that responses to the Unified Parkinson Disease Rating Scale Part II, which queries only about sialorrhea and choking/gagging during meals, and even more detailed questionnaires (Table 1) are unreliable markers of dysphagia.

The relationship between the prevalence of dysphagia in PD and the severity of the disease has received little attention. Only two studies report a correlation between disease severity and symptomatic dysphagia *(16,32)*. However, other investigators did not find a correlation, and further discerned that patients with the most advanced disease had fewer dysphagic symptoms than those less debilitated by PD *(17,31)*. These unanticipated results were posited to possible dementia, another complication of PD where prevalence increases with advancing disease. A similar argument is proposed for the underreporting of symptomatic dysphagia when compared to radiological results in patients with corticobasal degeneration *(38)*.

5. CLINICAL DYSPHAGIA

Neurological examination routinely incorporates a specific cranial nerve examination, but no review of swallowing capacity. A simple bedside screening test of swallowing, although no substitute for the rigorous examination performed by a clinical dysphagia specialist, provides a quick estimate of water-swallowing capacity *(39)*. Patients are asked to drink 150 cc of cold water as quickly and safely as possible. Observations include the number of swallows, time to empty the cup, and any aberrant swallowing behavior (e.g., coughing, gagging, or a posttest wet voice). Patients with PD require more swallows and are slower to complete the task than controls with both parameters declining with advancing disease *(40)*. However, a normal test does not exclude dysphagia, because only water swallowing is monitored.

Clinical dysphagia specialists conduct a detailed examination of cranial nerves 5, 7, 9, 10, and 12 as they relate to ingestion. However, they also analyze self-feeding by presenting a variety of food substances with varying textures, temperature, and tastes and record atypical feeding behaviors that might precipitate or exaggerate dysphagia. The more common feeding deficits in PD include reduced self-feeding capacity, abnormal neck and body postures while eating, impulsive feeding behaviors, difficulty regulating the quantity of food eaten, slow mastication, and hesitant swallow initiation *(17,41)*.

6. RADIOLOGICAL DYSPHAGIA

Numerous videofluoroscopic studies of food and liquid ingestion have been conducted in patients with PD. However, methodological and nomenclature differences have yielded incomplete and inconsistent observations of bolus movement (*see* Table 2). In early studies, patients only swallowed liquid barium while lying prone or standing erect *(6–11,42)*. Pre-esophageal bolus preparation and transit were largely ignored. More recent investigations administer a modified barium swallow (MBS) during which patients with PD sit erect and ingest not just liquid barium but also barium-impregnated foods of varying quantities and consistencies *(14,15,17,18,35,36,43–45)*. Unfortunately, the MBS is also an example of regional procedural blindness in that it scrutinizes oral preparatory, lingual, and pharyngeal phases of ingestion, but it ignores the esophageal phase.

6.1. Oral Preparatory Phase

The oral preparatory phase prepares food or liquids and positions the bolus on the tongue prior to lingual transfer. Once in the mouth, food is captured anteriorly by a firm lip seal, and compression of the posterior tongue posteriorly against the hard palate. The tongue squeezes food against the hard palate, then guides it onto the teeth for mastication with the cheeks. Once masticated, the tongue properly sizes and centers the bolus prior to the swallow, while any excess is temporarily squirreled between the teeth and cheeks. Prolongation of this phase is a generalized and commonly described abnormality in PD. More circumspect observations include one or several of the following: slow oral

Table 2
Abnormalities of Ingestion in Parkinson's Disease

Phases of ingestion				
Preoral	Oral preparatory	Lingual	Pharyngeal	Esophageal
↓ Movements to mouth	↓ Lip seal	↓ Peristalsis	↓ Peristalsis	
Impulsive feeding	↓ Bolus movement	Hesitant or delayed transfer	↓ Laryngeal elevation	Tertiary waves
Dysregulation of feeding rate	↓ Mastication	Premature transfer	↓ Hyoid elevation	Reverse peristalsis
	↓ Lingual-centering movements	Segmented bolus transfer	↓ Epiglotic tilting	↓ Transport
		Lingual tremor	Vallecular retention	↓ Emptying
		Lingual "freezing"	Pyriform sinus retention	↓ LES closure
		↓ Lingual seal	↓ Laryngeal closure	GE reflux hiatal hernia

↓, Slow or impaired. LES, lower esophageal sphincter; GE, gastroesophageal.

acceptance of the bolus, reduced bolus oral manipulation, inadequate or dysfunctional mastication, and poor bolus formation *(14,15,17,18,35,36)*. Less frequently observed aberrations include an insufficient lip seal (oral contents slip from the mouth) and lingual tremor *(15,17)*.

6.2. Lingual Phase

The lingual phase of ingestion is the first stage of the swallow. Although there are minor individual variabilties, the contraction of tongue blade or tongue dorsum forces the bolus against the hard palate and generates a lingual peristaltic wave that propels the bolus from the mouth into the oropharynx. During this phase, patients with PD manifest difficulty initiating the swallow, often displaying repetitive "pumping" movements *(14,15,17,36)*, approximating the leg hesitancies seen in freezing of gait. Segmented or "piecemeal" bolus swallowing is also common. These defective tongue movements may result in the bolus escaping over the tongue to invade the oropharynx and instigate a premature swallow *(14,15,17,36,45)*. An inefficient lingual phase also imparts a weakened bolus propulsive force, which, in turn, compromises pharyngeal motility.

6.3. Pharyngeal Phase

The pharyngeal phase begins nearly simultaneously with swallow initiation. The pharynx elevates and then contracts to surround the bolus, the hyoid bone and laryngeal cartilages rise, the epiglottis tilts to cover the laryngeal vestibule, the vocalis closes, and respiratory muscle activity pauses. A large majority of patients with PD evaluated for dysphagia manifest slow or uncoordinated pharyngeal transport *(15,18,36,43–45)*. The most common abnormalities include slowed pharyngeal peristalsis (>45%), bolus retention in the vallecular (>50%) and pyriform sinuses (>30%), and glottic aspiration (>15%; *18*). Because of its more proximate position to the laryngeal vestibule, spillage from pyriform sinus retention is more likely to cause laryngeal penetration or aspiration.

Although ignored in most studies of dysphagia in PD, epiglottic displacement is adversely affected in nearly 50% of patients *(18)*. When coupled with impaired extrinsic (laryngeal elevation) and intrinsic (vocal cord closure) laryngeal muscle movements during the swallow *(46)*, the risk of aspiration significantly increases. Those patients suffering from PD with more advanced disease are most likely to display three abnormalities of the pharyngeal swallow that increase bolus aspiration risk: pyriform sinus retention, absent epiglottic inversion, and defective true vocal cord closure.

The pharyngo-esophageal sphincter (PES) is the anatomic transition between the pharynx and esophagus. This sphincter is pulled open during the pharyngeal phase, allowing an unobstructed bolus transfer into the esophagus. Despite the opinion that dysphagia in PD is "…caused simply by clinical cricopharyngeal achalasia" *(47)* and several reports of PES dyssynergia with the advancing wave of pharyngeal peristalsis *(9,48)*, radiological studies of large numbers of patients with PD do not support PES dysfunction. Together, Eadie and Tyrer *(6)* and Leopold and Kagel *(18)* found only 1 of 143 patients with PD to have PES dysfunction. Manometric and electrophysiological evaluations of PES activity have also yielded contradictory results with either increased or normal PES pressures, respectively *(48–50)*. Likewise, these studies failed to discern any radiological PES dysfunction during videofluoroscopy.

6.4. *Esophageal Phase*

Once past the PES, the bolus traverses the length of the esophagus and exits through the lower esophageal sphincter (LES) into the stomach. Bolus movement during the final phase of ingestion is generated foremost by the continuing progression of pharyngeal peristalsis and supplemented by local neuromuscular networks that stimulate secondary peristalsis. Whether recorded during videofluoroscopy or inferred by esophageal manometry, more than 85% of patients with PD have demonstrated slow, uncoordinated, and ineffectual esophageal bolus transport *(18)*. Defective peristalsis ranges from minor slowing to aperistalsis *(7,11,18,51)*. Other esophageal aberrations include tertiary contractions, reverse peristalsis, "spasms" and patulency *(4,18,47,52)*. Delayed transport and reverse peristalsis are statistically more common in patients with more advanced PD *(19)*, a finding unconfirmed by esophageal manometry *(51,52)*.

The LES transitions bolus transport from the esophagus to the stomach. Functionality of the LES in PD has not been examined as extensively as other anatomic regions of ingestion. Those few such studies describe a prevalence of gastroesophageal (GE) reflux that ranges from 26–57% *(6,18)*. In patients studied by Eadie and Tyrer, GE reflux was three times more frequent than in control subjects *(6)*. Hiatal hernias are also often indicated, but their prevalence may be no more than that of control subjects *(53)*. In another study of esophageal motility in patients with PD (without a control population), both GE reflux and hiatal hernias were common, but no significant differences were uncovered based on disease severity *(18)*.

7. IMPLICATIONS OF DYSPHAGIA

Dysphagia consequences are usually both psychosocial and physical. As noted previously, symptomatic dysphagia often goes unrecognized by the patient with PD. However, observant family and friends may find aberrant feeding behavior disturbing and withdraw from, or become less tolerant of, the patient during meals. For those dysphagic patients with insight into their frailties, mealtimes may provoke more anxiety than provide satiety *(54)*. As dysphagia advances, patients or their caregivers reduce food selection for safety and time constraints *(55)*. Mealtimes serve for both enteral and emotional nutrition, and neither goal will be satisfied if meals are exceptionally prolonged by slowed feeding, mastication, and swallow initiation. The consequence of this spiral is a socially isolated and often malnourished patient.

The burden of advancing PD includes an increased aspiration risk or frank aspiration. Choking and coughing may be absent (the "silent aspirator") or minimal *(14)*. The absence of respiratory symptoms in patients with witnessed repeated aspiration during a MBS may suggest that dysphagia in PD is of little consequence *(43)*. However, this apparent disconnection may, in part, be caused by the artificial nature of MBS, during which patients sit with head and neck erect, contrary to daily meals, when many patients with PD eat with their head and neck anteroflexed *(17)*, a posture that prepositions pharyngeal and tracheal structures to self-protect the airway. Dysphagia progression eventuates in respiratory symptoms with pneumonia as the most common cause of death in PD *(56–58)*.

8. TREATMENT

8.1. Overview

There is no choir singing of concensus for the treatment of dysphagia in PD, for there are no words. As for paramedical therapies, even the notes are absent. A systematic review of paramedical therapies in PD by Deane et al. *(59)* did not find any nonpharmacologic dysphagia trials. Several drug studies do not directly address this question. Instead, some limited details can be extracted from their studies of dysphagia in PD that were designed to answer other questions *(15)*. Therefore, instead of overriding consensus for treatment, little more exists than results based on anecdotal data.

Minimal dysphagia with a relatively low risk of aspiration presents historically as isolated sialorrhea. Such patients often do not require specific intervention, and therapeutic decisions should be based on other PD symptoms or manifestations. More prominent drooling, even in the absence of additional dysphagic symptoms, is a sign of more seriously compromised ingestion. Treatment decisions then follow a more considered examination of ingestion by a MBS in addition to esophageal fluoroscopy, which is administered under the direction of an experienced clinical dysphagia specialist. Fiberoptic endoscopy during swallowing may also be informative.

8.2. Compensatory Techniques

During a diagnostic MBS, the dysphagia specialist also introduces various compensatory techniques and observes the responses. The result is a collection of facilitory and compensatory strategies taught to the patient and their caregiver, intended to remediate abnormalities in one or several phases of ingestion. Direct therapy methods may include changes in body positioning during meals, altering the quantity, taste, temperature, and texture of food permitted, and cued instructions to reduce the automaticity of meals by inserting repetitive cycles of mastication, breath holding, and chin tucking before swallowing to narrow the airway prior to swallow initiation. Swallows may be followed by intentional throat clearing, a more effortful supraglottic swallow *(60)*, and the Mendelsohn maneuver, a technique that prolongs laryngeal elevation during the swallow *(61)*. Indirect strategies are stimulation techniques and exercises to strengthen and quicken the swallow. Using the Mendelsohn maneuver with indirect therapies, Nagaya and coworkers reported that dysphagic patients with PD significantly reduced swallow initiation time after just one swallowing training session *(45)*. Cued swallowing can also shorten the duration of the oropharyngeal swallow *(62)*. Extrapolating from gait therapy research in PD *(63)*, cueing may redirect motor instructions to minimize disordered basal ganglia influences over the automatic and sequential components of ingestion.

Notwithstanding any other literature support, dysphagia therapy appears experientially successful in remediating dysphagia in patients with PD. However, because dysphagia may result in aspiration, subsequent pneumonia, or asphyxiation, researchers confront ethical barriers to the placebo-controlled studies usually necessary to determine treatment efficacy.

8.3. Levodopa

Drug treatment may diminish some aspects of impaired ingestion in PD, but the supportive literature is so sparse that it can suggest that dopaminergic pathways have little impact on swallowing *(44,64,65)*. However, accurate quantification of drug-induced ingestive changes is limited. Lingual tremor is uncommon (subsides during swallowing [*9,17*]) and is without known adverse affects. Deglutory muscle rigidity is immeasurable. Only the ingestive equivalent of bradykinesia can be witnessed at the bedside or during videofluoroscopy with few standards by which it can be judged *(41,64,66)*. Consequently, relative to scaled improvement of limb movement, even modest drug-induced benefits may be inconspicuous.

Any medication-related benefit should accrue primarily to the prepharyngeal phases of ingestion, those phases under the greatest volitional control. In the first publication of levodopa therapy for PD, Cotzias et al. *(67)* noted "striking" improvement in "drooling and dysphagia." Radiographical confirmation was not attempted. Levodopa therapy may improve jaw velocity and amplitude *(68)* and lessen swallow-related deficits in some patients with PD *(16,44,47,69–71)*, but levodopa-induced improvement of pharyngeal motility was not seen by Calne et al. *(42)*. However, their cohort may have been less affected, as no patients had vallecular or pyriform sinus stasis or aspiration, and prepharyngeal bolus transport was insufficiently documented.

8.4. Dopamine Agonists

Dopamine agonists also ameliorate some symptomatic and radiological swallowing abnormalities. Specifically bromocriptine has been reported to reduce drooling *(72)*. Also, apomorphine may produce some improvement in the oral preparatory and lingual phases *(73)*; off-period belching and associated esophageal motility may also improve *(74)*.

8.5. Anticholinergics

Anticholinergic agents and salivary gland botulinum toxin injections *(75)* can reduce salivary consistency or volume, but they have little positive impact on the motor act of ingestion. On a cautionary note, anticholinergic-induced xerostomia may further impair swallow initiation and therefore worsen ingestion. Finally, although particular drug treatment for dysphagia was not directly addressed, Clark and colleagues found that patients with PD experienced significant slowing of the swallow when medications were withdrawn *(40)*.

9. SUMMARY

In summary, the previous review provides testimony in PD to an ensemble of ingestive motor deficiencies, extending from lips to lower esophageal sphincter. It is doubtful that any of these abnormalities are specific for PD, because many have been reported in other bradykinetic-rigid syndromes *(38,76–78)*. However, the early appearance of significant dysphagia is exceptional in PD and should alert the clinician to an alternative diagnosis *(79)*. Once recognized, a detailed dysphagia evaluation should be considered.

REFERENCES

1. Parkinson J. An Essay on the Shaking Palsy. Whittingham and Bowland, London, 1817.
2. Eadie MJ. The pathology of certain medullary nuclei in Parkinsonism. Brain 1963;86:781–792.
3. Qualman SJ, Haupt HM, Yang P, Hamilton SR. Esophageal Lewy bodies associated with ganglia cell loss in achalasia. Similarity to Parkinson's disease. Gastroenterology 1984;87:848–856.
4. Penner A, Druckerman LJ. Segmental spasms of the esophagus and their relation to Parkinsonism. Am J Digest Dis 1942;9:282–286.
5. Brombart M. Clinical Radiology of the Esophagus. John Wright & Sons Ltd., Bristol, 1961.
6. Eadie MJ, Tyrer JH. Radiological abnormalities of the upper part of the alimentary tract in Parkinsonism. Aust Ann Med 1965;14:23–27.
7. Fischer RA, Ellison GW, Thayer WR, et al. Esophageal motility in neuromuscular disorders. Ann Int Med 1965;63:230–247.
8. Donner MW, Silbiger ML. Cinefluorographic analysis of pharyngeal swallowing in neuromuscular disorders. Am J Med Sci 1966;251:606–616.
9. Silbiger ML, Pikielney R, Donner MW. Neuromuscular disorders affecting the pharynx. Invest Radiol 1967;2:442–448.
10. Kiuchi S, Sasaki J, Arai T, Suzuki T. Functional disorders of the pharynx and esophagus. Acta Otolaryngol Suppl 1969;256:1–30.
11. Gibberd FB, Gleeson JA, Gossage AAR, Wilson RSE. Oesophageal dilatation in Parkinson's disease. J Neurol Neurosurg Psychiatry 1974;37:938–940.
12. Blonsky ER, Logemann JA, Boshes B, Fisher HB. Comparison of speech and swallowing function in patients with tremor disorders and in normal geriatric patients: a cinefluorographic study. J Gerontol 1975;30:299–303.
13. Kaye MD, Hoehn MM. Esophageal motor dysfunction in Parkinson's disease. In: Vantrappen G, ed. Proceedings of the 5th International Symposium on Gastrointestinal Motility. Typoff Press, Herentals, 1975.
14. Robbins JA, Logemann JAK, Kirshner HS. Swallowing and speech production in Parkinson's disease. Ann Neurol 1986;19:283–287.
15. Bushmann M, Dobmeyer SM, Leeker L, Perlmutter JS. Swallowing abnormalities and their response to treatment in Parkinson's disease. Neurology 1989;39:1309–1314.

16. Stroudley J, Walsh M. Radiological assessment of dysphagia in Parkinson's disease. Brit J Radiol 1991;64:890–893.
17. Leopold NA, Kagel MC. Prepharyngeal dysphagia in Parkinson's disease. Dysphagia 1996;11:14–22.
18. Leopold NA, Kagel MC. Pharyngo-esophageal dysphagia in Parkinson's disease. Dysphagia 1997;12:11–18.
19. Leopold NA, Kagel MC. Ingestion or deglutition? A proposed paradigm. Dysphagia 1997;12:202–206.
20. Wolfson VP, Laitman JT. Ultrasound investigation of fetal human upper respiratory anatomy. Anat Rec 1990;227:363–372.
21. Peleg D, Goldman JA. Fetal deglutition: a study of the anencephalic fetus. Eur J Obstet Gynecol Reproduc Biol 1978;8:133–136.
22. Nijland MJ, Day L, Ross MG. Ovine fetal swallowing: expression of preterm neurobehavioral rhythms. J Matern Fetal Med 2001;10:251–257.
23. Altschuler SM. Laryngeal and respiratory protective reflexes. Am J Med 2001;111(Suppl 8A):90S–94S.
24. Fay RA, Norgren R. Identification of rat brainstem multisynaptic connections to the oral motor nuclei using pseudorabies virus. I, Masticatory muscle motor system. Brain Res Brain Res Rev 1997;25:255–275.
25. Hattox AM, Priest CA, Keller A. Functional circuitry involved in the regulation of whisker movements. J Comp Neurol 2002;442:266–276.
26. Aziz Q, Rothwell JC, Barlow K, Thompson DG. Modulation of esophageal responses to magnetic stimulation of the human brain by swallowing and by vagal stimulation. Gastroenterology 1995;109:1437–1445.
27. Hamdy S, Aziz Q, Rothwell JC, et al. The cortical topography of human swallowing musculature in health and disease. Nat Med 1996;2:1217–1224.
28. Hamdy S, Mikulis DJ, Crawley A, et al. Cortical activation during human volitional swallowing: an event related fMRI study. Am J Physiol 1999;277:G219–G225.
29. Mosier K, Bereznaya I. Parallel cortical networks for volitional control of swallowing in humans. Exp Brain Res 2001;140:280–289.
30. Lieberman AN, Horowitz L, Redmond P, et al. Dysphagia in Parkinson's disease. Am J Med 1980;74:157–160.
31. Eadie MJ, Tyrer JH. Alimentary disorder in Parkinsonism. Aust Ann Med 1965;14:13–22.
32. Edwards LL, Pfeiffer RF, Quigley EMM, et al. Gastrointestinal symptoms in Parkinson's disease. Mov Disord 1991;6:151–156.
33. Bateson MC, Gibberd FB, Wilson RSE. Salivary symptoms in Parkinson disease. Arch Neurol 1973;29:274–275.
34. Pehlivan M, Yuceyar N, Ertekin C, et al. An electronic device measuring the frequency of spontaneous swallowing: digital phagometer. Dysphagia 1996;11:259–264.
35. Logemann J, Blonsky ER, Boshes B. Lingual control in Parkinson's disease. Trans Am Neurol Assoc 1973;98:276–278.
36. Bird MR, Woodward MC, Gibson EM, et al. Asymptomatic swallowing in elderly patients with Parkinson's disease: a description of findings on clinical examination and videofluoroscopy in sixteen patients. Age Aging 1994;23:251–254.
37. Potulska A, Friedman A, Krolicki L, et al. Swallowing disorders in Parkinson's disease. Neurol Neurochir Pol 2002;36:449–456.
38. Frattali CM, Sonies BC. Speech and swallowing disturbances in corticobasal degeneration. Adv Neurol 2000;82:153–160.
39. Nicklin J, Karni Y, Wiles CM. Measurement of swallowing time—a proposed method. Clin Rehab 1990;4:335–336.
40. Clarke CE, Gullaksen E, Macdonald S, Lowe F. Referral criteria for speech and language therapy assessment of dysphagia caused by idiopathic Parkinson's disease. Acta Neurol Scand 1998;97:27–35.
41. Atlin E, Norberg A, Axelsson K, et al. Aberrant eating behavior in elderly parkinsonian patients with and without dementia: analysis of videorecorded meals. Res Nurs Health 1989;12:41–51.
42. Calne DB, Shaw DG, Spiers ASD, Stern GM. Swallowing in Parkinsonism. Br J Radiol 1970;43:456–457.
43. Wintzen AR, Badrising UA, Roos RAC, et al. Influence of bolus volume on hyoid movements in normal individuals and patients with Parkinson's disease. Can J Neurol Sci 1994;21:57–59.
44. Fuh JL, Lee RC, Wang SJ, et al. Swallowing difficulty in Parkinson's disease. Clin Neurol Neurosurg 1997;99:106–112.
45. Nagaya M, Kachi T, Yamada T. Effect of swallowing training on swallowing disorders in Parkinson's disease. Scand J Rehab Med 2000;32:11–15.
46. Leopold NA, Kagel MC. Laryngeal motility during deglutition in patients with Parkinson's disease. Neurology 1997;48:373–375.
47. Palmer ED. Dysphagia in Parkinsonism. JAMA 1974;229:1349.
48. Ali GN, Wallace KL, Laundl TM, et al. Oral-pharyngeal dysfunction in patients with Parkinson's disease. Gastroenterol 1994;106(Abstract):A459.
49. Higo R, Tayama N, Watanabe T, Niimi S. Abnormal elevation of resting pressure at the upper esophageal sphincter of Parkinson's disease. Eur Arch Otorhinolaryngol 2001;258:552–556.
50. Ertekin C, Tarlaci S, Aydogdu I, et al. Electrophysiological evaluation of pharyngeal phase of swallowing in patients with Parkinson's disease. Mov Disord 2002;17:942–949.
51. Castell JA, Johnston BT, Colcher A, et al. Manometric abnormalities of the oesophagus in patients with Parkinson's disease. Neurogastroenterol Motil 2001;13:361–364.
52. Johnston BT, Colcher A, Li Q, et al. Repetitive proximal esophageal contractions: a new manometric finding and possible further link between Parkinson's disease and achalasia. Dysphagia 2001;16:186–189.
53. Edwards LL, Quigley EMM, Harned RK, et al. Characterization of swallowing and defecation in Parkinson's disease. Am J Gastroenterol 1994;89:15–25.

54. Ekberg O, Hamdy S, Woisard V, et al. Social and psychological burden of dysphagia: its impact on diagnosis and treatment. Dysphagia 2002;17:139–146.
55. McHorney CA, Bricker DE, Robbins J, et al. The SWAL-QOL outcomes tool for oropharyngeal dysphagia in adults: II. Item reduction and preliminary scaling. Dysphagia 2000;15:122–133.
56. Morgante L, Salemi G, Meneghini F, et al. Parkinson disease survival: a population-based study. Arch Neurol 2000;57:507–512.
57. Wermuth L, Stenager EN, Stenager E, Boldsen J. Mortality in patients with Parkinson's disease. Acta Neurol Scand 1995;92:55–58.
58. Beyer MK, Herlofson K, Arsland D, Larsen JP. Causes of death in a community-based study of Parkinson's disease. Acta Neurol Scand 2001;103:7–11.
59. Deane KHO, Ellis-Hill C, Jones D, et al. Systematic review of paramedical therapies for Parkinson's disease. Mov Disord 2002;17:984–991.
60. Kahrilas PJ, Logemann JA, Gibbons P. Food intake by maneuver; an extreme compensation for impaired swallowing. Dysphagia 1992;7:155–159.
61. Kahrilas PJ, Logemann JA, Krugler C, Flanagan E. Volitional augmentation of upper esophageal sphincter opening during swallowing. Am J Physiol 1991;260:G450–G456.
62. Pinnington LL, Muhiddin K, Ellis RE, Playford ED. Non-invasive assessment of swallowing and respiration in Parkinson's disease. J Neurol 2000;247:773–777.
63. Rubinstein TC, Giladi N, Hausdorff JM. The power of cueing to circumvent dopamine deficits: a review of physical therapy treatment of gait disturbances in Parkinson's disease. Mov Disord 2002;17:1148–1160.
64. Nilsson H, Ekberg O, Olsson R, Hindfelt B. Quantitative assessment of oral and pharyngeal function in Parkinson's disease. Dysphagia 1996;11:144–150.
65. Suchowersky O. Parkinson's disease: medical treatment of moderate to advanced disease. Curr Neurol Neurosci Rep 2002;2:310–316.
66. Cook IJ, Doods WJ, Dantas RO, et al. Timing of videofluoroscopic, manometric events and bolus transit during oral and pharyngeal phases of swallowing. Dysphagia 1989;4:8–15.
67. Cotzias GC, Papavasiliou PS, Gellene R. Modification of Parkinsonism—chronic treatment with l-dopa. New Engl J Med 1969;280:337–345.
68. Karlsson S, Persson M, Johnels B. Levodopa induced ON-OFF motor fluctuations in Parkinson's disease related to rhythmical masticatory jaw movements. J Neurol Neurosurg Psychiatry 1992;55:304–307.
69. Fonda D, Schwarz J, Clinnick S. Parkinsonian medication one hour before meal improves symptomatic swallowing: a case study. Dysphagia 1995;10:165–166.
70. Nowack WJ, Hatelid JM, Sohn RS. Dysphagia in Parkinsonism. Arch Neurol 1977;34:320.
71. Hunter PC, Crameri J, Austin S, et al. Response of Parkinsonian swallowing dysfunction to dopaminergic stimulation. J Neurol Neurosurg Psychiatry 1997;63:579–583.
72. Kartzinel R, Teychenne P, Gillespie MM, et al. Bromocriptine and levodopa (with or without carbidopa) in Parkinsonism. Lancet 1976;2:272–275.
73. Tison F, Wiart L, Guatterie M, et al. Effects of central dopaminergic stimulation by apomorphine on swallowing disorders in Parkinson's disease. Mov Disord 1996;11:729–732.
74. Kempster PA, Lees AJ, Crichton P, et al. Off-period belching due to a reversible disturbance of oesophageal motility in Parkinson's disease and its treatment with apomorphine. Mov Disord 1989;4:47–52.
75. Pal PK, Calne DB, Calne S, Tsui JK. Botulinum toxin A as treatment for drooling saliva in PD. Neurology 2000;54:244–247.
76. Kurihara K, Kita K, Hirayama K, Hara T. Dysphagia in multiple system atrophy—radiological and manometric study. Rinsho Shinkeigaku 1993;33:271–277.
77. Leopold NA. Dysphagia in drug-induced Parkinsonism. Dysphagia 1996;11:151–153.
78. Leopold NA, Kagel MC. Dysphagia in progressive supranuclear palsy: radiologic features. Dysphagia 1997;12:140–143.
79. Muller J, Wenning MJ, Verny M, et al. Progression of dysarthria and dysphagia in postmortem-confirmed parkinsonian disorders. Arch Neurol 2001;58:259–264.

8
Gastric Dysfunction

Tanya Gurevich, Amos D. Korczyn, and Nir Giladi

SUMMARY

Parkinson's disease (PD) is frequently regarded as a pure motor disorder. However, this degenerative illness affects also the autonomic as well as the enteric nervous systems. Impairment of gastric motility has been found in 70% of patients with PD. Neuropathological changes have been described in patients with PD in all parts of the nervous system responsible for gastric motility. Gastric motor dysfunction (delayed gastric emptying [GE]) is usually associated with early satiety, anorexia, abdominal fullness, nausea, and vomiting. Abnormalities in gastric myoelectric activity have been found in PD. Dysfunction of gastric motility may contribute to motor fluctuations in PD. Conversely, different medications used for the treatment of PD may exacerbate GE disturbances. Along with dopamine agonists, levodopa itself has been shown to slow gastrointestinal motility.

Treatment of gastroparesis is usually problematic. Dietetic interventions, in combination with the use of prokinetic medications, are recommended. Gastrostomy or jejunostomy feeding tubes may also be considered. Jejunostomy, which provides the possibility of direct levodopa infusions into the intestine, may be preferable in fluctuating patients with PD. Data are not yet available on the use of gastric electrical stimulation in PD. To date, there is no satisfactory therapeutic approach to gastroparesis, and the clinician needs considerable creativity to help the patient with PD overcome this disabling syndrome and its consequences.

Key Words: Parkinson's disease; gastric function; gastric emptying; motor fluctuations; levodopa pharmacokinetics.

1. INTRODUCTION

Parkinson's disease (PD) is a common degenerative illness affecting the central and autonomic as well as the enteric nervous system (ENS; *1*). Common gastrointestinal (GI) manifestations include sialorrhea, which probably reflects disordered swallowing, and more severe deglutition problems with consequent dysphagia, aspiration, and possible weight loss *(2–5)*.

Constipation is very frequent among patients with PD, often antedating motor manifestations of the disease *(6)*. Relatively little attention has been directed to dysfunction of the proximal part of the GI system, encompassing the esophagus and stomach. Gastric dysfunction may be important, not only because of its symptomatology, but also because it may affect drug absorption and, consequently, the motor manifestations of PD. Impairment of gastric motility has been reported to be present in 70% of patients with PD, especially in those with response fluctuations *(7)*. Conversely, among 146 consecutive patients with gastroparesis attending one gastroenterology clinic, the condition was related to PD in 7.5% *(8)*. Although considerable progress continues to be made in delineating many aspects of GI dysfunction in PD, therapeutic approaches to these symptoms are falling behind. A growing body of evidence indicates that GI symptoms primarily reflect direct involvement of the GI tract in the neurodegenerative process. GI symptomatology arises as a result of the PD effects on skeletal muscle

From: *Current Clinical Neurology*
Parkinson's Disease and Nonmotor Dysfunction
Edited by: R. F. Pfeiffer and I. Bodis-Wollner © Humana Press Inc., Totowa, NJ

function in the oropharynx, anorectum, and pelvic floor, but it is mainly caused by the direct involvement of the autonomic nervous system (ANS) and ENS in other portions of the GI tract *(9)*.

2. PHYSIOLOGY

Autonomic regulation of GI motor function consists of extrinsic control by the parasympathetic and sympathetic nervous systems and intrinsic control via the enteric plexuses *(10)*. The ENS has a key role in the generation and coordination of antral contractions and peristalsis, along with the regulation of gastric emptying (GE). The intrinsic innervation of the ENS consists of a network of neurons within the gut wall that are arranged in two principal plexuses: the myenteric plexus of Auerbach and submucosal plexus of Meissner. The intrinsic system is activated by vagal preganglionic fibers and inhibited by sympathetic pathways. The extrinsic innervation of the gut consists of parasympathetic vagal and sacral nerves (S2, S3, and S4) and the sympathetic outflow from the intermediolateral column of the spinal cord between the levels of the fifth thoracic and third lumbar segments. Extrinsic nerves are also intimately involved in the control of striated muscle portions of the esophagus and external anal sphincter.

3. PATHOLOGY AND PATHOPHYSIOLOGY

GI involvement in PD is a good example of the interaction between the central nervous system (CNS) and ANS. The demonstration of neuropathological abnormalities in the ENS analogous to those regarded as pathognomonic of the parkinsonian process in the brain suggests that the ENS, called "the little brain in the digestive system" *(11)*, and the CNS ("large brain") may demonstrate parallel pathological changes in many disease processes previously regarded as being confined to the CNS and somatic nervous systems *(9)*.

Lewy bodies, a pathological hallmark of PD, are widely distributed in Auerbach's and Meissner's plexuses in the GI tract of individuals with PD *(12,13)*. Recently, neurons that are immunoreactive for tyrosine hydroxylase have been also shown to exist in these plexuses in normal humans, and a possible relationship between these presumably catecholaminergic neurons and the occurrence of Lewy bodies in the ENS in PD has been suggested *(14)*.

Loss of neurons has been reported in the dorsal motor nucleus of the vagus (DMNV) in patients suffering from PD with autonomic failure *(15)*. This nucleus consistently contains Lewy bodies in PD, which are similar to other pigmented nuclei of the brainstem *(15,16)*. Moderate neuronal loss and Lewy bodies have been noted in the intermediolateral column of the spinal cord in patients with PD, including thoracolumbar sacral segments *(17,18)*. Lewy bodies also occur in sympathetic ganglia with or without obvious neuronal loss *(19)*.

Changes involving both the ANS and ENS are usually thought to underlie the GI dysfunction in PD *(20)*. However, gut dysfunction in PD may also be related to the degeneration of peripheral dopaminergic neurons, because endogenous dopamine may be involved in GI motility in several species, including humans *(21,22)*.

Therefore, neuropathological changes have been described in patients with PD in all parts of the nervous system accounting for gastric motility. Changes in any or all of these locations may affect gastric motility problems in this disease.

4. CLINICAL MANIFESTATIONS

Gastric motor dysfunction is a disorder of the upper gut and is typically characterized by delayed GE that may be linked with early satiety, anorexia, upper abdominal fullness, bloating, and sometimes pain, nausea, and vomiting. Nausea in patients with PD has been traditionally attributed to dopaminergic medications *(23,24)*. Double-blind studies with dopaminergic agonists indeed demonstrate that these drugs are associated with nausea *(25,26)*. However, the frequency of nausea in a group of patients with PD who were on these medications was reported to be similar to those who were untreated, suggesting that although dopaminergic medications are associated with nausea and vomiting, they cannot be the sole explanation for those symptoms in PD *(27)*.

Abnormalities in gastric myoelectric activity have been described in PD. Untreated patients with PD have significantly slower GE times when compared with controls *(28,29)*. In one study, electrogastrography (EGG) revealed dysrhythmias in 15 of 20 patients with PD; gastric motility was particularly impaired in patients with advanced PD *(30)*. Patients with PD had an abnormal EGG pattern that was similar to that of vagotomized patients in the acute stage *(20)*, showing reduced gastric electrical activity following a meal, implying the presence of vagal nerve dysfunction in PD.

5. GASTRIC MOTILITY AND MOTOR FLUCTUATIONS

Significant evidence suggests that in elderly people, particularly patients with PD, gastric transit time is slowed. This may translate into delayed absorption of drugs (e.g., levodopa; [*31*]). However, slower transit might also increase overall drug availability, but the initial response to the drug might be insignificant ("delayed on"). This effect could be enhanced by anticholinergic drugs (e.g., trihexyphenidyl [*32*]).

The mechanisms responsible for motor fluctuations in PD are not fully understood *(33)*. Pharmacokinetic factors, such as short half-life, peripheral *O*-methylation and facilitated transport across the blood–brain barrier, may be a source of unstable drug effects. However, erratic gastric motility may also contribute to the complex pharmacokinetics of levodopa *(34)*. Djaldetti et al. *(35)* described a patient with PD who had a smooth response to levodopa until she underwent vagotomy and pyloroplasty. Immediately after surgery, the patient began to complain that treatment with levodopa was markedly less effective; "delayed on" and "dose failure" phenomena appeared, indicating delayed GE.

Erratic gastric motility in patients with PD is also characterized by periods of effective contractions that induce efficient transit of food into the duodenum, which may in turn result in rapid uptake of levodopa that may also contribute to motor fluctuations. Although the "wearing off" phenomenon may be a result of changes in central pharmacokinetics caused by diminished presynaptic dopamine storage capacity, peripheral levodopa pharmacokinetics, especially erratic intestinal absorption of oral levodopa owing to delayed GE, may account for the "delayed on" and "dose failure" phenomena *(33,36)*. The main support for this hypothesis is that both "delayed on" and dose failure can often be prevented or ameliorated by taking levodopa before meals on an empty stomach, preferably in a crushed form with a generous amount of liquid, or when the stomach is bypassed and levodopa is administered via nasoduodenal or gastrojejunostomy tubes *(35,37)*. Kurlan et al. *(37)* assessed mobility and plasma levodopa concentrations in 10 patients with PD exposed to 5 modes of levodopa administration to clarify the influence of GE on levodopa-related motor fluctuations. They demonstrated that it is possible to produce steady plasma levodopa concentrations with a corresponding reduction in motor fluctuations by continuous intraduodenal administration of the drug *(38)*. Other enteral routes have produced a more variable plasma L-dopa concentration and clinical response *(37)*.

Cisapride, a prokinetic drug with cholinergic activity, increases gastric motility and has been shown to improve the "delayed on" and "dose failure" phenomena *(29)*. Taken together with the report of vagotomy-induced "delayed on" and "dose failure" *(35)*, it seems that the success of levodopa treatment depends partly on normal gastric motility, and stagnation of levodopa within the stomach from reduced gastric motility and prolonged transit time may affect the bioavailability of the drug. Age-related alteration in the activity of peripheral dopa decarboxylase in elderly patients may also contribute to erratic levodopa absorption in patients with PD.

An interesting perspective on motor fluctuations was recently proposed by Pierantozzi and colleagues *(39)*, who described six patients with PD in whom the area under the curve of levodopa plasma concentrations was augmented with prolongation of clinical benefit after *Helicobacter pylori* eradication. The authors suggested that *H. pylori*-activated gastric alterations may be responsible, at least in part, for the unpredictable absorption of oral levodopa in advanced PD.

Meal ingestion time in relation to the levodopa dose is an important determinant of drug absorption. Time to peak plasma levodopa concentration increased threefold (from 45 ± 23 to 134 ± 76 minutes; $p < 0.001$), when levodopa was administered after meals in the study of Baruzzi et al. *(40,41)*. At least in persons without PD, fatty food can slow GE *(41)*.

6. THE EFFECT OF ANTIPARKINSONIAN MEDICATIONS ON GASTRIC MOTILITY

The frailty of GI function in old age, particularly patients with PD, underlies the very frequent complaints of nausea, gastric fullness, or constipation following drug exposure *(42)*. Specifically, drugs with antimuscarinic or dopaminergic effects have been implicated.

Apomorphine facilitates swallowing in patients with PD *(43)*, but dopaminomimetic agents also inhibit GE, an effect blocked by metoclopramide, the dopamine antagonist *(44)*. Levodopa also slows GE to a similar extent in both elderly and young volunteers *(45)*. Dhasmana et al. *(46)* provided evidence that the decrease in GI motility elicited by dopamine and dopamine agonists occurs primarily through the activation of dopamine receptors involved in intestinal contractions. This peripheral GI effect of levodopa occurs despite cotreatment with a decarboxylase inhibitor, because some peripheral conversion to dopamine occurs within the stomach itself with activation of dopamine receptors leading to prolonged GE *(47,48)*. In one study, patients suffering from PD with response fluctuations had a significant delay in GE in comparison to those with a smooth response *(7)*.

Chronic exposure to levodopa may also modify the activity of the DMNV in the medulla oblongata. Several groups have shown that dopaminergic cells are present in the DMNV *(49–51)*. Alteration of the dopaminergic system of the DMNV could result in dopaminergic supersensitivity and possibly the enhancement of vagal activity to accelerate GE during the "on" state. In the study of Hardoff et al. *(28)*, GE and gastric motility were assessed in patients with PD at mild and moderate stages of the disease. Patients treated with levodopa for a relatively short time period who showed a smooth response to the drug had a slower GE time than did untreated patients. In contrast, after a longer duration of levodopa treatment and development of response fluctuations, patients had a dramatic shortening of GE–nearly to the rate recorded in healthy volunteers—when GE was measured during the "on" state induced by levodopa. Accelerated GE in a subgroup of treated patients with motor fluctuations (all with long-term exposure to levodopa) was also outlined by Murata and associates *(52,53)*. They demonstrated accelerated absorption of levodopa from the gut after prolonged exposure to levodopa in intact rats as well as in patients with PD. The effect of chronic levodopa treatment accelerating its own absorption from the gut was also reported by Abrahms et al. *(54)* and Muenter et al. *(55)* shortly after levodopa was introduced for the treatment of PD. Such an effect is supported by the clinical observation that taking medications during the "off" state can frequently result in a "delayed on" or a "no on" response (unpublished observations N. Giladi). Furthermore, a "delayed on" response, which is often associated with prolonged GE *(33)*, occurs most often after the first-morning levodopa dose, at which time the patient is typically "off" after 6–10 hours of fasting (and no medications). Yeh and colleagues *(56)* have shown that the second daily dose of levodopa has a significantly shorter absorption time. These results should encourage patients to take their medications while still "on" to accelerate levodopa absorption and avoid a delayed effect of the subsequent dose of levodopa.

It can be speculated that levodopa treatment initially slows down GE by its peripheral action on the gastric wall or pyloric function *(44)*, despite its favorable effects on other parkinsonian symptoms. Although the effect of other antiparkinsonian medications on gastrointestinal motility is likely largely overestimated *(57)*, nevertheless, this factor needs to be considered. In a study in rats, dopaminergic agents (i.e., apomorphine and bromocriptine) significantly slowed GI transit, an effect that was blocked by dopamine antagonists *(46)*.

Anticholinergic agents like trihexyphenidyl and benztropine may also impair GE. Trihexyphenidyl was shown to decrease levodopa absorption in rats *(58)*. Thus, the concomitant administration of trihexyphenidyl to patients receiving levodopa may decrease the therapeutic efficacy of levodopa by slowing its absorption *(59)*. On the contrary, trihexyphenidyl increased the proportion of levodopa absorbed in young volunteers in about 1 hour, which could be advantageous in some cases *(58)*.

Gastric relaxation invariably precedes nausea and emesis, as is seen with the classical emetic agent, apomorphine *(60)*. Other dopamine agonists, and possibly selegiline, may produce nausea and vomiting as side effects, not only by stimulating catecholamine receptors involved in the emetic response, but also via their direct dopaminergic effects in the GI tract *(48)*.

7. TREATMENT OF GASTROPARESIS IN PD

7.1. *Nonpharmacological Treatment*

Nonpharmacological treatment of gastroparesis in PD includes a diet that consists of small and frequent low-fat meals. Astarloa et al. *(61)* established the positive effect of a diet rich in insoluble fiber on plasma levodopa concentrations and motor function of patients with PD following a levodopa dose.

7.2. *Cholinergic Drugs*

Avoidance of anticholinergic medications may also be beneficial in the management of gastroparesis. The muscarinic cholinergic agent, bethanechol, enhances gastric contractions, but not in a coordinated way to stimulate GE and is therefore of limited value as a prokinetic agent *(62)*.

7.3. *Domperidone*

The most commonly used prokinetic medication in PD is the peripheral dopamine receptor antagonist, domperidone, and its use in patients with PD was first proposed by Agid et al. *(63)* and Quinn et al. *(64)*. In the study of Soykan and colleagues *(65)*, domperidone in a daily dose of 80 mg significantly reduced upper GI symptoms (nausea, vomiting, anorexia, abdominal bloating, heartburn, and regurgitation) and accelerated GE of a solid meal, but it did not interfere with response to antiparkinsonian treatment. Additionally, domperidone has an antiemetic effect, produced by its action on the chemoreceptor trigger zone. Domperidone is not available in the United States, but it is commonly used in other countries to manage GI symptoms. It is typically dosed orally at 10–20 mg three or four times daily. A suppository form is available as well.

7.4. *Cisapride*

Cisapride is another prokinetic drug that enhances GE by releasing acetylcholine from the myenteric plexus, acting on serotonin (5-HT_4) receptors. It also appears to antagonize 5-HT_3 receptors, resulting in GI smooth muscle contraction, which possibly contributes to its antiemetic effect *(66)*. Cisapride has no direct antidopaminergic effect and was shown to be effective and well-tolerated in fluctuating patients with PD, along with a significant shortening of the latency to "on" and reduction of the number of dose failures. This effect is related to improved pharmacokinetic parameters of levodopa *(29,67)*, but exacerbation of tremor has been reported *(68)*. The usual dose of cisapride is 10–20 mg four times daily, usually given 30 minutes before meals. Because of potential cardiac arrhythmias precipitated by numerous drug interactions and medical conditions, cisapride has been withdrawn from the open market in the United States and the United Kingdom.

7.5. *Erythromycin*

The motilin receptor agonist, erythromycin, may be effective in patients with gastroparesis, especially in relieving acute gastric stasis when given at a dose of 1–3 mg per kg intravenously every 8 hours. Oral dosing of 50–250 mg four times daily may also be effective *(11,62)*, but our literature search failed to reveal any studies on the use of erythromycin specifically as a prokinetic agent in PD.

7.6. Other Approaches

The use of prokinetic medications in combination with one another may be beneficial, but it has been minimally investigated and not at all in PD *(62)*. Despite dietary and pharmacological interventions, some patients will continue to have debilitating symptoms of gastroparesis. Such patients, including those with PD, may benefit from the appropriate use of dietary supplements *(69)*.

7.7. Enteral Feeding and Drug Administration

Eventually, in a small percentage of patients with PD, the placement of a gastrostomy or jejunostomy feeding tube may become necessary for the provision of optimal nutritional care *(62)*. In fluctuating patients with PD, jejunostomy may be preferable because it provides the possibility of direct infusion of levodopa into the intestine, thus reducing levodopa plasma level fluctuations. Intraduodenal administration of levodopa is thought to be an ideal model for the development of continuous-release levodopa preparations *(37,38)*. A jejunal pouch technique for levodopa delivery was proposed for the treatment of fluctuating patients with PD and successful experimental models in dogs and rhesus monkeys have been designed *(70,71)*.

7.8. Gastric Stimulation

Recent understanding of normal gastric electromechanical function and its abnormalities has led to the development of a gastric electrical stimulator, analogous to devices that stimulate other dysfunctional organs. It requires the surgical placement of electrodes into the gastric serosa. Patients activate the pacer in the immediate preprandial period and continue its operation for several hours after eating. Gastric electrical stimulation is associated with symptomatic relief, improvements in nutritional status, health resource utilization, and costs. It is approved by the Food and Drug Administration for patients with severe nausea and vomiting caused by gastroparesis, offering a new approach for patients with refractory gastroparesis when all other options have failed *(72,73)*. But no data are yet available on its use in PD. The methodology of neural electrical gastric stimulation consists of a microprocessor-controlled sequential activation of a series of annular electrodes that encircle the distal two-thirds of the stomach and induce propagated contractions, causing a forceful gastric emptying. The latter method is the most promising thus far, but it has only been applied in animals and would need to be tested further before it could be considered for patients with PD *(74)*.

7.9. Botulinum Toxin

Several other "nonstandard" methods have been proposed for the treatment of gastroparesis. Recently, three women with severe gastroparesis were treated with intrapyloric injections of botulinum toxin, and all were reported to have had significant symptomatic improvement *(75)*.

8. CONCLUSION

Gastroparesis is a well-recognized manifestation of PD, causing nausea and other symptoms, but also affecting drug absorption. Antiparkinsonian drugs may further exacerbate its GI manifestations. Currently, there is no efficient therapeutic method to gastroparesis, and clinicians will need a considerable amount to help the patient with PD overcome this disabling syndrome and its outcomes.

ACKNOWLEDGMENT

Esther Eshkol, Margot Feinstein and Lior Grodlinger are thanked for editorial assistance.

REFERENCES

1. Braak H, Braak E. Pathoanatomy of Parkinson's disease. J Neurol 2000;247(Suppl 2):II3–II10.
2. Edwards LL, Quigley EM, Pfeiffer RF. Gastrointestinal dysfunction in Parkinson's disease: frequency and pathophysiology. Neurology 1992;42:726–732.

3. Bagheri H, Damase-Michel C, Lapeyre-Mestre M, et al. A study of salivary secretion in Parkinson's disease. Clin Neuropharmacol 1999;22:213–215.
4. Chen H, Zhang SM, Hernan MA, et al. Weight loss in Parkinson's disease. Ann Neurol 2003;53:676–679.
5. Potulska A, Friedman A, Krolicki L, Spychala A. Swallowing disorders in Parkinson's disease. Parkinsonism Relat. Disord 2003;9:349–353.
6. Korczyn AD. Autonomic manifestations in Parkinson's disease. In: Nappi G, Caraceni T, eds. Morbo di Parkinson e Malattie Extrapiramidali. Edizione Mediche Italiane, Pavia, 1987, p. 210.
7. Djaldetti R, Baron J, Ziv I, Melamed E. Gastric emptying in Parkinson's disease: patients with and without response fluctuations. Neurology 1996;46:1051–1054.
8. Soykan I, Sivri B, Sarosiek I, et al. Demography, clinical characteristics, psychological and abuse profiles, treatment, and long-term follow-up of patients with gastroparesis. Dig Dis Sci 1998;43:2398–2404.
9. Quigley EM. Gastrointestinal dysfunction in Parkinson's disease. Semin. Neurol 1996;16:245–250.
10. Camilleri M. Autonomic regulation of gastrointestinal motility. In: Low PA, ed. Clinical Autonomic Disorders: Evaluation and Management, 2nd edition. Lippincott-Raven, Philadelphia, 1997;135–145.
11. Prather CM, Camilleri M. Gastrointestinal dysfunction: approach to management. In: Low PA, ed. Clinical Autonomic Disorders: Evaluation and Management, 2nd ed. Lippincott-Raven, Philadelphia, 1997;597–612.
12. Stadlan EM, Duvoisin R, Yahr M. The pathology of Parkinsonism. In: Proceedings of the Fifth International Congress of Neuropathology. Zurich, 1965; Excerpta Medica International Congress Series No. 100:569–571.
13. Wakabayashi K, Takahashi H. Neuropathology of autonomic nervous system in Parkinson's disease. Eur. Neurol 1997;38(Suppl 2):2–7.
14. Wakabayashi K, Takahashi H, Takeda S, Ohama E, Ikuta F. Lewy bodies in the enteric nervous system in Parkinson's disease. Arch. Histol. Cytol. 1989;52(Suppl):191–194.
15. Forno LS. Neuropathology of Parkinson's disease. J Neuropath Exp. Neurol 1996;55:259–272.
16. Hughes AJ, Daniel SE, Blankson S, Lees AJ. A clinicopathologic study of 100 cases of Parkinson's disease. Arch Neurol 1993;50:140–148.
17. Oppenheimer DR. Lateral horn cells in progressive autonomic failure. J Neurol Sci 1980;46:393–404.
18. Oyanagi K, Wakabayashi K, Ohama E, et al. Lewy bodies in the lower sacral parasympathetic neurons of a patient with Parkinson's disease. Acta Neuropathol (Berl) 1990;80:558–559.
19. Matthews MT. Autonomic ganglia in multiple system atrophy and pure autonomic failure. In: Bannister RG, Mathias CJ, eds. Autonomic Failure. A Textbook of Disorders of the Autonomic Nervous System. Oxford University Press, Oxford, 1992, p. 593.
20. Kaneoke Y, Koike Y, Sakurai N, et al. Gastrointestinal dysfunction in Parkinson's disease detected by electrogastroenterography. J Auton Nerv Syst 1995;50:275–281.
21. Van Nueten JM. Is dopamine an inhibitory modulator of gastric motility? Trends Pharmacol Sci 1980;1:233–235.
22. Willems JL, Buylaert WA, Lefebvre RA, Bogaert MG. Neuronal dopamine receptors on autonomic ganglia and sympathetic nerves and dopamine receptors in the gastrointestinal system. Pharmacol Rev 1985;37:165–216.
23. Hoehn MM, Yahr MD. Parkinsonism: onset, progression and mortality. Neurology 1967;17:427–442.
24. Pallis CA. Parkinsonism: natural history and clinical features. Br Med J 1971;3:683.
25. Korczyn AD, Brooks DJ, Brunt ER, et al. Ropinirole versus bromocriptine in the treatment of early Parkinson's disease: a 6-month interim report of a 3-year study. 053 Study Group. Mov Disord 1998;13:46–51.
26. Etminan M, Gill S, Samii A. Comparison of the risk of adverse events with pramipexole and ropinirole in patients with Parkinson's disease: a meta-analysis. Drug Saf 2003;26:439–444.
27. Edwards LL, Pfeiffer RF, Quigley EM, et al. Gastrointestinal symptoms in Parkinson's disease. Mov Disord 1991;6:151–156.
28. Hardoff R, Sula M, Tamir A, et al. Gastric emptying time and gastric motility in patients with Parkinson's disease. Mov Disord 2001;16:1041–1047.
29. Djaldetti R, Koren M, Ziv I, et al. Effect of cisapride on response fluctuations in Parkinson's disease. Mov Disord 1995;10:81–84.
30. Krygowska-Wajs A, Lorens K, Thor P, et al. Gastric electromechanical dysfunction in Parkinson's disease. Funct Neurol 2000;15:41–46.
31. Evans MA, Broe GA, Triggs EJ, et al. Gastric emptying rate and the systemic availability of levodopa in the elderly parkinsonian patient. Neurology 1981;31:1288–1294.
32. Roberts J, Waller DG, von Renwick AG, et al. The effects of co-administration of benzhexol on the peripheral pharmacokinetics of oral levodopa in young volunteers. Br J Clin Pharmacol 1996;41:331–337.
33. Sage JI, Mark MH. Basic mechanisms of motor fluctuations. Neurology 1994;44(7 Suppl 6):S10–S14.
34. Deleu D, Northway MG, Hanssens Y. Clinical pharmacokinetic and pharmacodynamic properties of drugs used in the treatment of Parkinson's disease. Clin Pharmacokinet 2002;41:261–309.
35. Djaldetti R, Achiron A, Ziv I, Melamed E. First emergence of "delayed-on" and "dose failure" phenomena in a patient with Parkinson's disease following vagotomy. Mov Disord 1994;9:582–583.

36. Kurlan R, Rothfield KP, Woodward WR, et al. Erratic gastric emptying of levodopa may cause "random" fluctuations of parkinsonian mobility. Neurology 1988;38:419–421.
37. Kurlan R, Nutt JG, Woodward WR. Duodenal and gastric delivery of levodopa in Parkinsonism. Ann Neurol 1988;23:589–595.
38. Sage JI, Sonsalla PK, McHale DM, et al. Clinical experience with duodenal infusion of levodopa for the treatment of motor fluctuations in Parkinson's disease. Adv Neurol 1990;53:383–386.
39. Pierantozzi M, Pietroiusti A, Sancesario G, et al. Reduced L-dopa absorption and increased clinical fluctuations in *Helicobacter pylori*-infected Parkinson's disease patients. Neurol Sci 2001;22:89–91.
40. Baruzzi A, Contin M, Riva R, et al. Influence of meal ingestion time on pharmacokinetics of orally administered levodopa in parkinsonian patients. Clin Neuropharmacol 1987;10:527–537.
41. Boulby P, Moore R, Gowland P, Spiller RC. Fat delays emptying but increases forward and backward antral flow as assessed by flow-sensitive magnetic resonance imaging. Neurogastroenterol Motil 1999;11:27–36.
42. Korczyn AD, Rubenstein AE. Autonomic nervous system complications of therapy. In: Silverstein A, ed. Neurological Complications of Therapy. Futura, New York, 1981, p. 405.
43. Tison F, Wiart L, Guatterie M, et al. Effects of central dopaminergic stimulation by apomorphine on swallowing disorders in Parkinson's disease. Mov Disord 1996;11:729–732.
44. Berkowitz DM, McCallum RW. Interaction of levodopa and metoclopramide on gastric emptying. Clin Pharmacol Ther 1980;27:414–420.
45. Robertson DR, Renwick AG, Macklin B, et al. The influence of levodopa on gastric emptying in healthy elderly volunteers. Eur J Clin Pharmacol 1992;42:409–412.
46. Dhasmana KM, Villalon CM, Zhu YN, Parmar SS. The role of dopamine (D_2), alpha and beta-adrenoceptor receptors in the decrease in gastrointestinal transit induced by dopamine and dopamine-related drugs in the rat. Pharmacol Res 1993;27:335–347.
47. Gancher ST, Nutt JG, Woodward WR. Peripheral pharmacokinetics of levodopa in untreated, stable and fluctuating parkinsonian patients. Neurology 1987;37:940–944.
48. Andrews PLR. Nausea, vomiting, and the autonomic nervous system. In: Mathias CJ, Bannister R, eds. Autonomic Failure: A Textbook of Clinical Disorders of the Autonomic Nervous System, 4th ed. Oxford University Press, New York, 1999:126–135.
49. Maqbool A, Batten TF, Berry PA, McWilliamm PN. Distribution of dopamine-containing neurons and fibres in the feline medulla oblongata: a comparative study using catecholamine-synthesizing enzyme and dopamine immunohistochemistry. Neuroscience 1993;53:717–733.
50. Loewy AD, Franklin MF, Haxhiu MA. CNS monoamine cell groups projecting to pancreatic vagal motor neurons: a transneuronal labeling study using pseudorabies virus. Brain Res 1994;638:248–260.
51. Ruggiero DA, Chau L, Anwar M, et al. Effect of cervical vagotomy on catecholaminergic neurons in the cranial division of the parasympathetic nervous system. Brain Res 1993;617:17–27.
52. Murata M, Kanazawa I. Repeated L-dopa administration reduces the ability of dopamine storage and abolishes the supersensitivity of dopamine receptors in the striatum of intact. rat. Neurosci Res 1993;16:15–23.
53. Murata M, Mizusawa H, Yamanouchi H, Kanazawa I. Chronic levodopa therapy enhances dopa absorption: contribution to wearing-off. J Neural Transm 1996;103:1177–1185.
54. Abrams WB, Coutinho CB, Leon AS, Spiegel HE. Absorption and metabolism of levodopa. JAMA 1971;218:1912–1914.
55. Muenter MD, Tyce GM. L-dopa therapy of Parkinson's disease: plasma L-dopa concentration, therapeutic response, and side effects. Mayo Clin Proc 1971;46:231–239.
56. Yeh KC, August TF, Bush DF, et al. Pharmacokinetics and bioavailability of Sinemet CR: a summary of human studies. Neurology 1989;39(11 Suppl 2):25–38.
57. Jost WH. Gastrointestinal motility problems in patients with Parkinson's disease. Effects of antiparkinsonian treatment and guidelines for management. Drugs Aging 1997;10:249–258.
58. Feldman S, Putcha L. Effect of anti-Parkinsonism drugs on gastric emptying and intestinal transit in the rat. Pharmacology 1977;15:503–511.
59. Algeri S, Cerletti C, Curcio M, et al. Effect of anticholinergic drugs on gastro-intestinal absorption of L-dopa in rats and in man. Eur J Pharmacol 1976;35:293–299.
60. Castro A, Mearin F, Larish J, Malagelada JR. Gastric fundus relaxation and emetic sequences induced by apomorphine and intragastric lipid infusion in healthy humans. Am J Gastroenterol 2000;95:3404–3411.
61. Astarloa R, Mena MA, Sanchez V, et al. Clinical and pharmacokinetic effects of a diet rich in insoluble fiber on Parkinson disease. Clin Neuropharmacol 1992;15:375–380.
62. Rabine JC, Barnett JL. Management of the patient with gastroparesis. J Clin Gastroenterol 2001;32:11–18.
63. Agid Y, Pollak P, Bonnet AM, et al. Bromocriptine associated with a peripheral dopamine blocking agent in treatment of Parkinson's disease. Lancet 1979;1:570–572.
64. Quinn N, Illas A, Lhermitte F, Agid Y. Bromocriptine and domperidone in the treatment of Parkinson disease. Neurology 1981;31:662–667.
65. Soykan I, Sarosiek I, Shifflett J, et al. Effect of chronic oral domperidone therapy on gastrointestinal symptoms and gastric emptying in patients with Parkinson's disease. Mov Disord 1997;12:952–957.

66. McCallum RW. Cisapride: a new class of prokinetic agent. The ACG Committee on FDA-related matters. American College of Gastroenterology. Am J Gastroenterol 1991;86:135–149.
67. Neira WD, Sanchez V, Mena MA, de Yebenes JG. The effects of cisapride on plasma L-dopa levels and clinical response in Parkinson's disease. Mov Disord 1995;10:66–70.
68. Sempere AP, Duarte J, Cabezas C, et al. Aggravation of parkinsonian tremor by cisapride. Clin Neuropharmacol 1995;18:76–78.
69. Cameron A, Rosenfeld J. Nutritional issues and supplements in amyotrophic lateral sclerosis and other neurodegenerative disorders. Curr Opin Clin Nutr Metab Care 2002;5:631–643.
70. Sage JI, Trooskin S, Schuh L, et al. Isolated jejunal pouches for levodopa delivery in parkinsonian patients with "on-off." Successful experimental model in dogs. Clin Neuropharmacol 1988;11:212–220.
71. Miller RW, Kurlan R, Wyatt JD, Gash DM. A jejunal pouch technique in the rhesus monkey and related clinical observations. J Med Primatol 1992;21:366–370.
72. McCallum RW, Chen JD, Lin Z, et al. Gastric pacing improves emptying and symptoms in patients with gastroparesis. Gastroenterology 1998;114:456–461.
73. GEMS Study Group. Long-term results of gastric stimulation four times higher than the slow wave frequency in patients with drug refractory gastroparesis. Gastroenterology 1999;116:G4131.
74. Bortolotti M. The "electrical way" to cure gastroparesis. Am J Gastroenterol 2002;97:1874–1883.
75. Lacy BE, Zayat EN, Crowell MD, Schuster MM. Botulinum toxin for the treatment of gastroparesis: a preliminary report. Am J Gastroenterol 2002;97:1548–1552.

9
Intestinal Dysfunction

Ronald F. Pfeiffer

SUMMARY

Intestinal involvement in Parkinson's disease (PD) has been known since James Parkinson's initial description of the disease in 1817. Relatively little attention has been directed toward small intestinal dysfunction in PD, but some evidence has accumulated that small intestinal motility may indeed be impaired in PD. However, the clinical consequences of any such dysfunction have not been clearly delineated. Much more information is available regarding colonic and anorectal dysfunction in the PD setting. Diminished bowel movement frequency, presumably reflecting colonic dysmotility with consequent slowed colonic transit, is present in a significant percentage of individuals with PD, reported figures ranging from 20 to 77%. Anorectal dysfunction, characterized by both excessive straining and a sense of incomplete emptying, develops even more frequently in PD, affecting more than 60% of patients with PD. Both central and enteric nervous system dysfunction may have a role in the generation of these intestinal and anorectal abnormalities. Recognition of two components of intestinal dysfunction in PD—slow-transit constipation and anorectal defecatory dysfunction—will hopefully open the therapeutic door to more specific and effective treatment for these troubling and occasionally disabling features of PD.

Key Words: Parkinson's disease; intestinal dysfunction; postprandial pattern; interdigestive pattern; colonic dysmotility; constipation; defecatory dysfunction; colon transit time; anorectal dysfunction; anorectal manometry.

1. INTRODUCTION

James Parkinson indicated quite clearly his awareness of intestinal dysfunction in the setting of Parkinson's disease (PD) in his remarkable 1817 treatise, *An Essay on the Shaking Palsy.* In addition to characterizing other gastrointestinal (GI) features of PD, his description of bowel dysfunction codifies in crystal clarity both constipation ("the bowels which had all along been torpid, now in most cases, demand stimulating medications of very considerable power") and defecatory dysfunction ("the expulsion of the feces from the rectum sometimes requiring mechanical aid"; [*1*]).

However, little else was placed in print regarding Parkinsonian intestinal dysfunction in the post-Parkinson neurological literature until 1965, when Eadie and Tyrer published their analysis of GI dysfunction in 107 patients with Parkinsonism. Of these, 76 had been diagnosed with idiopathic PD, whereas the majority of the remainder carried a diagnosis of postencephalitic Parkinsonism *(2)*. A group of comparably aged persons with "acute orthopedic" disorders served as controls. Constipation (no distinction was made between decreased frequency and dysfunctional defecation), along with other GI features, such as difficulty chewing, drooling, dysphagia, and frequent "heartburn," were noted to be present more often in individuals with Parkinsonism than in controls.

Then in 1991, when Edwards and colleagues published their survey of 98 patients with PD and 50 comparably aged spousal controls *(3),* additional information regarding GI dysfunction in PD became

From: *Current Clinical Neurology*
Parkinson's Disease and Nonmotor Dysfunction
Edited by: R. F. Pfeiffer and I. Bodis-Wollner © Humana Press Inc., Totowa, NJ

available. The GI features they identified closely parallel those described by both Eadie and Tyrer and Parkinson himself, including disordered salivation (drooling), dysphagia, nausea, constipation (decreased bowel movement frequency), and defecatory dysfunction (difficulty with the actual act of defecation). In a series of subsequent reports that focus largely (although not exclusively) on bowel dysfunction in PD, these authors further investigated, cataloged, and characterized this surprisingly common, yet complex and troublesome aspect of PD *(4–12)*. Recent years have witnessed a sustained and ever-growing literature on the subject of intestinal dysfunction in PD with the primary focus clearly on colonic and anorectal abnormalities. This bowel-focused literature is reviewed in this chapter, along with a brief review of the scarce literature regarding small intestinal function in PD.

2. SMALL INTESTINE

2.1. *Anatomy and Physiology*

The intestine is divided into two primary components—the small and large intestine (or colon)—which possess definite similarities, but also serve clearly different functions. In adults, the small intestine reaches the rather astounding length of approximately 6 m *(13)* and is divided into three segments: duodenum, jejunum, and ileum. The small intestine is responsible for absorption of nutrients, salt, and water. Motility within the small intestine is produced by contractions of the circular and longitudinal muscle layers that compose the intestinal walls. Interstitial cells of Cajal, which are part of the enteric nervous system (ENS), generate electrical slow waves that serve a pacemaker function and migrate in an aborad direction. When spike bursts are superimposed on a slow wave, actual muscle contraction occurs, which then travels for an undetermined (but probably short) distance in either direction along the small intestine.

Two distinct patterns of small intestinal motor function have been identified *(14)*. The fed (postprandial) pattern, which appears within 10 to 20 minutes following a meal, is characterized by more segmental, and consequently less propulsive, contractions that assist in the mixing of digestive enzymes with the chyme and maximize mucosal contact, thus promoting nutrient absorption. The second pattern, the fasting (interdigestive) pattern, appears 4 to 6 hours after a meal and is divided into three phases. First is a period of relative motor quiescence, followed by increasingly prominent contractions in the subsequent two phases that presumably serve to "flush" solid residues from the small intestine into the colon, preventing bezoar formation and minimizing bacterial accumulation within the small intestine. This complex pattern of small intestinal motility is under the direct control of the ENS, but it is modulated by both autonomic and hormonal influences.

2.2. *Small Intestinal Dysfunction in PD*

Little attention has been focused on whether any changes in small intestinal function occur in the setting of PD. Thorough assessment of small intestinal function is rendered very difficult because of its inaccessibility and length; undoubtedly, this has discouraged dedicated investigation. However, some information is available.

Orocecal transit time was shown to be markedly prolonged in 15 patients with PD when compared with 15 age- and sex-matched control individuals *(15)*. Yet, it must be recognized that this investigative method is a measure of combined gastric and small intestinal transit and does not assess small intestinal function in isolation. Small intestinal manometry has also been employed in the study of patients with PD, and abnormalities in small intestinal motor patterns have been demonstrated *(16)*. Small intestinal dilatation has also been observed radiographically *(17)*. In the laboratory, disruption of the migrating myoelectric complex has been documented in rats following administration of 1-methyl-4-phenyl-1,2,3,6-tetrahydropyridine (MPTP), along with the reduction in jejunal myenteric plexus dopamine levels *(18)*. Studies that evaluate whether similar changes occur in PD have not been undertaken.

The clinical consequences of small intestinal dysfunction in PD, if it indeed occurs, have not been systematically investigated. Some individuals with PD experience a very uncomfortable abdominal bloating sensation, which is sufficiently severe at times to compel the anguished individual to loosen trousers, even when they are clearly not even tight. This typically develops during "off" periods and resolves with the re-emergence of levodopa benefit. It is conceivable that this uncomfortable sensation might be related to small intestinal dysmotility, but no study has actually addressed this issue. If there is an association, agents that accelerate small intestinal transit time (e.g., the serotonin-4 receptor agonist prucalopride; *19*) might provide symptomatic relief for patients with these symptoms. Another potential consequence of delayed small intestinal transit might be an alteration in intestinal nutrient absorption. However, this also has not been studied.

3. COLON

3.1. Anatomy and Physiology

The colon, approximately 1.0 to 1.5 m in length in adults, is composed of the same two muscle layers—circular and longitudinal—found in the small intestine *(13,20)*. The ileocecal valve, which divides the colon from the small intestine, is not a true sphincter but still effectively regulates colonic filling and prevents colo-ileal reflux. The colon stores material marked for excretion and performs an important role in the regulation of fluid, electrolyte, and short-chain fatty acid absorption. It can increase fluid absorption up to fivefold in appropriate circumstances. As in the stomach and small intestine, ICCs perform a pacemaker function in the generation of pressure waves that regulate colonic motility. Motor control of colonic motility is mostly mediated directly through the ENS with modulation via the autonomic nervous system. Parasympathetic innervation of the ascending and transverse colon is vagal in origin, whereas the descending and rectosigmoid regions receive their innervation by the pelvic nerves. Sympathetic supply to the colon originates in the thoracic spinal cord and reaches the colon via the inferior mesenteric and pelvic plexuses. Sympathetic activity produces the vasoconstriction of mucosal and submucosal blood vessels, downregulates motility, and inhibits secretion (thus, limiting water loss); parasympathetic activity increases enteric motor activity and colonic motility *(20)*.

3.2. Colonic Dysfunction in PD

To the lay public, constipation is a somewhat nonspecific term that may connote both decreased bowel movement frequency (usually with hard stool) and difficulty completing a bowel movement, often with excessive straining, sometimes with inability to evacuate fecal contents entirely, and occasionally with associated pain *(21)*. However, these two problems are actually quite different, with distinctive physiology and clinical characteristics; hence, a separate classification and discussion of each is needed to fully understand bowel dysfunction in PD. Decreased bowel movement frequency is primarily a consequence of colonic dysmotility and is discussed in this section, whereas defecatory dysfunction is primarily an anorectal anomaly and is discussed in the following section.

Divergence between the public concept and formal medical definition of what constitutes normal bowel movement frequency has also evolved in recent years, representing a source of confusion and sometimes consternation, both within the literature and inside the clinic. In the past, it was standard to label anything less frequent than a daily bowel movement as abnormal, constituting constipation, and this continues to be the concept embraced by many patients, particularly the elderly. The current formal medical boundary of constipation (or colonic inertia), however, has been redefined as fewer than three bowel movements weekly. Recently, some investigators have employed an even more strict definition of constipation as one or fewer evacuations per week *(22,23)*. Clinicians realize that not all patients are willing to accept the medical establishment's wisdom in this regard. To further complicate matters, the observation has also been made that estimations of bowel movement frequency reported by patients often conflict with their own diary records, typically in the direction of underestimating frequency *(24)*.

Recognition of this change in what actually constitutes normal bowel movement frequency is important when reviewing reports in the medical literature of constipation in PD. Estimates of the percentage of patients with PD experiencing constipation have descended from the 50–67% range of earlier reports to levels of 20–29% in more current publications. In 1958, Schwab and England reported the presence of constipation in two-thirds of their patients *(25)*, whereas in 1965, Eadie and Tyrer noted that 51% of their study sample of patients with PD did not have daily bowel movements, compared with 13% of their controls with orthopedic disease *(2)*. They also reported that over 50% of their patients were using laxatives on a regular basis. In notable contrast, using a definition of constipation as fewer than three bowel movements per week, Edwards and colleagues reported in 1991 that the presence of constipation in only 29% of their 98 patients with PD in comparison to 10% of their spousal controls *(3)*. Siddiqui and colleagues found its presence in only 20% of patients with PD in their 2002 survey report *(26)*. In contrast, in a group of patients with PD studied recently by Stocchi and colleagues, bowel movement frequency of fewer than three times per week was described by 77% of the 17 patients *(27)*. The explanation for this divergence is not readily apparent.

In survey studies, the presence of constipation in PD has correlated with disease duration and severity *(2,28)*. However, in clinical practice, it is not unusual for patients with PD to recollect the development of some degree of bowel dysfunction even prior to the appearance of more typical motor features of PD *(7)*. Constipation occuring early in the course of PD has also been documented by Bassotti and colleagues *(22)*.

Derived from data accumulated in the Honolulu Heart Program study, a recent report has propelled this a step further by suggesting that diminished bowel movement frequency may actually constitute a risk factor for PD development *(29)*. An association was documented between the frequency of bowel movements and risk of developing PD. Men who reported a bowel movement frequency of less than one per day were found to have a risk of developing PD that was 2.7 times greater than men who had daily bowel movements and fourfold higher than those with two or more bowel daily movements. Although these findings may simply reflect the fact that the appearance of constipation can precede the emergence of conventional PD motor features, it is worth noting that a bowel movement frequency of less than one per day does not actually even represent constipation by current definition. Therefore, other hypothetical explanations might (and perhaps should) also be advanced. Perhaps rapid transit of material through the GI tract, implied by frequent bowel movements, limits the exposure to, and absorption of, toxic substances capable of damaging dopaminergic neurons. Further studies investigating this possibility might prove to be very interesting and informative.

Considerable evidence has now accumulated that implicates slowed colon transit of fecal material as the physiological basis for decreased bowel movement frequency in PD. Employing radiopaque markers, colon transit studies have indicated that as many as 80% of persons with PD may have abnormally prolonged transit times *(30)*. Jost and Schimrigk initially reported an average colon transit time (CTT) of 5 to 7 days (120–168 hours) in a group of 20 persons with PD *(30)*, and in a subsequent study of 22 subjects in whom CTT could be measured, the average time was 130 hours *(31)*. Edwards and colleagues also documented slowed CTT in a study of 13 participants with PD, but the CTT they documented was considerably shorter than that noted by Jost and Schimrigk, finding a mean of 44 hours when compared with 20 hours in spousal controls *(6)*. A more recent study further confirms that CTT is slowed in PD, but the times reported (82.4 minutes in patients with PD and 39 minutes in controls) appear to be incorrectly labeled in minutes instead of hours *(32)*. Therefore, despite the variance in average CTT in published reports, there seems to be ample agreement that CTT is prolonged in PD. The reason for the widely varying CTTs reported by various investigators is not clearly evident.

In addition to the earlier survey studies, another study by Jost and Schimrigk in recently diagnosed patients with PD seems to support the idea that constipation becomes more severe as PD progresses. In this study, the average CTT in patients with PD was 89 hours *(33)* in comparison to the considerably longer CTTs reported in their earlier studies cited previously, which included individuals with more advanced disease.

Prolongation of CTT in untreated individuals strongly suggests that it develops as part of the disease process itself; yet, the demonstration by Ashraf and colleagues shows that not all persons with prolonged CTT experience clinically symptomatic constipation. This evidence seems to indicate that delayed CTT may not be the sole determining factor for stool frequency *(34)*. Other factors certainly may have a role in the genesis of constipation in some individuals, but it is not clear what these factors might be. Medications—not only anticholinergic drugs but also levodopa and dopaminergic agonists—may be responsible for diminished bowel movement frequency in some individuals, but not all individuals with PD who experience constipation are receiving these medications.

The pathophysiologic basis of constipation in PD has not been definitively defined. Evidence has accumulated for both central and peripheral mechanisms; it is very probable that both are involved.

Animal studies that employ dopaminergic agents have demonstrated that activation of central D1 and D2 receptors stimulates colonic motility by increasing colonic spike bursts *(35)*. In these studies performed in rats, Bueno and colleagues found that intracerebroventricular injection of the selective D1 agonist, (+)SCH 23390, the selective D2 agonist, quinpirole, and dopamine itself increased the frequency of colonic spike bursts (indicating increased colonic motility) by 54.8, 68.7, and 48.7%, respectively. Additional evidence favoring a central site of action was provided by the absence of any change in colonic spike burst frequency when these agents were injected intraperitoneally. It has been suggested that CNS influences on both bladder and colonic function may be coordinated through Barrington's nucleus (also known as the pontine micturition center), which lies adjacent to, or possibly within *(36)*, the locus coeruleus in the pons *(32,37–39)*. Utilizing the pseudorabies virus, Pavcovich and colleagues were able to demonstrate transynaptic labeling from the distal colon of neurons in Barrington's nucleus *(37)*. Using similar techniques, other investigators have identified additional sites within the CNS as being potentially involved with the central regulation of colonic function, including neurons within the dorsal motor nucleus of the vagus, nucleus of the solitary tract, nucleus ambiguous, and area postrema *(39)*. Also, it appears that the colonic connections with Barrington's nucleus travel via bulbospinal pathways, whereas connections with the other medullary nuclei are mediated through vagal pathways *(39)*.

Evidence favoring a peripheral basis for slowed colonic transit in PD has arisen in recent years as well. Numerous investigators have noted changes within the ENS in PD. In 1987, Kupsky and colleagues were the first to document the presence of Lewy bodies in the colonic myenteric and submucosal plexuses of individuals with PD *(40)*. This was subsequently confirmed by several other groups *(41–43)*, who found Lewy bodies in both dopaminergic neurons and in those containing vasoactive intestinal peptide. Using immunohistochemical methods, Singaram and colleagues *(43)* studied colon tissue removed from 11 persons with PD, 9 at the time of colectomy undertaken for intractable constipation, and 2 at autopsy. Lewy bodies were primarily evident in myenteric neurons and only rarely in the submucosal plexus. With immunohistochemical methods, Singaram and colleagues were also able to demonstrate a very striking reduction in the number of dopaminergic neurons in the colonic myenteric plexus of patients with PD in comparison to both healthy controls and individuals with idiopathic constipation *(43)*.

Other abnormalities within colonic tissue have also been documented in individuals with constipation owing to problems other than PD. Serotonin receptor immunoreactivity was recently found to be reduced in colonic tissue (specifically, the left colon) of patients who underwent subtotal colectomy for treatment of colonic inertia when compared with those where colectomy was performed for colon carcinoma *(44)*. Other studies of patients with chronic idiopathic intestinal pseudo-obstruction or slow transit constipation have shown a marked pan-colonic loss of ICC, which are believed to function as pacemaker cells in the gut *(45,46)*. Whether these abnormalities are also present in patients with PD suffering from constipation is unknown.

3.3. *Treatment of Colonic Dysmotility*

The treatment of slow-transit constipation in PD can be difficult and frustrating, both for the patient and physician. Formal studies in this patient population are largely lacking with the consequence that treatment is mostly based on clinical experience rather than rigorous clinical investigation *(47)*. In fact, treatment of Parkinsonian constipation has generally simply mirrored practices that are employed in treating idiopathic constipation, and only recently some clinical trials focusing on patients with PD have been carried out. Increased dietary fiber reduces CTT in normal individuals *(48),* most likely by increasing bulk within the colonic lumen. In their survey study, Edwards and colleagues *(3)* had each participant complete a food frequency dietary questionnaire that permitted calculation of the average daily intake of dietary components, including fiber. They found that the mean daily fiber intake in patients with PD was noticeably lower (11 g in untreated patients; 14 g in those on anti-Parkinsonian therapy) than the 15 to 20 g generally recommended *(3,49).* However, no distinction was made between constipated and nonconstipated individuals regarding fiber intake. In one of the few formal controlled clinical trials performed to date in PD patients, psyllium was found to be effective in increasing stool weight and frequency, but did not alter CTT *(34).* Improved motor function, presumably reflecting increased levodopa bioavailability, has also been documented with increased fiber intake *(50).* Fiber supplementation can also be achieved by concoctions of high-fiber foodstuffs (e.g., a combination of applesauce, unprocessed wheat bran, and prune juice) consumed on a daily basis. It is important to couple increased fiber consumption with adequate fluid intake in treating constipation. A 15-g daily fiber intake, along with at least 1.5 L of water, has been recommended *(49).* Adding a stool softener (e.g., docusate) can also be useful.

If increased fiber and fluid intake does not sufficiently control constipation, an osmotic laxative, such as lactulose or sorbitol, can be a very useful next step. These agents increase colonic osmotic pressure, which results in increased water content, and consequently bulk of, the stool. A 30-mL lactulose dose once or twice daily can be used initially with subsequent downward titration of dosage if necessary. Because sorbitol is less expensive than lactulose, it might be considered as a cost-effective alternative *(51).* More recently, the effectiveness of polyethylene glycol electrolyte-balanced solutions has been demonstrated in patients with PD *(52,53).* Its routine use in large volumes as a colon-cleansing agent prior to colonoscopy is well-established, but in PD it can be administered on a regular or even daily basis in much smaller amounts than those used in conjunction with colonoscopy.

Patients often turn to irritant laxatives, such as senna-containing compounds, which are available without prescription for relief from constipation. These compounds are often effective, but daily use should be discouraged because of concern regarding potential myenteric plexus injury as a consequence of extended use, even though such damage has not actually been definitively proven. When other measures fail, enemas can be administered as necessary to the patient suffering from PD with severe constipation.

The value of prokinetic agents in the treatment of slow-transit constipation is uncertain. Cisapride was reported to be beneficial in initial short-term studies in patients with PD, but it was less convincingly effective in long-term studies *(54,55).* Moreover, cisapride is no longer available because of the potential risk of cardiotoxicity. Prucalopride, a serotonin-4 agonist, has more recently been shown to be effective as a prokinetic agent in patients with severe chronic constipation *(19,56),* but its effect in individuals with PD has not been specifically reported. Anecdotal reports have described the efficacy of the cholinomimetic agents, pyridostigmine *(57)* and neostigmine *(58),* in the treatment of constipation in PD, but no formal studies of these compounds have been reported. In these reports, pyridostigmine was taken orally, whereas neostigmine was administered intravenously. The efficacy of neurotrophin-3 in a small double-blind study of patients suffering from PD with constipation has been reported in abstract form *(59).* Misoprostol, an analog of prostaglandin, can stimulate colonic motility, particularly in the left colon, and has been reported to be effective in alleviating chronic constipation. However, it has not been specifically studied in patients with PD *(60).* Colchicine has also been anecdotally reported to be effective in treating constipation in PD *(61).*

Potentially life-threatening complications of slow-transit constipation in PD include megacolon *(17,49,62,63),* intestinal pseudoobstruction, volvulus, and even bowel perforation *(3,8,62,63).* Surgical treatment in the form of colectomy may be necessary in such situations.

4. ANORECTUM

4.1. Anatomy and Physiology

The rectum is a storage reservoir in which feces are held until a convenient opportunity occurs to evacuate its contents. The internal and external anal sphincter muscles are tonically contracted, thus preventing leakage of rectal matter as feces accumulate. The longitudinal smooth muscle layer, which in the colon had been concentrated into the muscle bands called *taenia,* spreads out in the rectum into an encircling sheath. The internal anal sphincter (IAS) consists of smooth muscle that is continuous with the circular muscle layer of the rectum *(20).* In contrast, the external anal sphincter (EAS) is a band of striated muscle distal to the IAS. The IAS is under autonomic control via the pelvic plexus; the EAS is controlled by motor neurons in the sacral spinal cord through the pudendal nerve. The puborectalis muscle is also thought by many to contribute to the maintenance of fecal continence by means of tonic contraction that pulls the rectum anteriorly, forming an anorectal angle of approximately 90–95 degrees that impedes rectal emptying *(64,65).* The anorectal angle formed by puborectalis contraction may be especially important for the retention of semisolid (as opposed to liquid) material *(66).* The erect position may provide an additional contribution to the maintenance of fecal continence by further sharpening the anorectal angle to about 80 degrees *(65).* Although it should be noted that the importance of this anorectal angle in the maintenance of continence is not universally accepted *(64,67).*

The act of defecation is characterized by relaxation of the two anal sphincters and the puborectalis muscle, which results in a straightening or opening of the anorectal angle. Also, it is defined by contraction of the glottic, diaphragmatic, and abdominal wall muscles, which elevates intra-abdominal pressure and encourages evacuation of the rectal contents.

4.2. Anorectal Dysfunction in PD

Anorectal dysfunction, characterized by excessive straining, often with a sense of incomplete evacuation and sometimes pain, is actually the more prevalent form of bowel dysfunction in PD. Edwards and colleagues *(3)* differentiated between decreased bowel movement frequency and defecatory dysfunction and noted the latter in 67% of patients with PD, compared with only 29% who reported decreased bowel movement frequency. As with slow-transit constipation, anorectal dysfunction can also appear early in the course of PD *(22).*

Clinical neurophysiological and radiographical studies have shed considerable light on the pathophysiological basis for disordered defecation in PD. The act of defecation is not solely dependent on sphincter and puborectalis relaxation, but also demands the coordinated contraction of numerous additional muscles and muscle groups while the sphincters relax to effectively accomplish evacuation. It is now clear from studies, such as anorectal manometry, anorectal electromyography, and defecography, that this does not always occur in individuals with PD, and dyscoordination may actually be the rule. In one study, abdominopelvic (or pelvic floor) dyssynergia was present in over 60% of patients with PD *(22).*

Lower basal sphincter pressure and difficulty maintaining sphincter pressure have been documented during anorectal manometry in patients with PD, as have some more distinctive abnormalities, including unusual phasic contractions of the sphincter muscles during voluntary contraction and a "paradoxical" hypercontractile response of the external anal sphincter and puborectalis muscles on rectosphincteric (rectoanal inhibitory) reflex testing, where sphincter relaxation (rather than contraction) is expected *(6,68,69).* These abnormalities of anorectal muscle function appear to be distinctive for PD, not simply a general reflection of constipation. Ashraf and colleagues studied 15 patients with PD, 9 persons with idiopathic constipation, and 8 control individuals and found these abnormalities only in the patients with PD *(70).*

Failure of the EAS and puborectalis muscles to relax during attempted defecation, producing functional outlet obstruction, was originally observed in patients with PD by Mathers and colleagues *(71,72)* and subsequently confirmed by others *(6).* It has been suggested that this is a focal dystonic phenomenon *(71,72).* Moreover, fluctuation in the severity of the anorectal abnormalities in response to dopaminergic medications has been documented with deterioration during "off" periods and improvement in function when patients are "on" *(68)*. However, paradoxical sphincter and puborectalis contraction during attempted defecation may also occur in healthy controls, leading some investigators to question its correlation with difficult defecation *(73,74)*.

Evaluation of defecation with rectoanal videomanometry has provided objective confirmation of the subjective sense of incomplete emptying during defecation that is experienced in many patients with PD by demonstrating that incomplete defecation with the presence of significant postdefecation residuals is common in PD *(32)*. Dynamic transperineal ultrasound has recently been reported to be a simple and accurate method for evaluating the pelvic floor in individuals with defecatory dysfunction *(75)*. This technique has not yet been applied in the study of patients who have PD.

4.3. Treatment of Anorectal Dysfunction

It is important to recognize and differentiate anorectal difficulties from colonic inertia when assessing bowel dysfunction in patients with PD. Although softening the stool by various measures will make it easier to expel, such measures do not correct the fundamental defect in muscular coordination that produces the problem. In fact, laxatives and other measures that hasten the arrival of stool to the rectum may sometimes accentuate the problem, creating a situation that might be likened to a frantic crowd trying to leave a burning building through a narrow, or even blocked, exit. Unfortunately, the array of treatment options for anorectal dysfunction is somewhat limited.

Some evidence suggests that dopaminergic medications may improve anorectal function in individuals with PD. As noted previously, improvement in anorectal manometric and electromyographic measures of anorectal function during "on" periods with deterioration during "off" episodes has been described *(68)*. Additionally, Mathers and colleagues found some degree of improvement in both electromyographic and proctographic measures of anorectal function following apomorphine injections in most of the patients they studied *(72)*, as did Edwards and colleagues in some (but not all) of the eight patients who had PD, they studied with apomorphine *(76)*. Occasional patients on levodopa will also report that it is easier for them to have a bowel movement when they are "on" than when they are "off."

Albanese and colleagues have pioneered yet another approach to treat outlet obstruction-type constipation in PD, successfully injecting botulinum toxin into the puborectalis muscle under transrectal ultrasonographic guidance *(77,78)*. In their recently reported full study *(78)*, 18 patients received the injections and were evaluated by means of anorectal manometry, defecography, and electromyography at baseline and at 1 and 2 months following the injections. Resting anal tone and maximum voluntary contraction were unchanged, but anal tone during straining was reduced, and the anorectal angle during straining was widened. The duration of benefit was not clearly defined, but improvement in test parameters was still evident at the 2-month mark. In their earlier case report *(77)*, improvement had waned by 12 weeks. Although these results are encouraging, the risk for producing fecal incontinence is present with this procedure, and perianal thrombosis has also been reported *(79)*.

Behavioral techniques, such as defecation training and biofeedback measures, have been successfully employed in the treatment of outlet obstruction constipation *(80,81)*, but they have not been specifically examined in patients who have PD. Sacral nerve stimulation is a technique that might also conceivably have some application in patients with PD, but this also has not yet been evaluated. Surgical treatment (e.g., colectomy) is rarely necessary in patients with PD.

5. CONCLUSION

As awareness of the nonmotor features of PD has grown in recent years, it has become quite clear that intestinal dysfunction poses a significant problem for a considerable number of patients with PD. Understanding of the pathophysiological basis for this dysfunction is expanding, and more effective management measures are evolving. Recognition and definition of the two components of Parkinsonian bowel dysfunction—slow-transit constipation and anorectal defecatory dysfunction—is beginning to foster the development of more effective management measures. However, much more remains to be learned.

REFERENCES

1. Parkinson J. An Essay on the Shaking Palsy. Whittingham and Rowland, London, 1817.
2. Eadie MJ, Tyrer JH. Alimentary disorder in Parkinsonism. Aust Ann Med 1965;14:13–22.
3. Edwards LL, Pfeiffer RF, Quigley EMM, et al. Gastrointestinal symptoms in Parkinson's disease. Mov Disord 1991;6:151–156.
4. Edwards LL, Quigley EMM, Hofman R, Pfeiffer RF. Gastrointestinal dysfunction in Parkinson's disease: frequency and pathophysiology. Neurology 1992;42:726–732.
5. Edwards LL, Quigley EMM, Hofman R, Pfeiffer RF. Gastrointestinal symptoms in Parkinson's disease: 18 month follow-up study. Mov Disord 1993;8:83–86.
6. Edwards LL, Quigley EMM, Harned RK, et al. Characterization of swallowing and defecation in Parkinson's disease. Am J Gastroenterol 1994;89:15–25.
7. Pfeiffer RF, Quigley EMM. Gastrointestinal motility problems in patients with Parkinson's disease: epidemiology, pathophysiology and guidelines for management. CNS Drugs 1999;11:435–438.
8. Quigley EMM. Gastrointestinal dysfunction in Parkinson's disease. Semin Neurol 1996;16:245–250.
9. Quigley EMM. Epidemiology and pathophysiology of gastrointestinal manifestations in Parkinson's disease. In: Corazziari E, ed. NeUroGastroenterology. deGruyter, Berlin, 1996, pp. 167–178.
10. Pfeiffer RF. Gastrointestinal dysfunction in Parkinson's disease. Clin Neurosci 1998;5:136–146.
11. Quigley EMM. Gastrointestinal features. In: Factor SA, Weiner WJ, eds. Parkinson's Disease. Diagnosis and Clinical Management. Demos, New York, 2002, pp. 87–93.
12. Pfeiffer RF. Gastrointestinal dysfunction in Parkinson's disease. Lancet. Neurol 2003;2:107–116.
13. Keljo DJ, Gariepy CE. Anatomy, histology, embryology, and developmental anomalies of the small and large intestine. In: Feldman M, Friedman LS, Sleisenger MH, eds. Sleisenger and Fordtran's Gastrointestinal and Liver Disease, 7th ed. Saunders, Philadelphia, 2002, pp. 1643–1663.
14. Andrews JM, Dent J. Small intestinal motor physiology. In: Feldman M, Friedman LS, Sleisenger MH, eds. Sleisenger and Fordtran's Gastrointestinal and Liver Disease, 7th ed. Saunders, Philadelphia, 2002, pp. 1665–1678.
15. Davies KN, King D, Billington D, Barrett JA. Intestinal permeability and orocaecal transit time in elderly patients with Parkinson's disease. Postgrad Med J 1996;72:164–167.
16. Bozeman T, Anuras S, Hutton T, Mikeska C. Small intestinal manometry in Parkinson's disease. Gastroenterology 1990;99:(Abstract)1202.
17. Lewitan A, Nathanson L, Slade WR. Megacolon and dilatation of the small bowel in Parkinsonism. Gastroenterology 1952;17:367–374.
18. Eaker EY, Bixler GB, Dunn AJ, et al. Chronic alterations in jejunal myoelectric activity in rats due to MPTP. Am J Physiol 1987;253:G809–G815.
19. Emmanuel AV, Roy AJ, Nicholls TJ, Kamm MA. Prucalopride, a systemic enterokinetic, for the treatment of constipation. Aliment Pharmacol Ther 2002;16:1347–1356.
20. Cook IJ, Brookes SJ. Motility of the large intestine. In: Feldman M, Friedman LS, Sleisenger MH, eds. Sleisenger and Fordtran's Gastrointestinal and Liver Disease, 7th ed. Saunders, Philadelphia, 2002, pp. 1679–1691.
21. Stark ME. Challenging problems presenting as constipation. Am J Gastroenterol 1999;94:567–574.
22. Bassotti G, Maggio D, Battaglia E, et al. Manometric investigation of anorectal function in early and late stage Parkinson's disease. J Neurol Neurosurg Psychiatry 2000;68:768–770.
23. Bassotti G, Germani U, Fiorella S, et al. Intact colonic motor response to sudden awakening from sleep in patients with chronic idiopathic (slow-transit) constipation. Dis Colon Rectum 1998;41:1550–1556.
24. Ashraf W, Park F, Lof J, Quigley EM. An examination of reliability of reported stool frequency in the diagnosis of idiopathic constipation. Am J Gastroenterol 1996;91:26–32.
25. Schwab RS, England AC. Parkinson's disease. J Chron Dis 1958;8:488–509.
26. Siddiqui MF, Rast S, Lynn MJ, et al. Autonomic dysfunction in Parkinson's disease: a comprehensive symptom survey. Parkinsonism Relat Disord 2002;8:277–284.
27. Stocchi F, Badiali D, Vacca L, et al. Anorectal function in multiple system atrophy and Parkinson's disease. Mov Disord 2000;15:71–76.
28. Sakakibara R, Shinotoh H, Uchiyama T, et al. Questionnaire-based assessment of pelvic organ dysfunction in Parkinson's disease. Auton Neurosci 2001;92:76–85.
29. Abbott RD, Petrovitch H, White LR, et al. Frequency of bowel movements and the future risk of Parkinson's disease. Neurology 2001;57:456–462.
30. Jost WH, Schimrigk K. Constipation in Parkinson's disease. Klin Wochenschr 1991;69:906–909.
31. Jost WH, Schimrigk K. The effect of cisapride on delayed colon transit time in patients with idiopathic Parkinson's disease. Wien Klin Wochenschr 1994;106:673–676.
32. Sakakibara R, Odaka T, Uchiyama T, et al. Colonic transit time and rectoanal videomanometry in Parkinson's disease. J Neurol Neurosurg Psychiatry 2003;74:268–272.
33. Jost WH, Schrank B. Defecatory disorders in de novo parkinsonians—colonic transit and electromyogram of the external anal sphincter. Wien Klin Wochenschr 1998;110:535–537.

34. Ashraf W, Pfeiffer RF, Park F, et al. Constipation in Parkinson's disease: objective assessment and response to psyllium. Mov Disord 1997;12:946–951.
35. Bueno L, Gue M, Fabre C, Junien JL. Involvement of central dopamine and D1 receptors in stress-induced colonic motor alterations in rats. Brain Res Bull 1992;29:135–140.
36. Ding YQ, Zheng HX, Wang DS, et al. Localization of Barrington's nucleus in the pontine dorsolateral tegmentum of the rabbit. J Hirnforsch 1999;39:375–381.
37. Pavcovich LA, Yang M, Miselis RR, Valentino RJ. Novel role for the pontine micturition center, Barrington's nucleus: evidence for coordination of colonic and forebrain activity. Brain Res 1998;784:355–361.
38. Valentino RJ, Miselis RR, Pavcovich LA. Pontine regulation of pelvic viscera: pharmacological target for pelvic visceral dysfunctions. Trends Pharmacol Sci 1999;20:253–260.
39. Vizzard MA, Brisson M, de Groat WC. Transneuronal labeling of neurons in the adult rat central nervous system following inoculation of pseudorabies virus into the colon. Cell Tissue Res 2000;299:9–26.
40. Kupsky WJ, Grimes MM, Sweeting J, et al. Parkinson's disease and megacolon: concentric hyaline inclusions (Lewy bodies) in enteric ganglion cells. Neurology 1987;37:1253–1255.
41. Wakabayashi K, Takahashi H, Ohama E, Ikuta F. Parkinson's disease: an immunohistochemical study of Lewy-body containing neurons in the enteric nervous system. Acta Neuropathol 1990;79:581–583.
42. Wakabayashi K, Takahashi H, Ohama E, et al. Lewy bodies in the visceral autonomic nervous system in Parkinson's disease. In: Narabayashi H, Nagatsu T, Yanagisawa N, Mizuno Y, eds. Parkinson's Disease. From Basic Research to Treatment, Advances in Neurology, vol. 60. Raven Press, New York, 1993, pp. 609–612.
43. Singaram C, Ashraf W, Torbey C, et al. Dopaminergic defect of enteric nervous system in Parkinson's disease patients with chronic constipation. Lancet 1995;346:861–864.
44. Zhao RH, Baig MK, Thaler KJ, et al. Reduced expression of serotonin receptor(s) in the left colon of patients with colonic inertia. Dis Colon Rectum 2003;46:81–86.
45. Lyford GL, He CL, Soffer E, et al. Pan-colonic decrease in interstitial cells of Cajal in patients with slow transit constipation. Gut 2002;51:496–501.
46. Jain D, Moussa K, Tandon M, et al. Role of interstitial cells of Cajal in motility disorders of the bowel. Am J Gastroenterol 2003;98:618–624.
47. Wiesel PH, Norton C, Brazzelli M. Management of faecal incontinence and constipation in adults with central neurological diseases. Cochrane Database Syst Rev 2001;4:CD002115.
48. Müller-Lissner SA. Effect of wheat bran on weight of stool and gastrointestinal transit time: a meta-analysis. Br Med J 1988;296:615–617.
49. Corazziari E, Badiali D. Management of lower gastrointestinal tract dysfunction. Semin Neurol 1996;16:289–296.
50. Astarloa R, Mena MA, Sanchez V, et al. Clinical and pharmacokinetic effects of a diet rich in insoluble fiber on Parkinson's disease. Clin Neuropharmacol 1992;15:375–380.
51. Lederle FA, Busch DL, Mattox KM, et al. Cost-effective treatment of constipation in the elderly: a randomized double-blind comparison of sorbitol and lactulose. Am J Med 1990;89:597–601.
52. Corazziari E, Badiali D, Habib FI, et al. Small volume isosmotic polyethylene glycol electrolyte balanced solution (PMF-100) in treatment of chronic nonorganic constipation. Dig Dis Sci 1996;41:1636–1642.
53. Eichhorn TE, Oertel WH. Macrogol 3350/electrolyte improves constipation in Parkinson's disease and multiple system atrophy. Mov Disord 2001;16:1176–1177.
54. Jost WH, Schimrigk K. Cisapride treatment of constipation in Parkinson's disease. Mov Disord 1993;8:339–343.
55. Jost WH, Schimrigk K. Long-term results with cisapride in Parkinson's disease. Mov Disord 1997;12:423–425.
56. Coremans G, Kerstens R, De Pauw M, Stevens M. Prucalopride is effective in patients with severe chronic constipation in whom laxatives fail to provide adequate relief. Results of a double-blind, placebo-controlled clinical trial. Digestion 2003;67:82–89.
57. Sadjadpour K. Pyridostigmine bromide and constipation in Parkinson's disease. JAMA 1983;249:1148.
58. Koornstra JJ, Klaver NS, ter Maaten JC, et al. Neostigmine treatment of acute pseudo-obstruction of colon (Ogilvie syndrome). Ned Tijdschr Geneeskd 2001;145:586–589.
59. Pfeiffer RF, Markopoulou K, Quigley EM, et al. Effect of NT-3 on bowel function in Parkinson's disease. Mov Disord 2002;17(Abstract):S223–S224.
60. Roarty TP, Weber F, Soykan I, McCallum RW. Misoprostol in the treatment of chronic refractory constipation: results of a long-term open label trial. Aliment Pharmacol Ther 1997;11:1059–1066.
61. Sandyk R, Gillman MA. Colchicine ameliorates constipation in Parkinson's disease. J R Soc Med 1984;77:1066.
62. Caplan LH, Jacobson HG, Rubinstein BM, Rotman MZ. Megacolon and volvulus in Parkinson's disease. Radiology 1965;85:73–79.
63. Rosenthal MJ, Marshall CE. Sigmoid volvulus in association with Parkinsonism. Report of four cases. J Am Geriatr Soc 1987;35:683–684.
64. Madoff D, Williams JG, Caushaj PF. Fecal incontinence. N Engl J Med 1992;326:1002–1007.
65. Altomare DF, Rinaldi M, Veglia A, et al. Contribution of posture to the maintenance of anal continence. Int J Colorectal Dis 2001;16:51–54.

66. Hajivassiliou CA, Carter KB, Finlay IG. Anorectal angle enhances faecal continence. Br J Surg 1996;83:53–56.
67. Parks AG. Anorectal incontinence. Proc R Soc Med 1975;68:681–690.
68. Ashraf W, Wszolek ZK, Pfeiffer RF, et al. Anorectal function in fluctuating (on-off) Parkinson's disease: evaluation by combined anorectal manometry and electromyography. Mov Disord 1995;10:650–657.
69. Normand MM, Ashraf W, Quigley EM, et al. Simultaneous electromyography and manometry of the anal sphincters in parkinsonian patients: technical considerations. Muscle Nerve 1996;19:110–111.
70. Ashraf W, Pfeiffer RF, Quigley EMM. Anorectal manometry in the assessment of anorectal function in Parkinson's disease: a comparison with chronic idiopathic constipation. Mov Disord 1994;9:655–663.
71. Mathers SE, Kempster PA, Swash M, Lees AJ. Constipation and paradoxical puborectalis contraction in anismus and Parkinson's disease: a dystonic phenomenon? J Neurol Neurosurg Psychiatry 1988;51:1503–1507.
72. Mathers SE, Kempster PA, Law PJ, et al. Anal sphincter dysfunction in Parkinson's disease. Arch Neurol 1989;46:1061–1064.
73. Voderholzer WA, Neuhaus DA, Klauser AG, et al. Paradoxical sphincter contraction is rarely indicative of anismus. Gut 1997;41:258–262.
74. Schouten WR, Briel JW, Auwerda JJ, et al. Anismus: fact or fiction? Dis Colon Rectum 1997;40:1033–1041.
75. Beer-Gabel M, Teshler M, Schechtman E, Zbar AP. Dynamic transperineal ultrasound vs. defecography in patients with evacuatory difficulty: a pilot study. Int J Colorectal Dis 2004;19:60–67.
76. Edwards LL, Quigley EMM, Harned RK, et al. Defecatory function in Parkinson's disease: response to apomorphine. Ann Neurol 1993;33:490–493.
77. Albanese A, Maria G, Bentivoglio AR, et al. Severe constipation in Parkinson's disease relieved by botulinum toxin. Mov Disord 1997;12:764–766.
78. Albanese A, Brisinda G, Bentivoglio AR, Maria G. Treatment of outlet obstruction constipation in Parkinson's disease with botulinum neurotoxin A. Am J Gastroenterol 2003;98:1439–1440.
79. Jost WH, Schanne S, Mlitz H, Schimrigk K. Perianal thrombosis following injection therapy into the external anal sphincter using botulinum toxin. Dis Colon Rectum 1995;38:781.
80. McKee RF, McEnroe L, Anderson JH, Finlay IG. Identification of patients likely to benefit from biofeedback for outlet obstruction constipation. Br J Surg 1999;86:355–359.
81. Dailianas A, Skandalis N, Rimikis MN, et al. Pelvic floor study in patients with obstructive defecation: influence of biofeedback. J Clin Gastroenterol 2000;30:176–180.

10
Impaired Sexual Function

Cheryl Waters and Janice Smolowitz

SUMMARY

The incidence of impaired sexual function in adults with Parkinson's disease (PD) is greater than in the general population. Studies have examined different aspects of sexual function among adults with PD and their partners. Comparison groups have included healthy adults matched for age and gender, as well as age-matched controls with chronic, non-neurological disease with motor impairment. Impaired sexual function in PD is most likely multifactorial. Depression, physical disability, and autonomic dysfunction may contribute to the increased prevalence of erectile dysfunction (ED) in PD. Given this multifactorial basis, clinicians should routinely assess patient needs. In studies of men with PD, treatment with sildenafil significantly improved sexual satisfaction. Also, erection has been reported as a side effect of subcutaneous apomorphine treatment of resistant motor fluctuations. As a treatment for ED, sublingual apomorphine is available in Europe. For women with PD, therapeutic interventions and impaired sexual function have not been described. Further research is required to develop treatment for adults with PD and sexual dysfunction.

Key Words: Erectile dysfunction; hyposexuality; sexual dysfunction; reduced libido; sexual dissatisfaction; decreased sexual activity; impaired sexual function.

1. INTRODUCTION

Sexuality has been described as a holistic phenomenon that is different from and more than its physiological components *(1–3)*. Sexuality and sexual function are affected by the interaction of physiological, emotional, intellectual, spiritual, social, and cultural influences *(1–3)*. Sexual behavior and function change during the life cycle. Advancing age is correlated with a decline in sexual activity *(4,5)*. Sexuality is affected by life events, such as illness, which require lifestyle changes *(6)*. Sexual function may be altered by chronic illnesses, e.g., diabetes mellitus, heart disease, hypertension, and depression *(7)*. The presence of impaired sexual function has been found in adults with Parkinson's disease (PD; *8–17*) and will be the focus in this chapter. Reports on sexual function in the general population are briefly discussed to provide an overview of the research on patients who have PD with impaired sexual function. Its physiology is briefly explained as a basis for potential therapeutic interventions.

2. SEXUAL DYSFUNCTION IN THE GENERAL POPULATION

As mentioned previously, sexual dysfunction may result from emotional and physical illnesses, as well as increasing age, affecting relationships and quality of life *(7,18,19)*. In men, "the persistent inability to achieve or maintain an erection sufficient for satisfactory sexual performance" is defined as erectile dysfunction (ED; *20*). According to the National Health and Social Life Survey (NHSLS), a national probability study that included 1410 men between the ages of 18 and 59, the prevalence rates for ED were 7% for men 18 to 29, 9% for men 30 to 39, 11% for men 40 to 49, and 18% for men 50 to

From: *Current Clinical Neurology*
Parkinson's Disease and Nonmotor Dysfunction
Edited by: R. F. Pfeiffer and I. Bodis-Wollner © Humana Press Inc., Totowa, NJ

59 *(18)*. In the Massachusetts Male Aging study update, which included 847 noninstitutionalized men between the ages of 40 and 70, the prevalence of ED was 8% for men 40 to 49, 16% for men 50 to 59, and 37% for men 60 to 69 *(21)*. The age-adjusted risk of ED was higher for men with diabetes, heart disease, hypertension, and men with lower education. Studies conducted in the Netherlands, Spain, Germany, and Australia have reported prevalence rates of ED between 11% and 33.9% *(22–25)*.

Masters and Johnson characterized four sequential phases in the sexual response cycle: excitement, plateau, orgasm, and resolution *(26)*. A three-phase model consisting of desire, arousal, and orgasm was subsequently developed *(27)*. Female sexual impairment affects 30 to 50% of women in the United States and increases with age *(28–30)*. The NHSLS, which included 1749 women, found that 43% experienced sexual dysfunction *(18)*. Age and relationship status were strongly associated with sexual satisfaction: older women and singles more frequently reported sexual difficulty, and sexual arousal and lubrication diminished with age. A correlation was also found with socioeconomic status and educational level. The study indicated that low desire was more common in women with comorbid medical and psychiatric disorders.

3. SEXUAL DYSFUNCTION IN ADULTS WITH PD

Research examining this subject is limited. Studies have reported different aspects of sexual function and related variables using validated, self-report questionnaires and interviews in men and women with PD, couples with one spouse affected by PD, men with PD, and women with PD. Comparison groups have included healthy adults matched for age and gender, as well as age-matched controls with chronic, non-neurological disease with motor impairment. As yet, there are no studies with quantitative measures that objectively evaluate sexual function.

Three studies have analyzed sexual function in men and women with PD. One study included a comparison group of healthy adults matched for age and gender. Of this group, 36 men and 14 women with idiopathic PD and no evidence of mental deterioration completed a structured questionnaire that addressed sexual activity, function, and libido *(8)*. Mean age of participants was 57.9 years (standard deviation [SD] 10.1 years); mean disease duration was 7.01 years (SD 3.9 years). Sixty-eight percent of participants reported decreased sexual activity, and 26% described decreased libido. ED was reported in 38.8% of men and described more frequently in men over 61 years old.

To determine whether adults with PD differed in sexuality from similarly aged healthy adults, 121 adults with PD and 126 controls matched for age and gender participated in a study that compared opinions about public sexual attitudes, emotion from personal sexual practice, personal sexual function, and general health perception *(9)*. Adults with PD were recruited from a PD self-support organization and physicians' patient lists, and the controls were enlisted for participation from a community registry. A physician investigator examined the adults with PD and reviewed their medical records. The physician completed the motor portion of the Unified Parkinson's Disease Rating Scale (UPDRS; *31*) and the Hoehn and Yahr *(32)* score. Participants were interviewed about disease variables and sociodemographical data. In the presence of an investigator, participants completed a 33 item multiple-choice self-report questionnaire that addressed various aspects of sexuality *(33)*, a depression scale *(34)*, and the Wechsler Adult Intelligence scale *(35)* to measure the influence of education.

All subjects reported they were currently involved in heterosexual relationships. Frequency of intercourse did not differ between adults with PD and the controls. The average age of adults with PD was 45 years. Adults with PD reported greater disagreement with present attitudes about sexuality than did controls. Significantly more adults with PD were unemployed and depressed, and this group indicated greater dissatisfaction with their personal sexual lives than controls. Greater sexual discontent was described by adults with PD and concomitant depression than by nondepressed adults with PD. In men with PD, a higher level of dissatisfaction was reported in comparison to women. Depressed, unemployed adults with PD were more often unhappy with their current sexual relationship, felt lonely more often, and were less able to enjoy flirtation. The subjects with PD were less satisfied with their lives, felt older than their stated age, and perceived their health to be poorer than the controls.

Interviews with 25 patients with PD (15 men and 10 women) younger than age 56 were conducted to describe sexual function in a sample of young adults with PD *(10)*. The interview and physical examination were conducted by a female neurologist. Interview content discussed libido, sexual activity, orgasm, penile/vaginal sensibility, and changes in sexual activity owing to motor symptoms. Women were interviewed regarding vaginal dryness and pain, whereas ED was discussed with men. Both men and women were questioned about the influence of urinary incontinence on their sex lives and their partner's acceptance of their physical disability. Depression was measured with the Beck Depression Inventory (BDI; *36*).

The mean age of participants was 50.3 years, and the mean age of disease onset was 44.7 years. Libido changes were not statistically different between men and women, although women reported more marked changes in libido. More women reported changes in sexual activity than men. Causes of sexual dysfunction reported by men included ED (n = 3), reduced libido after the initiation of medication (n = 2), change in orgasm (n = 2), and lack of partner's acceptance (n = 1). Causes of sexual dysfunction reported by women included declined libido after the initiation of medication (n = 4), change in orgasm (n = 3), vaginal dryness (n = 3), sexual dysfunction from rigidity (n = 5), and lack of partner's acceptance (n = 1). Urinary incontinence was reported by four women and four men. Specifically, one woman reported major depression on the BDI; she was not sexually active. Of the participants in this sample, 55% of optimally treated patients with PD reported changes in sexual function.

There have been two studies that described the perceptions of patients and spouses pertaining to the affected partner's sexual ability and aspects of the couple's relationship *(11,12)*. Thirty-six men and 14 women with PD, along with their spouses, were recruited from a movement disorders clinic to participate in an investigation of the relationship of autonomic nervous system (ANS) dysfunction, depression, medication, motor disabilities, and sexual difficulties *(11)*. Patients and their spouses completed separate, self-report questionnaires and the Geriatric Depression Scale *(37)* as well as a questionnaire that addressed degree of sexual interest, arousal, and performance skills *(38)*. They also answered questions about medical history, medications, and symptoms of increased sweating, constipation, or urinary difficulty to evaluate ANS function. ANS dysfunction was defined as the minimum of two of the following symptoms: increased sweating, constipation, or urinary difficulty. Spouses completed a questionnaire regarding sexual interest, arousal, and performance of the affected spouse, as well as their own sexual interests.

Patient mean age was 67.3 years, and the mean duration of disease was 6.96 years. Of male patients, 88% stated that their sexual frequency had decreased since the PD diagnosis, and 44% reported reduced sexual interest and drive. Fifty-four percent were not able to achieve an erection; only 14% were able to maintain an erection. Depression was present in 19%, and sexual dysfunction was indicated in 1.7% of these patients. ANS dysfunction was prevalent in 69%, and of these, 70% reported problems with sexual function.

In female patients, 79% stated that their sexual frequency had decreased since diagnosis, 71% reported a decline in sexual interest, and 38% were unable to achieve orgasm. Vaginal dryness during intercourse was found in 38%, whereas 67% felt it was more difficult to be aroused. Frequency of orgasm was reduced since diagnosis in 75%. Depression was present in only one woman.

Of all the couples, 78% shared the same bed. A reduction in the affected partner's sexual interest was noted by 54% of the spouses, and 54% of spouses reported loss of interest in having sexual relations with their partner affected by PD.

Young-onset patients with PD and their spouses that attended a weekend residential meeting in the United Kingdom were surveyed to estimate the prevalence of sexual dysfunction in patients with PD and their partners. Participants were asked to describe the nature of sexual difficulties experienced, and the relationship between sexual dysfunction, psychological morbidity, psychosocial stress, physical disability, and ANS dysfunction *(12)*. A total of 44 couples attended the meeting; 34 couples and 4 spouses of patients who had PD participated in the study. Questionnaires were completed by 23 male and 11 female patients. Data describing age of PD onset, current medications, and physical disability were collected independently from the patient and partner. Sexual function was assessed by the

Golombok Rust Inventory of Sexual Satisfaction *(39),* a 28-item survey with male and female forms. Marital function was assessed using the Golombock Rust Inventory of Marital Status *(40).* Depression and anxiety in patients and spouses were reviewed with the BDI *(36)* and the State Trait Scale Anxiety Inventory *(41).* Patients completed an acceptance of illness scale *(42)* and their spouses completed a caregiver strain index *(43).* ANS dysfunction was rated on a questionnaire, and three neurologists rated the likelihood of ANS dysfunctionbased on these answers.

Male patients (mean age 51.9 years; SD 8.9 years) were notably older and had a later onset of disease than female patients (mean age 44.7 years; SD 7.2 years). A statistically significant difference was not found in the duration of illness or degree of disability for male and female patients. Sexual dissatisfaction and the perception that sexual problems existed were primarily in couples where the patient was male. Marital dissatisfaction was highest in male patients and their partners. BDI scores were highest in the male and female patient groups: 36% of the female patients and 29% of the male patients were depressed. Of female spouses, 15% were depressed, and female spouses demonstrated significantly greater trait anxiety than male spouses, ($p < 0.01$). Major differences were not demonstrated in caregiver strain and acceptance of illness. Regarding ANS, 39% of male and 54% of female patients were rated with possible or probable dysfunction.

Singer reported on ANS dysfunction, including sexual dysfunction, in 48 men with PD *(13,14).* The patients with PD were compared with 32 healthy elderly men. ED affected 60.4% of men with PD versus 37.5% of controls. ED was not associated with other autonomic features, duration of levodopa therapy, or age.

One study has compared the role of sexual function in men with PD with men who had arthritis *(15).* Sexual function and its relationship to age, PD severity, and depression was described in 41 married men with PD. The comparison group consisted of 29 married men with arthritis. Men with a history of dementia, illnesses, or use of medications known to cause impotence were excluded from participation. Men with PD were recruited from three neurology clinics; men with arthritis were recruited from arthritis clinics at the same three hospitals. Providers of participants who had PD rated the patients' stage of disease using the Hoehn and Yahr scale *(32)* and Columbia Parkinson scale *(44).* Providers of patients with arthritis rated severity of disease using the Functional Capacity in Rheumatoid Arthritis Scale *(45).* Participants completed the Zung Depression Scale *(46)* and Sexual Functioning Questionnaire *(47).*

The two groups were well-matched for age, but they differed in duration of disease. The average duration of PD was 6 years in comparison to 15 years for patients with arthritis. Similarities were found between the two groups. Total scores for sexual functioning and subscores for desire, arousal, orgasm, satisfaction, and frequency of sex per month did not differ significantly between the two groups. Age was notably related to total sexual function score (PD, $r = -0.40$, $p < 0.05$; arthritis, $r = -0.39$, $p < 0.05$). Sexual dysfunction increased with severity of illness, and without depression, was found in both groups.

One report has exclusively addressed sexual function in women with PD *(16),* where 27 married women with PD and 27 age-matched married women without history of neurological disease participated in the study. Data was collected by a medical student. Demographic information included age, years with PD, ethnicity, educational and employment status, onset and cessation of menstruation, hormone replacement therapy, and concomitant illness. Women with PD were assessed for presence of ANS dysfunction, as evidenced by the presence of significant postural hypotension, and history of urinary or fecal incontinence. To establish severity of disease, according to the Hoehn and Yahr scale *(32),* neurological examinations of women with PD were conducted when they were in the "on" motor state. All participants completed the Brief Index of Sexual Functioning for Women (BISF-W; *48*) and BDI *(36).* The BISF-W is a 22-item questionnaire that measures sexual interest/desire, sexual activity, and satisfaction.

Women with PD and women in the control group differed in employment and ethnicity: 22% of patients with PD were employed, 67% were retired, and 11% were unable to work; 37% of control group participants were employed and 63% were retired. Of the 27 patients who had PD, there were 23 Caucasians, 2 Asians, and 2 Hispanics. In the control group, 19 Caucasians, 1 Asian, 3 Hispanics, 3 African-Americans, and 1 woman described herself as "other." Approximately 50% of both samples were sexually active. Patients who had PD reported less satisfaction with their sexual relationship than the control group. Women with PD reported greater anxiety or inhibition during sex ($p = 0.04$), more difficulty with vaginal tightness ($p = 0.03$), and more problems with involuntary urination ($p = 0.03$). Patients with PD were less satisfied with their partners than the controls ($p = 0.005$). Also, patients with PD were significantly more depressed than community controls. In women with PD, the Hoehn and Yahr stage of disease was mildly correlated with change in satisfaction and change in sexual activity. In both groups, age was associated with change in sexual satisfaction and sexual activity.

4. PHYSIOLOGY OF SEXUAL FUNCTION

4.1. *Physiology of Penile Erection*

Primary regulation of penile erection is provided by the central and peripheral nervous system *(49,50)*. Integration for central control of erection appears to occur in the medial preoptic area (MPOA) of the hypothalamus, where sensory impulses from the amygdala that have input from the cortical association areas are received *(7)*. Stimuli to the MPOA include proerectile dopamine-mediated signals and inhibitory norepinephrine-mediated signals. The MPOA provides neural input to the paraventricular nucleus (PVN) of the hypothalamus. Descending pathways from the PVN may have proerectile action through oxytocin-mediated pathways. Neural connections between the MPOA and the brainstem are provided by periaqueductal gray matter, which may have proerectile activity. Neurons from the PVN project to the thoracic and lumbosacral nuclei related with erection *(49)*. Reflex erections are mediated through T12-S3 cord levels *(7,51)*, and the penis is innervated by the sympathetic nervous system at T11-L2 *(7)*. Sympathetic input is antierectile, whereas parasympathetic and somatic nervous system innervation of the penis is mediated through the S2-S4 segments and is proerectile. Autonomic input to the penis is integrated in the inferior hypogastric plexus. The cavernous nerves originate in the inferior hypogastric plexus. The lesser cavernous nerves travel along the penis to supply the erectile tissue of the corpus spongiosum and urethra, and the greater cavernous nerves innervate the helicine arteries and erectile tissue. Fibrous tissue encases intercavernous nerves, preventing compression during erection. Branches of the intercavernous nerves travel with the prostatevesicular artery branches. Stimuli from the perineum and lower urinary tract mucosa are conveyed by the sacral reflex arc. Branches of the pudendal nerves, ilioinguinal nerve, and the dorsal penile nerves provide sensory input from the glans penis and skin and penile root *(7,51,52)*.

In the flaccid state, sympathetic neural activity is predominant, minimizing blood flow into the sinus cavernosa *(7)*. Intracorporeal smooth muscle is in a semicontracted state. Maintenance of this state is the result of intrinsic myogenic activity, adrenergic neurotransmission, and endothelium-derived-contracting factors. For smooth muscle cell contraction to occur, adequate local levels of neurotransmitters, expression of receptors, integrity of the transduction mechanism, ion channel homeostasis, interactions between contractile proteins, and effective communication over gap junctions all must be present.

Sexual stimulation causes parasympathetic neural activity to dominate, resulting in increased blood flow into the sinuses of the corpora cavernosa, smooth muscle relaxation, and achievement of erection *(7)*. Nitric oxide (NO) is the main neurotransmitter mediating penile erection. During nonadrenergic, noncholinergic neurotransmission, NO is released from the endothelium of the corpora cavernosa. NO activates soluble guanylyl cyclase within the muscle cells, which raises the intracellular concentration of cyclic guanosine monophosphate (cGMP). cGMP activates a protein kinase, causing hyperpolarization of the muscle cell membrane, sequestration of intracellular calcium, and calcium channel inhibition that blocks calcium influx. Smooth muscle relaxation, dilation of arterial vessels, and increased blood flow into the sinuses of the corpora cavernosa result from the decrease in cytosolic calcium concentration.

4.2. Hormonal and Neurogenic Mediators of Female Sexual Function

Two physiologic changes occur during the female sexual response cycle: vasocongestion of the external and internal genitalia and breasts and myotonia throughout the body *(53)*. Hormones and neurogenic mediators regulate female sexual function *(5)*. Estradiol levels affect cells throughout the nervous system and influence nerve transmission. Estrogen causes vasodilatation, resulting in increased vaginal, clitoral, and urethral arterial blood flow, which prevents atherosclerotic compromise of pelvic arteries and arterioles and also maintains sexual response. With aging and menopause, women experience decreased sexual desire, less frequency of sexual activity, and a reduction in sexual responsiveness. A correlation between the presence of sexual complaints and estradiol levels below 50 pg/mL has been demonstrated *(54)*. Estrogen regulates vaginal NO synthase, the enzyme responsible for production of NO *(5)*. NO is involved in the modulation of vaginal relaxation and secretory processes. NO has been identified in clitoral cavernosal smooth muscle and may be a mediator of clitoral cavernosal and vaginal wall smooth muscle relaxation. Aging results in decreased vaginal NO levels and increased vaginal wall fibrosis. In women, low testosterone levels are associated with a decline in sexual arousal, genital sensation, libido, and orgasm. The neurogenic mechanisms that modulate vaginal and clitoral smooth muscle tone as well as vaginal and clitoral vascular muscle relaxation are undetermined. Preliminary studies suggest the involvement of vasoactive intestinal polypeptide and NO.

5. THERAPEUTIC INTERVENTIONS

In both men and women, impaired sexual function can be caused by psychogenic factors, organic factors, and aging *(5,7)*. Organic causes are categorized as vascular, neurogenic, hormonal, disease-related, and drug-induced. In men, psychogenic causes of ED include depression, performance anxiety, relationship problems, and psychosocial distress *(23–25)*. Alternatively, in women, issues related to self esteem, body image, relationship with partner, and ability to communicate sexual needs affect sexual function *(5)*.

Impaired sexual function in PD is most likely multifactorial, where depression, physical disability, and autonomic dysfunction may contribute to the increased incidence of ED in PD *(55)*. Given the multiple factors for impaired sexual function, the needs of patients, partners, and couples should be individually assessed. The World Health Organization definition of sexual health as "the integration of the somatic, emotional, intellectual, and social aspects of sexual being, in ways that are positively enriching and that enhances personality, communication, and love" *(56)* can guide therapeutic intervention.

5.1. Diagnosis and Treatment of Erectile Dysfunction in Men With PD

5.1.1. Nonpharmacological Measures

Recommendations for the diagnosis and treatment of ED were developed by the First International Consultation on ED *(57)*. Diagnostic evaluation has been described *(7,57)*, and a stepped approach to treatment is recommended. When possible, prescribed medications associated with ED should be discontinued *(57,58)*. First-line therapy includes lifestyle modification, psychological counseling, androgen replacement therapy, and oral therapy *(57)*. Lifestyle modification includes smoking cessation, avoidance of substance abuse, adequate nutrition, physical activity, and sleep. In men with PD, there is limited discussion of first-line pharmacological therapies. Treatments with testosterone gel *(59)* and sildenafil *(60,61)* have been described. Erection has been reported as a side effect of subcutaneous apomorphine treatment of motor-resistant fluctuations with PD *(55)*.

5.1.2. Testosterone

Testosterone is thought to stimulate libido in the central nervous system *(62)*. Erections in response to erotic visual stimuli may be partially androgen-dependent *(63)*. Animal and human studies have found that low-normal range concentrations of testosterone are sufficient to maintain sexual activity *(64)*. Testosterone deficiency is found in 20 to 25% of men over age 60 *(59)*. Testosterone deficiency can result in depression, fatigue, decreased libido, and decreased work performance. Okun et al. *(59)* retrospectively analyzed the effect of testosterone replacement therapy in five men with PD and evidence of plasma testosterone deficiency. The men had not clinically improved with antidepressants and anti-Parkinsonian medication. Four of the men were initially screened with the St. Louis Testosterone Deficiency Questionnaire (SLTDQ; *65*). Men who met SLTDQ criteria were screened for total and free testosterone levels. Prostate-specific antigen and digital rectal exam were performed to exclude the presence of prostate cancer. The UPDRS motor score was recorded. Patients with testosterone levels less than 70 pg/mL with no medical contraindications were treated with a topical application of testosterone gel. Patients reported decrease in fatigue, depression, anxiety, and improved sexual function 1 month later. To assess the prevalence of testosterone deficiency, total testosterone levels for 68 men enrolled in a PD registry were sent for evaluation, and 35% had evidence of plasma testosterone deficiency. The risk of testosterone deficiency increased 2.8-fold per decade.

5.1.3. Sildenafil

Sildenafil, a selective inhibitor of cGMP-specific phosphodiesterase type 5, enhances the effect of NO release into the corpora cavernosa from nonadrenergic noncholinergic nerves of the parasympathetic system and vascular endothelium during sexual stimulation *(7)*. Sildenafil potentiates the hypotensive effect of nitrates and is absolutely contraindicated in men using nitrates *(66)*. Sildenafil may be hazardous in men with borderline low blood pressure, borderline low cardiac volume or medications that can prolong its half-life *(67)*. Adverse effects include headache, flushing, nasal congestion, dyspepsia, abnormal vision, diarrhea, and dizziness *(7)*. To optimize the treatment outcome, sildenafil should be ingested on an empty stomach. Excessive alcohol consumption should be avoided.

Studies of men with various etiologies of ED have reported improved function with sildenafil *(66)*. To evaluate the efficacy and safety of sildenafil in men with PD and ED, 10 men participated in an 8-week open-label pilot study *(60)*. The BDI *(36)*, UPDRS *(31)*, and a Sexual Health Inventory-M version (SHI-M) questionnaire *(68)* were administered prior to treatment and at the conclusion of the treatment period. Four 50-mg doses of sildenafil were prescribed for use in four sexual encounters during the first month. At the conclusion of the first month, participants had telephone conversations with a urologist and movement disorder neurologist. Participants were then permitted to increase the dose to 100 mg for each of the four sexual encounters during the second month. All participants took eight doses of medication during the study period. Four men increased the dose to 100 mg during the second month. A statistically significant improvement in total SHI-M scores was demonstrated ($p = 0.01$). Significant improvement was demonstrated in overall sexual satisfaction, satisfaction with sexual desire, achievement of erection, maintenance of erection, and orgasm. One patient reported a headache during three encounters. There were no reports of syncope or presyncope.

In a randomized, double-blind, placebo-controlled, crossover study of sildenafil *(61)*, 24 men with ED, 12 with PD, and 12 with multiple system atrophy (MSA) participated. Participants completed the International Index of Erectile Function questionnaire *(69)* and a quality-of-life questionnaire, and partners completed a brief questionnaire. The starting dose for the active drug was 50 mg. Dosage was titrated up to 100 mg or down to 25 mg at follow-up visits, depending on efficacy and tolerability. Of the 12 men with PD, 10 completed the study, and 9 of the 10 men reported a good response to sildenafil. Eight men titrated up to 100 mg; One man titrated down to 25 mg. Although one man reported lack of efficacy, most of the participants with PD reported significant improvement in the ability to achieve and maintain erection, along with improvement in sex life with sildenafil. Partners' questionnaire responses confirmed the patients' reports. Men with PD demonstrated minimal change in blood pressure (BP). Six men with MSA were studied before recruitment was stopped. Four men received placebo first. Three men with MSA experienced significant postural fall in BP with symptoms of orthostatic hypotension 1 hour after receiving sildenafil. Patients with MSA reported improved sexual function and quality of sex life after taking sildenafil. The authors recommended the measurement of lying and standing BP as well as education about symptoms of hypotension before prescribing sildenafil for men with early Parkinsonism, which may be difficult to distinguish from MSA.

5.1.4. Apomorphine

Apomorphine is a D1/D2 receptor agonist used to treat resistant motor fluctuations in adults with PD *(71)*. Under experimental conditions, the parenteral administration of apomorphine produces erectile responses in humans and rats *(71,72)*. Apomorphine-induced erections are likely the result of stimulation of central D-2 dopamine receptors and are inhibited by the selective D2 antagonist, sulpiride *(73)*. Domperidone, a peripheral dopamine antagonist, does not inhibit apomorphine-induced erections or the yawning that accompanies the erection *(74)*. Animal studies suggest there is a link between the hypothalamic pathways involved in erection and yawning *(75)*.

Apomorphine-induced erections in men with PD have been reported. O'Sullivan and Hughes *(55)* surveyed 15 men who attended a movement disorder neurology clinic and used intermittent subcutaneous injections of apomorphine to treat PD complicated by motor fluctuations. Results reported 5 of the 15 men with erection as a side effect of treatment. Erections coincided with apomorphine administration. Four of the men had experienced ED before beginning apomorphine treatment, and two of the men had improvement in their sexual relationship with their partner as a result of treatment. The only patient that had not experienced ED prior to beginning apomorphine treatment reported undesirable arousal associated with the erections.

In a placebo-controlled trial of men with no discernable organic etiology for ED, buccal administration of apomorphine was found to be significantly more effective than placebo, as demonstrated by rigidity testing *(76)*. In 11 patients, 64% indicated successful intercourse for up to 7 months. Both 2- and 4-mg doses of rapidly acting sublingual apomorphine were studied and found to be effective in men with ED with controlled coronary artery disease, hypertension, diabetes mellitus, and prostate hypertrophy *(66)*. Adverse effects included nausea, dizziness, and somnolence. Sublingual apomorphine is available in Europe *(7)*, but in the United States, it is still under investigation *(78)*.

5.1.5. Other Treatment Methods

According to the First International Council on Erectile Dysfunction, second-line therapy includes vacuum constriction devices, intracavernosal injection, and transurethral therapy *(57)*. Third-line therapy utilizes penile prosthesis and revascularization. Reports evaluating the efficacy of these treatment modalities in men with PD were not identified in the literature review.

Levodopa and alternate current (AC)-pulsed electromagnetic field density stimulation are not recognized treatments for ED. However, their effect on sexual function has been described *(78,79)*. Hypersexuality is a rarely reported side effect of levodopa therapy in men with PD *(80,81)*. Levodopa was evaluated in a clinical trial of 21 healthy men without ED *(78)*. Subjects ingested 800 mg of levodopa for 7 days. Sleep-related penile tumescence was monitored. Erectile responses significantly improved from baseline, and no adverse effects were reported. The results provide support for a central dopaminergic erection-mediation pathway.

Sandyk *(79)* reported on two men with PD and ED, ages 70 and 73, respectively, who experienced sexual arousal and nocturnal erections after receiving treatment for PD with transcranial administrations of AC-pulsed electromagnetic fields (EMFs) of 7.5 picotesla flux density. EMF treatment was administered after the men received their usual anti-Parkinson medication when they were in the "on" state. The first patient received EMF treatment for 2 consecutive days. During the first treatment, he felt relaxed and yawned. He reported a decrease in parkinsonian symptoms after the treatment. In the evening, he experienced sexual arousal and awakened during the night with several repetitive spontaneous erections that lasted 15 to 20 minutes. During the second treatment, he experienced sexual arousal and had nocturnal erections during the subsequent three nights. The second patient had Hoehn and Yahr stage IV PD. He had two successive EMF treatments for 4 days and reported sexual arousal associated with nocturnal erection.

5.2. *Diagnosis and Treatment of Women With PD and Impaired Sexual Function*

A diagnostic framework and classification system for female sexual dysfunction has identified four categories of dysfunction *(82)*. This classification system is consistent with DSM IV: Diagnostic and Statistical Manual of Mental Disorders of the American Psychiatric Association and International Classification of Diseases-10 categories *(83)*. The four major categories of female sexual dysfunction described in this classification system include disorders of sexual desire, sexual arousal, orgasm, and sexual pain. Sexual desire disorders include hypoactive sexual desire disorder and sexual aversion disorder. Dyspareunia and vaginismus are some types of sexual pain disorders. The four classifications are subtyped as lifelong versus acquired, generalized versus situational, and organic versus mixed. The etiologies may be multifactorial.

A comprehensive approach to the evaluation of sexual function should include a complete medical history, physical examination, pelvic examination, and hormonal profile as indicated *(5)*. Recommendations for physiologic testing have been described *(5)*. Therapeutic interventions for the treatment of impaired sexual function in women with PD were not identified in this literature review.

6. CONCLUSION

The incidence of impaired sexual function in adults with PD is greater than the general population *(8–17)*. Further clinical and basic science research in this area is required for the development of therapeutic interventions.

REFERENCES

1. Allen ME. A holistic view of sexuality and the aged. Holist Nurs Pract 1987;1:76–83.
2. Woods NF. Toward a holistic perspective of human sexuality: alterations in sexual health and nursing diagnoses. Holist Nurs Pract 1987;1:1–11.
3. Johnson BK. Older adults and sexuality: A multidimensional perspective. J Gerontol Nurs 1996;22:6–15.
4. Singer C, Weiner WJ. Erectile and ejaculatory disturbance: overview of diagnosis and treatment. In: Sexual Dysfunction: a Neuromedical Approach, Futura, Armonk, NY, 1994, pp. 45–59.
5. Berman JR, Berman L, Goldstein I. Female sexual dysfunction: incidence, pathophysiology, evaluation, and treatment options. Urology 1999;54:385–391.
6. Woods NF. Human Sexuality in Health and Illness, 2nd ed. C.V. Mosby, St. Louis, MO, 1972.
7. Shabsigh R, Anastasiadis AG. Erectile dysfunction. Annu Rev Med 2003;54:153–168.
8. Burguera JA, Garcia Reboll L, Martinez Agullo E. Sexual dysfunction in Parkinson's disease. Neurologia. 1994;9:178–181.
9. Jacobs H, Vieregge A, Vieregge P. Sexuality in young patients with Parkinson's disease: a population based comparison with healthy controls. J Neurol Neurosurg Psychiatry 2000;69:550–552.
10. Wermuth L, Stenager E. Sexual problems in young patients with Parkinson's disease. Acta Neurol Scand 1995;91:453–455.
11. Koller WC, Vetere-Overfeld B, Williamson A, et al. Sexual dysfunction in Parkinson's disease. Clinical Neuropharmacol 1990;13:461–463.
12. Brown RG, Jahanshahi M, Quinn N, Marsden CD. Sexual function in patients with Parkinson's disease and their partners. J Neurol Neurosurg Psychiatry 1990;53:480–486.
13. Singer C, Weiner WJ, Sanchez-Ramos J, Ackerman M. Sexual function in patients with Parkinson's disease. J Neurol Neurosurg Psychiatry 1991;54:942.
14. Singer C, Weiner WJ, Sanchez-Ramos J. Autonomic dysfunction in men with Parkinson's disease. Eur Neurol 1992;32:134–140.
15. Lipe H, Longstreth WT. Jr., Bird T. D, Linde M. Sexual function in married men with Parkinson's disease compared to married men with arthritis. Neurology 1990;40:1347–1349.
16. Welsh M, Hung L, Waters CH. Sexuality in women with Parkinson's disease. Mov Disord 1997;12:923–927.
17. Lambert D, Waters C. Sexual dysfunction in Parkinson's disease. Clin Neurosci 1998;5:73–77.
18. Laumann EO, Paik A, Rosen RC. Sexual dysfunction in the United States: prevalence and predictors. JAMA 1999;281:537–544.
19. Jonler M, Moon T, Brannan W, et al. The effect of age, ethnicity and geographical location on impotence and quality of life. Br J Urol 1995;75:651–655.
20. NIH Consensus Development Panel on Impotence. NIH Consensus Conference: Impotence. JAMA 1992;270:83–90.
21. Johannes CB, Araujo AB, Feldman HA, et al. Incidence of erectile dysfunction in men 40–69 years old: longitudinal results from the Massachusetts male aging study. J Urol 2000;163:460–463.
22. Blanker MH, Bohnen AM, Groeneveld FP, et al. Correlates for erectile and ejaculatory dysfunction in older Dutch men: a community based study. J Am Geriatr Soc. 2001;49:436–442.

23. Martin-Morales A, Sanchez-Cruz JJ, Saenz de Tejada I, et al. Prevalence and independent risk factors for erectile dysfunction in Spain: results of the Epidemiologia de la Disfuncion Erectil Masculina Study. J Urol 2001;166:569–575.
24. Braun M, Wassmer G, Klotz T, et al. Epidemiology of erectile dysfunction: results of the "Cologne Male Survey." Int J Impot Res 2000;12:305–311.
25. Chew KK, Earle CM, Stuckey BG, et al. Erectile dysfunction in general medicine practice: prevalence and clinical correlates. Int J Impot Res 2000;12:41–45.
26. Masters W, Johnson V. Human Sexual Response. Little Brown and Company, Boston, MA, 1966.
27. Kaplan HS. The New Sex Therapy. Brunner/Mazel Inc., New York, 1974.
28. Spector IP, Carey MP. Incidence and prevalence of the sexual dysfunctions: a critical review of the empirical literature. Arch Sex Behav 1990;19:389–408.
29. Rosen RC, Taylor JF, Leiblum SR, Bachmann GA. Prevalence of sexual dysfunction in women: results of a survey study of 329 women in an outpatient gynecological clinic. J Sex Marital Ther 1993;19:171–188.
30. Read S, King M, Watson J. Sexual dysfunction in primary medical care: prevalence, characteristics, and detection by the general practitioner. J Public Health Med 1997;19:387–391.
31. Fahn S, Elton RI, Members of the UPDRS Development Committee. Unified Parkinson's disease Rating Scale. In: Fahn S, Marsden CD, Goldstein M, eds. Recent Developments in Parkinson's Disease II. Macmillan, Florham Park, 1987, pp. 153–163.
32. Hoehn M, Yahr MD. Parkinsonism: onset, progression and mortality. Neurology 1967;17:427–442.
33. Schneider HD. Sexualverhalten in der zweiten Lebenshalfte: Ergebnisse sozialwissenschaftlicher Forschung. Kohl-hammer Verlag, Stuttgart, 1980.
34. Zerssen D Von, Koeller DM. Paranoid-Depressivitats-Skala. Beltz Test, Weinheim, 1976.
35. Wechsler D. Handanweisung zum Hamburg-Weschler-Intelligenztest fur Erwachsene (HAWIE). Hans Huber Verlag, Bern, 1982.
36. Beck AT, Beamesderfer A. Assessment of depression: the depression inventory. Mod Probl Pharmacopsychiatry 1974;7:151–169.
37. Yesavage JA, Brink TL, Rose TL, et al. Development and validation of a geriatric depression screening scale: a preliminary report. J Psychiatric Res 1982–1983;17:37–49.
38. Othmer E, Othmer SC. Evaluation of sexual dysfunction. J Clin Psychiatry 1987;48:191–193.
39. Rust J, Golombok S. The Golombok Rust Inventory of Sexual Satisfaction. NFER-Nelson, Windsor, 1986.
40. Rust J, Bennun I, Crowe M, Golombok S. The Golombok-Rust inventory of marital state. Sex Marital Ther 1988;1:55–60.
41. Spielberger CD, Gorsuch RL, Lushene RE. Manual for the State-Trait Anxiety Inventory. Consulting Psychologists Press, Palo Alto, CA, 1970.
42. Felton BJ, Revenson TA. Coping with chronic illness: a study of illness controllability and the influence of coping strategies on psychological adjustment. J Consult Clin Psychol. 1984;52:343–353.
43. Robinson BC. Validation of a Caregiver Strain Index. J Gerontol 1983;38:344–348.
44. Yahr MD, Duvoisin RC, Schear MJ, et al. Treatment of Parkinsonism with levodopa. Arch Neurol 1969;21:343–354.
45. Steinbrocker O, Traeyer CH, Batterman RC. Therapeutic criteria in rheumatoid arthritis. JAMA 1949;140:659–662.
46. Zung WW. A self-rating depression scale. Arch Gen Psychiatry 1965;12:63–70.
47. Watts RJ. Sexual functioning, health beliefs, and compliance with high blood pressure medications. Nurs Res 1982;31:278–283.
48. Taylor JF, Rosen RC, Leiblum SR. Self-report assessment of female sexual function: psychometric evaluation of the Brief Index of Sexual Functioning for Women. Arch Sex Behav 1994;23:627–643.
49. Giuliano FA, Rampin O, Benoit G, Jardin A. Neural control of penile erection. Urol Clin North Am 1995;22:747–766.
50. Burnett AL. Neurophysiology of erectile function and dysfunction. In: Hellstrom WJG, ed. The Handbook of Sexual Dysfunction. The American Society of Andrology, San Francisco, CA, 1999, pp. 12–17.
51. Saenz de Tejada I. Anatomy physiology, and pathophysiology of erectile dysfunction. In: Jardin A, Wagner G, Khoury S, eds. Erectile Dysfunction. Plymbridge Distrib., Plymouth, UK, 2000, pp. 65–102.
52. Goldstein I. Male sexual circuitry. Working Group for the Study of Central Mechanisms in Erectile Dysfunction. Sci Am 2000;283:70–75.
53. McCarty T, Fromm L, Weiss-Roberts L, et al. In: Copeland L, ed. Textbook of Gynecology. Saunders, Philadelphia, PA, 2000, pp. 475–485.
54. Sarrel PM. Sexuality and menopause. Obstet Gynecol 1990;75(4 Suppl):26S–30S.
55. O'Sullivan JD, Hughes AJ. Apomorphine-induced penile erections in Parkinson's disease. Mov Disord 1998;13:536–539.
56. World Health Organization. Education and treatment in human sexuality: the training of health professionals. Report of the WHO Meeting. Technical Report Services, 1975, no. 572.
57. Jardin A, Wagner G, Khoury S, et al. Recommendations of the first international consultation on erectile dysfunction. In: Jardin A, Wagner G, Khoury S, et al. eds. Erectile Dysfunction. Plymbridge Dist., Plymouth, UK, 2000, pp. 711–726.
58. Rosen RC, Lane RM, Menza M. Effects of SSRIs on sexual function: a critical review. J Clinical Pharmacol 1999;19:67–85.
59. Okun MS, McDonald WM, DeLong MR. Refractory nonmotor symptoms in male patients with Parkinson disease due to testosterone deficiency: a common unrecognized comorbidity. Arch Neurol 2002;59:807–811.
60. Zesiewicz TA, Helal M, Hauser RA. Sildenafil citrate (Viagra) for the treatment of erectile dysfunction in men with Parkinson's disease. Mov Disord 2000;15:305–308.

61. Hussain IF, Brady CM, Swinn MJ, et al. Treatment of erectile dysfunction with sildenafil citrate (Viagra) in Parkinsonism due to Parkinson's disease or multiple system atrophy with observations on orthostatic hypotension. J Neurol Neurosurg Psychiatry 2001;71:371–374.
62. Cohan P, Korenman SG. Erectile dysfunction. J Clin Endocrinol Metab 2001;86:2391–2394.
63. Carani C, Scuteri A, Marrama P, Bancroft J. The effects of testosterone administration and visual erotic stimuli on nocturnal penile tumescence in normal men. Horm Behav 1990;24:435–441.
64. Bhasin S. The dose-dependent effects of testosterone on sexual function and on muscle mass and function. Mayo Clin Proc 2000;75(Suppl):S75–S76.
65. Morley JE, Charlton E, Patrick P, et al. Validation of a screening questionnaire for androgen deficiency in aging males. Metabolism 2000;49:1239–1242.
66. Padma-Nathan H, Giuliano F. Oral drug therapy for erectile dysfunction. Urol Clin North Am 2001;28:321–334.
67. Wespes E, Amar E, Hatzichristou D, et al. Guidelines on erectile dysfunction. Eur Urol 2002;41:1–5.
68. Rosen RC, Cappelleri JC, Smith MD, et al. Development and evaluation of an abridged 5-item version of the International Index of Erectile Dysfunction (IIEF-5) as a diagnostic tool for erectile dysfunction. Int J Impot Res 1999;11:319–326.
69. Rosen RC, Riley A, Wagner G, Osterloh IH, Kirkpatrick J, Mishra A. The international index of erectile function (IIEF): a multidimensional scale for assessment of erectile dysfunction. Urology 1997;49:822–830.
70. Steiger MJ, Quinn NP, Marsden CD. The clinical use of apomorphine in Parkinson's disease. J Neurol 1992;239:389–393.
71. Gower AJ, Berendsen HG, Princen MM, Broekkamp CLE. The yawning-penile erection syndrome as a putative model for dopamine autoreceptor activity. Eur J Pharmacol 1984;103:81–89.
72. Lal S, Laryea E, Thavundayil JX, et al. Apomorphine induced penile tumescence in impotent patients – preliminary findings. Prog Neuropsychopharmacol Biol Psychiatry 1987;11:235–242.
73. Nair NP, Lal S, Iskandar HI, et al. Effect of sulpiride, an atypical neuroleptic, on apomorphine-induced growth hormone secretion. Brain Res Bull 1982;8:587–591.
74. Lal S, Nair NP, Iskandar HL, et al. Effect of domperidone on apomorphine-induced growth hormone secretion in normal men. J Neural Transm 1982;54:75–84.
75. Argiolas A, Melis MR, Mauri A, Gessa GL. Paraventricular nucleus lesion prevents yawning and penile erection induced by apomorphine and oxytocin but not ACTH in rats. Brain Res 1987;421:349–352.
76. Heaton JP, Morales A, Adams MA, et al. Recovery of erectile function by the oral administration of apomorphine. Urology 1995;45:200–206.
77. Burnett AL. Oral pharmacotherapy for erectile dysfunction: current perspectives. Urology 1999;54:392–400.
78. Horita H, Sato Y, Adachi H, et al. Effects of levodopa on nocturnal penile tumescence: a preliminary study. J Androl 1998;19:619–634.
79. Sandyk R. AC pulsed electromagnetic fields-induced sexual arousal and penile erections in Parkinson's disease. Int J Neurosci 1999;99:139–149.
80. Uitti R. J, Tanner C. M, Rajput A. H, et al. Hypersexuality with antiparkinsonian therapy. Clin Neuropharmacol 1989;12:375–383.
81. Weinman E, Ruskin PE. Levodopa dependence and hypersexuality in older Parkinson disease patients. Am J Geriatr Psychiatry 1995;3:81–83.
82. Basson R, Berman J, Burnett A, et al. Report of the international consensus development conference on female sexual dysfunction: definitions and classifications. J Urol 2000;163:888–893.
83. American Psychiatric Association: DSM-IV Diagnostic and statistical manual of mental disorders, edition 4. American Psychiatric Press, Washington, DC, 1994.

11
Urological Dysfunction

Carlos Singer

SUMMARY

Symptoms of urinary dysfunction occur frequently with Parkinson's disease (PD), particularly men. Irritative symptoms, encompassing frequency, urgency, and urge incontinence, are reported in 57 to 83% of patients with PD. Obstructive symptoms, such as hesitancy and weak urinary stream, may be present in 17 to 27% of individuals. Detrusor hyperreflexia is the urodynamic correlate of irritative urinary symptoms. Detrusor areflexia is uncommon in PD; when present, anticholinergic drugs are most often responsible. Coexistent obstructive uropathies may complicate the clinical picture in patients with PD and could produce both obstructive and irritative effects. Urinary dysfunction with PD may also be the result of dysfunctional infravesicular mechanisms like sphincter bradykinesia. Irritative urinary symptoms owing to PD are often responsive to anticholinergic drugs, whereas catheterization may be necessary if the symptoms are obstructive in nature.

Key Words: Urinary dysfunction; irritative; obstructive; sphincter bradykinesia; detrusor hyperreflexia; anticholinergic drugs; pontine micturition center.

1. INTRODUCTION

Patients with Parkinson's disease (PD) commonly present with urinary complaints. The treating neurologist should have a basic knowledge of the most frequent patterns of presentation to provide advice on their significance and guide the patient regarding available treatments. This chapter has been organized around sections that summarize key issues of this subject.

2. GENDER PREVALENCE OF UROLOGICAL SYMPTOMS

The earliest series originated from groups of parkinsonian patients who were being selected for basal ganglia surgery *(1,2)*. Urological symptoms were present in 38% (11/29) of Murnaghan's series *(1)* and 71% (44/62) of Porter and Bors' series (all male). There were no comparisons with controls.

Lemack and colleagues selected 80 men and 39 women with mild-to-moderate PD (Hoehn and Yahr < stage 3) and performed a questionnaire-based assessment using the American Urological Association Symptom Index in men and the Urogenital Distress Inventory-6 in women *(3)*. Men scored higher than age-matched controls with similar values to those of men with symptomatic benign prostatic hyperplasia. Results were less clear with PD women, who scored higher than nonage-matched volunteers, but lower than an age-matched female group presenting for urological evaluation, and yet free of neurological disease.

Two series have investigated the prevalence of specific urological symptoms in patients with PD and compared them to controls *(4,5)*. Significantly higher prevalence figures in PD were found for urinary urgency *(4,5)*, sensation of incomplete bladder emptying *(4)*, nocturia *(5)*, daytime frequency, and urge incontinence. Estimates for obstructive symptoms (hesitancy and weak stream) exhibited the

From: *Current Clinical Neurology*
Parkinson's Disease and Nonmotor Dysfunction
Edited by: R. F. Pfeiffer and I. Bodis-Wollner © Humana Press Inc., Totowa, NJ

Table 1
Prevalence of Urological Symptoms in Two Populations of Patients With PD

Urinary symptoms	Singer et al. *(4)*	Sakakibara et al., *(13)*
Urinary urgency	46% (Men)	54% (Men) 42% (Women)
Sensation of incomplete bladder emptying	42% (Men)	
Nocturia		63% (Men) 53% (Women)
Daytime frequency		16% (Men) 28% (Women)
Urge incontinence		70% (Men) 28% (Women)

* Determined to be significantly higher than a control population.

most discrepancy between men and women *(5)*, perhaps reflecting overlap with prostatic disease (*see* Table 1).

3. IRRITATIVE VERSUS OBSTRUCTIVE SYMPTOMS

The most frequently investigated urinary symptoms are usually grouped either as *irritative* (frequency, urgency and urge incontinence) or *obstructive* (hesitancy and weak urinary stream). Irritative symptoms invariably predominate by a large margin. Proportions for irritative compared to obstructive symptomatology range from 73% versus 27% to 83% versus 17% *(1,6,7)*. Pavlakis et al. reported a distribution of 57% irritative, 23% obstructive, and 20% mixed symptomatology in a group of 30 patients with PD *(8)*.

Obstructive symptoms are not consistently reported, as illustrated by at least three reports *(2,9,10)*. Alternatively, more careful attention to nonmotor symptoms during the "off" state may uncover a higher prevalence of urinary symptomatology *(11)* and possibly a different proportionality of irritative in comparison to obstructive types.

4. APPEARANCE AND PROGRESSION OF UROLOGICAL SYMPTOMS

Limited information exists regarding predisposing factors for the presence of urinary symptoms in PD. Both the duration and severity of disease may be influential. Chandiramani et al. reported an average lapse of 5. 75 years between the onset of motor symptoms and onset of urological symptoms *(10)*. In their study of 70 urologically symptomatic patients with PD, Araki et al. reported that their symptom index scores increased with disease severity *(12)*.

Sakakibara and colleagues *(13)* studied ^{123}I-β-CIT single-photon emission computed tomography scans of seven patients who have PD with urinary dysfunction and compared them to four patients with PD free of urinary symptoms. The uptake was significantly reduced in the former group, again suggesting a link between severity of the nigrostriatal dopaminergic deficit and presence of urinary symptomatology.

5. URODYNAMIC CORRELATION OF DETRUSOR HYPERREFLEXIA

Detrusor hyperreflexia is a cystometric finding characterized by the presence of involuntary detrusor contractions in response to bladder filling that the patient is unable to inhibit. These contractions generate pressure values that exceed 15 cm of water *(8,14,15)*.

Some authors have reported a very close clinical correlation of irritative symptoms with detrusor hyperreflexia in PD *(6,12)*. The prevalence of detrusor hyperreflexia found among urologically symptomatic patients with PD ranges from 45 to 100% *(1,2,6–8,12,16–18)*. Such prevalence figures roughly parallel those reported for irritative symptoms in PD (*see* Section 3.). The information on factors predisposing to detrusor hyperreflexia in PD also seems to parallel the information on irritative symptoms (*see* Section 4.). Stocchi et al. *(19)* analyzed 30 patients with PD and found that those with detrusor hyperreflexia had more severe and longer duration of disease. Araki et al. *(12)* studied 70 patients with PD who had been referred for urological evaluation and were free of obstructive etiologies. Of these patients, 67% (47/70) had pure hyperreflexia with the majority (42/47) in intermediate to advances stages of the disease (Hoehn and Yahr stage 3 or higher).

6. DETRUSOR AREFLEXIA

Detrusor areflexia is a cystometrographic finding with decreased sensation during filling and increased bladder capacity *(2,6)* (≥600 mL), along with a desire to void first experienced at a high-filling volume *(20)*. The postvoid residual volume is higher than 100 mL *(20)*. Detrusor areflexia results in hesitancy and weak urinary stream.

Detrusor areflexia is uncommon in PD. Incidence figures for detrusor areflexia in series of urologically symptomatic patients *(1,6,8,18,20)* have ranged from 0% (0/9; *18*) through 11% *(12)* to 27% (4/15; *6*). Stocchi et al. *(19)* did not find detrusor areflexia in any of their 30 patients who had PD—symptomatic or asymptomatic—who were studied with urodynamics where anticholinergics had been withheld.

6.1. *Medication Effects and Other Etiologies*

Anticholinergic drugs are the most common cause of detrusor areflexia in patients with PD according to some authors *(15)*. In fact, the concurrent use of anticholinergics is frequently mentioned in reported findings of detrusor areflexia in PD *(1,2,7,8)*.

However, in some instances, detrusor areflexia may be found in patients with PD in the absence of anticholinergic medication. One example is the study by Raz of urologically symptomatic patients with PD, where the confounding effect of anticholinergics was eliminated by withdrawing them 1 week prior to the urodynamic investigations *(6)*. In such cases, the clinician should consider multiple system atrophy as an alternative diagnosis to PD (*see* Section 10.), concurrent obstructive uropathy (*see* Section 7.), and "myogenic" areflexia.

Myogenic areflexia was originally described as the result of muscle fiber injury caused by overdistention, which is itself a consequence of obstruction *(21)*. Recently, a myopathic process of the bladder wall has also been proposed to be present in the absence of obstruction. Araki et al. have invoked this theory to explain findings in 6 of their 70 patients referred for urological evaluation *(12)*. These patients—all stage 4 in the Hoehn and Yahr scale—had hyperreflexia that was associated with impaired contractile function in the absence of obstructive etiologies. A similar process has been reported in the elderly *(22)*.

7. IMPACT OF COEXISTENT OBSTRUCTIVE UROPATHIES

Obstructive uropathies (i.e., benign prostatic hypertrophy in males and stenosis of the bladder neck in females) have been recognized as causes of both irritative and obstructive symptoms in the general population *(21)*. The association of irritative symptoms with obstructive uropathies may also be the product of detrusor hyperreflexia that is indistinguishable from the purely neurogenic type.

Certain investigations have pointed to obstructive uropathies as the sole or contributing causes of urinary symptoms in some patients who have PD *(7,8,16,18)*. Estimates of prevalence vary from 17% to 33% *(7,8,18)*. However, correlation with specific obstructive symptoms is not always outlined with sufficient clarity *(7,8,18)*.

8. DYSFUNCTION OF INFRAVESICAL MECHANISMS

PD may also course with dysfunctional infravesical mechanisms (DIVM). A full urodynamic evaluation includes measurement of infravesical mechanisms, such as urethral pressure profile, urinary flow,

Table 2
List of Dysfunctional Infravesical Mechanisms Reported in the Literature

Dysfunction	References
Elevated urethral pressure profile	Murnaghan *(1)*
	Raz *(6)*
Decreased urinary flow	Berger et al. *(7)*
	Berger et al. *(23)*
Sphincter bradykinesia	Pavlakis et al. *(8)*
	Galloway *(17)*
	Andersen et al. *(16)*
	Andersen et al. *(14)*
Pseudodyssynergia	Pavlakis et al. *(8)*
Sphincter "tremor"	Galloway *(17)*
Vesicosphincter dyssynergia	Andersen et al. *(16)*
	Andersen et al. *(14)*
	Araki et al. *(12)*
Involuntary asymptomatic sphincteric activity	Berger et al. *(7)*
	Berger et al. *(23)*

and sphincter EMG recording during bladder filling and bladder emptying. DIVMs encompass dysfunctions of the striated urethral sphincter and the pelvic floor, either occurring alone or in combination. Different kinds of DIVMs have been described (*see* Table 2). They have been inconsistently reported and in variable numbers *(1,8,16,19)*; sometimes they are not found at all *(18)*. The descriptions are sometimes poorly characterized and may not be confirmed again in other reports. Correlation with clinical symptomatology is frequently inadequate or lacking *(1,8,16)*; therefore, the clinical significance of DIVMs is unclear.

8.1. Sphincter Bradykinesia, Pseudodyssynergia, and Vesicosphincter Dyssynergia

The most frequent DIVM is known as sphincter bradykinesia, consisting of delayed relaxation of the striated urethral sphincter and pelvic floor. There is a normal guarding reflex with an increase in striated muscle activity during bladder filling before the onset of detrusor contraction. Sphincter bradykinesia is an abnormality where involuntary EMG activity persists through at least the initial part of the expulsive phase of the CMG *(8)*.

In one series *(8)*, 11% (3/28) of patients who have PD had sphincter bradykinesia. In another study, Galloway *(17)* reported that 42% (5/12) of his urologically symptomatic patients were unable to relax the external urethral sphincter with voiding, which was associated with low flow rates. Andersen et al. *(16)* studied 24 urologically symptomatic patients with Parkinsonism (the term "Parkinson's disease" is not used). The same authors revised their data in a subsequent article *(14)* and reported electromyographic findings in these 24 patients with PD. The authors did not specify whether all 24 patients were symptomatic. Of these patients, 21% (5/24) had impaired sphincter control, defined as poor ability to contract or relax the sphincter on command.

Pseudodyssynergia has been reported less frequently than sphincter bradykinesia. Pseudodyssynergia has been defined as "an attempt at continence by voluntary contraction of the pelvic musculature during an involuntary detrusor contraction" *(21)*. Pavlakis et al. *(8)* reported pseudodyssynergia in 2 patients, part of a group of 10 in whom the maximum flow rate was decreased. The clinical role of this phenomenon could not be defined because of coexistent prostatic obstruction. Sphincter "tremor" was described in 11 of 12 patients in another series *(17)*. Neither pseudodyssynergia nor sphincter "tremor" have been confirmed in subsequent reports.

Vesicosphincter dyssynergia is a DIVM also reported less often than sphincter bradykinesia. Whereas Pavlakis et al. called attention to the absence of vesicosphincter dyssynergia *(8)*, Andersen et al. *(14,16)* reported two patients with an abnormality they initially called "dyssynergia" *(16)* but later labeled "spasticity" *(14)*. In a series of 70 PD patients referred for prological evaluation *(12)* who were free of obstructive etiologies, Araki et al. found two patients (3%) who had both hyperreflexia and detrusor-sphincter dyssynergia (2/70).

Berger and colleagues *(7,23)* studied 29 patients with PD (24 men and 5 women) who were urologically symptomatic. In 61% (14/23) of patients tested, they documented sporadic involuntary electromyographic activity of the external sphincter during *involuntary* detrusor contractions, but in none did this cause obstruction. They labeled this phenomenon "involuntary sphincteric activity." Because this phenomenon was not associated with radiographic or manometric evidence of obstruction at the level of the membranous urethra, the authors concluded that it did not meet criteria for the definition of detrusor-sphincter dyssynergia. This activity is reminiscent of pseudodyssynergia in that both occur in response to involuntary detrusor contractions, but pseudodyssynergia is seen as a *voluntary* act.

9. DOPAMINERGIC MEDICATION

Dopaminergic medication likely improves voiding by facilitating relaxation of the striated sphincter and increasing bladder contractility. Raz demonstrated a decrease in the urethral pressure profile (UPP) after treatment with levodopa in 10 patients who had PD with urological symptoms *(6)*. An increase in UPP occurred in patients whose treatment with levodopa was interrupted for 1 week (number of patients not specified).

In a series of 30 patients with PD, 11 displayed delayed or incomplete perineal floor relaxation *(19)*. All experienced greatly improved perineal muscle control after subcutaneous injection of apomorphine (4 mg), a dopamine agonist. There was no effect on detrusor hyperactivity. In another series of 10 patients who had PD with urinary symptoms *(24)*, urodynamic studies were performed before and after the subcutaneous administration of apomorphine. Voiding efficiency improved after apomorphine injection with an overall decrease in bladder outflow obstruction. There was an increase in the mean and maximum flow rates in nine patients and reduction in postmicturition residual volume in six. This was accompanied by fluoroscopic evidence of widening of the urethra at the level of the distal sphincter mechanism. Of additional interest was that three patients were unable to void during the "off" state, despite considerable discomfort and a feeling of bladder fullness, as a consequence of decreased detrusor contractility *(24)*. After apomorphine injection voiding detrusor pressure in these three patients increased while calculated bladder outflow resistance fell, resulting in considerable improvement in voiding. No information was provided as to whether these patients were on anticholinergic drugs. The investigators concluded that because their patients were all premedicated with domperidone, a peripheral dopamine antagonist, the effects of apomorphine on both smooth and striated musculature of the lower urinary tract must be mediated by changes in the central dopaminergic transmission *(24)*.

Uchiyama et al. *(25)* reported the effects of a single dose of 100 mg levodopa on urinary function in 18 patients who had PD with severe end-of-dose wearing-off. Patients were on levodopa and dopamine agonists, but not on anticholinergics. There was an increase in detrusor contractility; alternatively, there was an increase in urethral obstruction. However, the net effect favored the increase in bladder contractility. The result was a decrease in residual volume, that is, an improvement in voiding efficiency.

9.1. Effects of Dopaminergic Medication on Detrusor Activity

Fitzmaurice et al. *(18)* reported on nine urologically symptomatic patients who had PD with detrusor hyperreflexia. The effects of levodopa were variable. Six patients had less severe detrusor hyperreflexia when off (including one patient whose hyperreflexia disappeared), whereas three were better when on levodopa. A description of the impact of treatment on the actual symptoms was not provided.

Detrusor function during the filling (storage) phase was not consistently altered by apomorphine in another study *(24),* in which detrusor hyperreflexia improved in some cases and deteriorated in others.

In their study of 18 patients with PD who had severe wearing off, Uchiyama et al. *(25)* showed an unpredictable effect on bladder function during filling. Urinary urgency (with or without detrusor hyperreflexia or low-compliance bladder) was aggravated in nine patients (50%), alleviated in three (17%), and unchanged in six (33%).

10. DIAGNOSIS OF MULTIPLE SYSTEM ATROPHY

Early and prominent urinary symptoms and "obstructive" symptoms (in the absence of obstruction) are clues to the diagnosis of multiple system atrophy (MSA). Chandiramani et al. *(10)* performed a retrospective study of 52 patients with MSA and 41 patients with PD. Of MSA patients, 60% (31/52) had urinary symptoms preceding or coinciding with diagnosis of the disease. There were 16 patients who reported frequency, urgency, or incontinence before the onset of Parkinsonism, and 15 patients developed urinary symptoms at the same time as Parkinsonism. In contrast, in 94% of patients with PD, the urogenital symptoms clearly followed the neurological diagnosis by a few years. Two other series, identified in a review by Fowler, also confirm a 60% prevalence of *early* urinary symptoms in MSA *(26).* In one series *(10),* patients with MSA were more likely to suffer from troublesome incontinence (73%). They were also more likely to have elevated postvoid residuals than patients with PD (66% versus 16%, respectively). Among the males with MSA, 93% had erectile dysfunction (ED), including 48% in whom this complaint preceded the MSA diagnosis. Although ED can also be seen in PD, the proportion of early ED is less *(27).* In the series of Chandiramani et al. *(10),* all 11 men with MSA who underwent transurethral prostatectomy (TURP) were incontinent postoperatively (*see* Section 15.).

Fowler *(26)* has proposed the following five urogenital criteria as implied in the diagnosis of MSA: (1) urinary symptoms preceding or presenting with Parkinsonism; (2) ED preceding or presenting with Parkinsonism; (3) urinary incontinence; (4) significant postmicturition residue (>100 mL); and (5) worsening bladder control after urological surgery. However, none of these criteria are specific, and the clinician has to view their presence in context with the remaining clinical features.

11. SPHINCTER EMG

In the appropriate context sphincter EMG may differentiate MSA from PD. Stocchi et al. *(19)* found EMG to provide important differentiating data between MSA and PD. The main feature that differentiated 32 MSA patients from 30 patients with PD was abnormal sphincter EMG in 75% (24/32) of the MSA patients when compared with none of the patients who had PD. Vodušek conducted a comprehensive review of the subject *(28).* He concluded that anal sphincter EMG abnormalities could distinguish MSA from PD during the first 5 years after the onset of symptoms and signs if other causes for sphincter denervation (e.g., surgery) had been ruled out. However, with such criteria, as Vodušek readily admits, sphincter EMG offers a low sensitivity.

12. VOIDING DYSFUNCTION IN PD

Voiding dysfunction results from the loss of the inhibitory effect that the basal ganglia exert on the pontine micturition center. This inhibitory effect is likely mediated by D1 receptors and results in a "quiet" bladder during the filling phase. The experimental studies performed by Lewin et al. in cats have proven pivotal to the understanding of the pathogenesis of voiding dysfunction in PD *(29,30).* Lewin et al. stimulated the thalamus and different sites of the basal ganglia and found that the stimulation was inhibitory of detrusor contractions. Inhibition ranged from prolongation of the intercontraction interval of the detrusor to occasional complete suppression of detrusor contractions with the activity only resuming after stimulation was stopped. Interestingly, stimulation of the red nucleus, subthalamic nucleus, and substantia nigra was more inhibitory than stimulation of the thalamus.

Current beliefs propose that impulses from a cortical micturition center in the mesial frontal lobes *(19)* travel to the pontine-mesencephalic reticular formation. This pathway is thought to be influenced by the basal ganglia, thalamic nuclei, and anterior vermis of the cerebellum *(8,14)*. Micturition may also be influenced by the anterior cingulate gyrus, locus ceruleus, and nucleus tegmento lateralis dorsalis *(19)*.

Studies in conscious rats suggest that D1 receptors (linked to stimulation of adenylate cyclase; *31*) tonically *inhibit* the micturition reflex *(32)*. Administration of mixed D1/D2 agonists in anesthetized MPTP-lesioned monkeys increased their pathologically reduced bladder volume threshold *(33)* and could be antagonized by pretreatment with a D1 antagonist. This inhibitory effect of the D1 receptors presumably would be exerted via the forebrain system *(31)*, perhaps through potentiation of the GABAergic system in the basal ganglia *(33)*. The loss of D1 activation in PD may therefore underlie the bladder overactivity present during the storage phase in PD.

13. EFFECTS OF ANTICHOLINERGIC DRUGS

Irritative symptoms are responsive to anticholinergic drugs. However, exclusion of obstructive uropathy prior to symptomatic treatment is advisable. Oxybutynin and tolterodine are among the more frequently used anticholinergic drugs in the symptomatic treatment of irritative symptoms. Other agents include propantheline bromide, hyoscyamine, and flavoxate *(34)*. The oxybutynin dose ranges from 2.5 mg at bedtime to 5 mg TID. Side effects include hesitancy, weak urinary stream, dry mouth, difficulty with visual accommodation, constipation, and aggravation of glaucoma.

Some experts have suggested using extended-release forms of anticholinergics to prevent high-serum levels during therapy with the notion that this may reduce the likelihood of cognitive dysfunction *(35)*. Examples include tolterodine LA at doses of 2 to 4 mg once daily and oxybutynin LA at doses of 5 to 30 once daily *(36)*. More recently, oxybutynin transdermal has been released *(36)*. This route avoids first-pass metabolism, resulting in a lower concentration of its active metabolite. Because this metabolite has a higher affinity in vitro for parotid cells than for bladder cells, it may explain the lower incidence of dry mouth reported with transdermal oxybutynin *(36)*.

If therapy with a single anticholinergic agent proves to be suboptimal, the tricyclic antidepressant, imipramine hydrochloride, can be used in combination, as it has a different receptor site profile *(21)*.

14. TREATMENT OF OBSTRUCTIVE SYMPTOMS

Treating obstructive symptoms is based on ruling out structural causes of obstruction first, followed by ensuring bladder emptying by either intermittent or permanent catheterization. Combination treatment with anticholinergics and attempts to optimize dopaminergic treatment are also recommended. The successful treatment of obstructive symptoms of hesitancy and weak urinary stream begins with a careful drug history, searching for medications with an anticholinergic effect. Urodynamic studies should follow that investigate for the presence of detrusor areflexia, DIVM, or an obstructive uropathy.

A frequent clinical setting for the development of detrusor areflexia in PD occurs when symptomatic detrusor instability (hyperreflexia) is treated with anticholinergic drugs. This may produce the urodynamic findings of involuntary bladder contractions associated with incomplete emptying, secondary to unsustained detrusor contractions *(21)*. In that case, management consists in combining anticholinergics with clean, intermittent catheterization by oneself or others *(21)*. Successful management also helps in preventing recurrent urinary tract infections.

Another possible cause of obstructive symptoms is DIVM. In cases of external urethral sphincter bradykinesia or pseudodyssynergia with high-voiding pressures (>90-cm H_2O), some investigators recommend both anticholinergics and intermittent catheterization (similar to treatment employed for mixed detrusor hyperreflexia with incomplete bladder emptying) because persistent high pressures are certain to result in damage to the bladder and, ultimately, to the upper urinary tract *(21)*. Sphincter bradykinesia has also been shown to be responsive to dopaminergic treatment *(6,19,24)*, whereas pseudodyssynergia may be correctable with biofeedback *(8)*.

Patients with MSA are also more likely to have poor bladder compliance and sphincter insufficiency *(23)*. This could result in episodes of incontinence, including both overflow and stress incontinence (in addition to hesitancy and weak stream). Intermittent catheterization, with or without anticholinergics (i.e., oxybutynin), may be the initial treatment *(10,23)*. In some cases, desmopressin spray may be used *(10)*. Because of motor dysfunction, treatment may evolve to permanent indwelling catheterization or suprapubic cystostomy *(23,35)*. Stress incontinence in females can be treated with urethral suspension or a sling procedure, but if there is concurrent detrusor hyperreflexia, the consequence may be suboptimal *(35)*.

15. SURGICAL TREATMENT FOR PROSTATIC OBSTRUCTION

Surgical relief of prostatic obstruction (or other obstructive uropathies) is advisable, but the resolution of urinary symptoms following surgery is unpredictable. Resolution of the detrusor instability can be expected in 60 to 70% of patients postoperatively if the instability is the result of prostatic obstruction *(21)*. Therefore, the patient should be advised that such operations (i.e., prostatectomy) are primarily indicated for relief of obstruction and to avoid the need of catheterization *(7)*, but they may not eliminate the often coexistent irritative symptoms.

Berger et al. *(7)* reported persistence of urge incontinence in eight men with PD who had undergone prostatic surgery with evidence of detrusor hyperreflexia in seven patients. They could not find any urodynamic parameters that would predict preoperatively whether a hyperreflexic bladder will stabilize after successful relief of the obstruction *(7)*. If urge incontinence persists after surgery, anticholinergic therapy can be added. If it still persists, condom catheter drainage may be necessary. There are no urodynamic parameters capable of estimating preoperatively which hyperreflexic bladder will stabilize after successful obstruction relief.

Urologists should be aware of the necessity to rule out MSA prior to surgery. In the series of Chandiramani et al. *(10)*, postoperative results were very different for PD and MSA patients. Three of the five PD patients who underwent TURP reported a good result. Despite oral oxybutynin, one patient with an adequate flow rate had persistent urgency but improved considerably after intravesical oxybutynin. Another patient had a large postvoid residual after TURP and was indicated to have an atonic bladder of unknown etiology. All 11 men with MSA who experienced TURP were incontinent postoperatively. Nine (82%) had problems immediately, and two (18%) became incontinent within 1 year. Similarly, five anti-incontinence procedures in three women were unsuccessful.

16. DEEP-BRAIN STIMULATION SURGERY

It is reasonable to expect improvement of urological symptoms in those patients undergoing deep-brain stimulation surgery, but more studies are necessary. Murnaghan *(1)* reported results of basal ganglia surgery on urological symptoms and findings in 29 patients with PD. In the analysis, 8 patients complained of bladder disturbances, and 11 had abnormal cystometrograms. There were 11 patients who had cystometrograms performed pre- and postoperatively; only 5 were unchanged postoperatively. Normal bladder function was converted into hyperreflexic bladder in two of four patients examined before and after stereotaxic lesions of the thalamic nuclei, whereas stereotactic lesions of the posterior limb of the internal capsule normalized three of four uninhibited bladders. Murnaghan concluded that thalamotomy may be associated with increased bladder tonus and pallidotomy with decreased bladder tonus. Capsulotomy may reduce tonus, but bladder sensation may be affected *(1)*.

In 1971, Porter and Bors *(2)* also reviewed the effects of thalamotomy on bladder function. They studied the impact of uni- and bilateral thalamotomy on 49 patients with PD (11 of whom had normal function). They found that neurogenic bladder dysfunction was more frequently seen in clinically bilateral cases. It was only after bilateral stereotaxic surgery that improvement of bladder function could be consistently documented.

The same authors then followed up on the status of 40 patients over a long term (4–8 months after their last operation, unilateral or bilateral). These patients had somatic manifestations that had been "significantly improved" after the surgery (no quantification provided). These results indicated that the neurogenic bladder of the parkinsonian patient was responsive to surgical therapy, although the response was not as prompt or successful as treatment of somatic manifestations. Furthermore, the subjective response of the individual was often more pronounced than the objective evidence of improvement.

The authors also postulated that thalamotomy improved the postvoid residual volume by relaxing the bladder floor and—especially in the "hypoactive bladder"—by increasing the activity of the detrusor muscle *(2)*. This analysis is consistent with the findings of Murnaghan *(1)*. It would have been of interest to learn if the use of anticholinergics had decreased postoperatively as a possible alternative explanation to the decline in postvoid residual.

Andersen et al. *(16)* examined 44 patients with Parkinsonism, including 8 who had undergone thalamotomy. None of the eight patients had normal bladder function. The authors concluded that stereotactic operations on the thalamus could produce uninhibited bladder contractions with a subsequent risk of urological disturbances.

To date, there is only one report of the effect of basal ganglia surgery on Parkinsonian voiding dysfunction that stems from the "new era" that began in the 1990s *(37)*. The investigators studied five patients who had undergone bilateral implantation of subthalamic nucleus electrodes. These patients had not been assessed urologically preoperatively. Instead, they were studied urodynamically 4 to 9 months postsurgery with comparisons made between the stimulator-on and -off states. (There was no mention made as to being "on" or "off" levodopa during the procedures.) The authors found consistent improvement in bladder capacity (bladder volume at which urinary leakage was observed; or if leakage did not occur, bladder volume at unbearable desire to void) and reflex volume (bladder volume at initial hyperreflexic detrusor contraction).

REFERENCES

1. Murnaghan GF. Neurogenic disorders of the bladder in Parkinsonism. Brit J Urol 1961;33:403–409.
2. Porter RW, Bors E. Neurogenic bladder in Parkinsonism: effect of thalamotomy. J Neurosurg 1971;34:27–32.
3. Lemack GE, Dewey Jr RB, Roehrborn CG, et al. Questionnaire-based assessment of bladder dysfunction in patients with mild to moderate Parkinson's disease. Urology 2000;56:250–254.
4. Singer C, Weiner WJ, Sanchez-Ramos JR. Autonomic dysfunction in men with Parkinson's disease. Eur Neurol 1992;32:134–140.
5. Sakakibara R, Shinotoh H, Uchiyama T, et al. Questionnaire-based assessment of pelvic organ dysfunction in Parkinson's disease. Auton Neurosci 2001;92:76–85.
6. Raz S. Parkinsonism and neurogenic bladder. Experimental and clinical observations. Urol Res 1976;4:133–138.
7. Berger Y, Blaivas JG, DeLaRocha ER, Salinas JM. Urodynamic findings in Parkinson's disease. J Urol 1987;138:836–883.
8. Pavlakis AJ, Siroky MB, Goldstein I, Krane RJ. Neurourologic findings in Parkinson's disease. J Urol 1983;129:80–83.
9. Niimi Y, Ieda T, Hirayama M, et al. Clinical and physiological characteristics of autonomic failure with Parkinson's disease. Clin Auton Res 1999;9:139–144.
10. Chandiramani VA, Palace J, Fowler CJ. How to recognize patients with Parkinsonism who should not have neurological surgery. Brit J Urol 1997;80:100–104.
11. Raudino F. Non motor off in Parkinson's disease. Acta Neurol Scand 2001;104:312–313.
12. Araki I, Kitahara M, Tomoyuki O, Kuno S. Voiding dysfunction and Parkinson's disease: urodynamic abnormalities and urinary symptoms. J Urol 2000;164:1640–1643.
13. Sakakibara R, Shinotoh H, Uchiyama T, et al. SPECT imaging of the dopamine transporter with [^{123}I]-β-CIT reveals marked decline of nigrostriatal dopaminergic function in Parkinson's disease with urinary dysfunction. J Neurol Sci 2001;187:55–59.
14. Andersen JT. Disturbances of bladder and urethral function in Parkinson's disease. Int Urol Nephrol 1985;1:35–41.
15. Martignoni E, Pacchetti C, Godi L, et al. Autonomic disorders in Parkinson's disease. J Neural Transm Suppl 1995;45:11–19.
16. Andersen JT, Hebjorn S, Frimodt-Moller C, et al. Disturbances of micturition in Parkinson's disease. Acta Neurol Scand 1976;53:161–170.

17. Galloway NTM. Urethral sphincter abnormalities in Parkinsonism. Brit J Urol 1983;55:691–693.
18. Fitzmaurice H, Fowler CJ, Rickards D, et al. Micturition disturbance in Parkinson's disease. Brit J Urol 1985;57:652–656.
19. Stocchi F, Carbone A, Inghilleri M, et al. Urodynamic and neuro-physiological evaluation in Parkinson's disease and multiple system atrophy. J Neurol Neurosurg Psychiatry 1997;62:507–511.
20. Andersen JT, Bradley WE. Cystometric, sphincter and electromyelographic abnormalities in Parkinson's disease. J Urol 1976;116:75–78.
21. Sotolongo JR. Voiding dysfunction in Parkinson's disease. Semin Neurol 1988;8:166–169.
22. Resnick NM, Yalla SV. Detrusor hyperactivity with impaired contractile function. An unrecognized but common cause of incontinence in elderly patients. JAMA 1987;257:3076–3081.
23. Berger Y, Salinas JN, Blaivas JG. Urodynamic differentiation of Parkinson disease and the Shy-Drager syndrome. Neurourology and Urodynamics 1990;9:117–121.
24. Christmas TJ, Chapple CR, Lees AJ, et al. Role of subcutaneous apomorphine in parkinsonian voiding dysfunction. Lancet 1998;2:1451–1453.
25. Uchiyama T, Sakakibara R, Hattori T, Yamanishi T. Short-term effect of a single levodopa dose on micturition disturbance in Parkinson's disease patients with wearing-off phenomenon. Mov Disord 2003;18:573–578.
26. Fowler CJ. Urinary disorders in Parkinson's disease and multiple system atrophy. Funct Neurol 2001;16:277–282.
27. Singer C, Weiner WJ, Ackerman M, Sanchez-Ramos J. Sexual dysfunction in early Parkinson's disease. Neurology 1990;40(Suppl 1):221.
28. Vodušek DB. Sphincter EMG and differential diagnosis of multiple system atrophy. Mov Disord 2001;16:600–607.
29. Lewin RJ, Porter RW. Inhibition of spontaneous bladder activity by stimulation of the globus pallidus. Neurology 1965;15:1049–1052.
30. Lewin RJ, Dillard GU, Porter RW. Extrapyramidal inhibition of the urinary bladder. Brain Res 1967;4:301–307.
31. Yokoyama O, Komatsu K, Ishiura Y, et al. Overactive bladder—experimental aspects. Scand J Urol Nephrol Suppl 2002;210:59–64.
32. Seki S, Igawa Y, Kaidoh K, et al. Role of dopamine D1 and D2 receptors in the micturition reflex in conscious rats. Neurourol Urodyn 2001;20:105–113.
33. Yoshimura N, Mizuta E, Yoshida O, Kuno S. Therapeutic effects of dopamine D1/D2 receptor agonists on detrusor hyperreflexia in 1-methyl-4-phenyl-1,2,3,6-tetrahydropyridine-lesioned parkinsonian cynomolgus monkeys. J Pharmacol Exp Therap 1998;286:228–233.
34. Anonymous. Tolterodine for overactive bladder. Med Lett Drugs Ther 1998;40:101–102.
35. Siroky MB. Neurological disorders. Cerebrovascular disease and Parkinsonism. Urol Clin North Am 2003;30:27–47.
36. Anonymous. Oxybutynin transdermal (Oxytrol) for overactive bladder. Med Lett Drugs Ther 2003;45:38–39.
37. Finazzi-Agro E, Peppe A, D'Amico A, et al. Effects of subthalamic nucleus stimulation on urodynamic findings in patients with Parkinson's disease. J Urol 2003;169:1388–1391.

12
Cardiovascular Autonomic Dysfunction

David S. Goldstein

SUMMARY

Patients with Parkinson's disease (PD) often have signs or symptoms indicating impaired reflexive cardiovascular regulation, including orthostatic intolerance from orthostatic hypotension. Orthostatic hypotension in PD has been thought to be a side effect of treatment with levodopa. However, recent studies have shown that virtually all patients with PD and orthostatic hypotension, regardless of levodopa treatment, have abnormal blood pressure responses to the Valsalva maneuver and markedly decreased baroreflex-cardiovagal gain. In contrast, only a minority of patients without orthostatic hypotension have abnormal Valsalva responses, and baroreflex-cardiovagal gain is often approximately normal. Plasma levels of the sympathetic neurotransmitter, norepinephrine, are lower in patients who have PD with rather than without orthostatic hypotension, suggesting a relatively smaller complement of sympathetic nerves. Almost all patients with PD and orthostatic hypotension have significantly reduced sympathetic noradrenergic innervation of the left ventricular myocardium, and most of those without orthostatic hypotension also have diffuse or localized loss of cardiac sympathetic innervation. These findings contrast with those in multiple system atrophy (MSA) with orthostatic hypotension, which can be difficult to distinguish clinically from PD. In MSA with orthostatic hypotension, sympathetic neurocirculatory failure occurs without evidence of sympathetic denervation of the heart. Therefore, PD involves not only a central catecholaminergic lesion, with the loss of dopamine cells of the nigrostriatal system, but also a peripheral catecholaminergic lesion, with the loss of postganglionic norepinephrine cells of the sympathetic nervous system, especially in the heart. The functional consequences of cardiac sympathetic denervation in PD, relationship between central dopaminergic and peripheral noradrenergic pathologies, and the bases for cardioselective sympathetic denervation in PD without orthostatic hypotension remain unknown.

Key Words: Autonomic nervous system; norepinephrine; sympathetic nervous system; orthostatic hypotension.

1. INTRODUCTION

Patients with PD frequently have symptoms or signs of autonomic failure *(1,2)*. Symptoms include constipation, urinary incontinence, orthostatic or postprandial lightheadedness, heat or cold intolerance, and erectile dysfunction. Among the signs are slurred speech and difficulty swallowing, altered saliva production, decreased bowel sounds, and orthostatic hypotension *(3)*. The latter occurs commonly in PD *(4–11)*. Because of increased susceptibility to falls and other accidental trauma, orthostatic hypotension in this setting can be not only disabling but also life-threatening. Despite the availability of effective treatments, disorders of cardiovascular regulation in PD remain underappreciated *(12)*.

2. ORTHOSTATIC HYPOTENSION INDEPENDENT OF LEVODOPA TREATMENT

According to a long-held notion, orthostatic hypotension in PD results from treatment with levodopa *(13)*. If levodopa caused orthostatic hypotension in PD, then patients with orthostatic hypoten-

From: *Current Clinical Neurology*
Parkinson's Disease and Nonmotor Dysfunction
Edited by: R. F. Pfeiffer and I. Bodis-Wollner © Humana Press Inc., Totowa, NJ

sion would be expected to be using levodopa, whereas those without orthostatic hypotension would not. Therefore, a higher proportion of patients with orthostatic hypotension would be taking levodopa therapy than patients without it. Recent work has failed to support these predictions *(14)*. Patients with PD and orthostatic hypotension do not differ from those without orthostatic hypotension, in levodopa treatment or actual plasma levodopa concentrations. Perhaps most convincingly, orthostatic hypotension can occur in patients with PD who have never taken levodopa or discontinued levodopa treatment in the remote past. Nevertheless, as discussed below (in Section 5) such patients have physiologic evidence of baroreflex failure and decreased cardiovascular innervation by sympathetic nerves, which can explain the orthostatic hypotension.

Orthostatic hypotension in patients with Parkinsonism has also been attributed to another diagnosis, such as striatonigral degeneration or the parkinsonian form of MSA *(15)*. As described later, these explanations also often do not suffice because of the intact sympathetic cardiovascular innervation found in most or all patients with these alternative diagnoses.

Whether sympathetic denervation in the body as a whole explains orthostatic hypotension in PD has been unclear. Findings based on ^{123}I-metaiodobenzylguanidine (MIBG) scanning have led to the views that in PD, cardiac sympathetic denervation occurs independently of orthostatic hypotension or other manifestations of autonomic failure and that the denervation is selective for the heart *(16–19)*. In contrast, patients with PD and orthostatic hypotension have lower mean plasma levels of norepinephrine, the sympathetic neurotransmitter, during supine rest than do patients without orthostatic hypotension, supporting the notion of relatively more generalized sympathetic denervation *(14,20–22)*.

Patients with PD and orthostatic hypotension have both markedly decreased baroreflex-cardiovagal gain and attenuated orthostatic increments in plasma norepinephrine levels. These findings point to disruption of baroreflexes, which would be expected to contribute to orthostatic hypotension.

Even in the setting of carbidopa treatment, which inhibits conversion of levodopa to dopamine outside the central nervous system, levodopa increases plasma levels of both dopamine and its deaminated metabolite, dihydroxyphenylacetic acid *(23–26)*. Exogenously administered dopamine at relatively low doses is well-known to produce vasodilation by stimulating dopamine receptors on vascular smooth muscle cells and possibly by inhibiting norepinephrine release from sympathetic nerves *(27–29)*. Dopamine also augments natriuresis and diuresis, which promotes depletion of extracellular fluid and blood volumes. Accordingly, in the setting of decreased cardiovascular sympathetic innervation and baroreflex failure, vasodilation and hypovolemia elicited by dopamine produced from levodopa might decrease the blood pressure, both during supine rest and when standing in patients with PD. Thus, orthostatic intolerance and orthostatic hypotension may occur in patients with PD while taking levodopa/carbidopa or dopamine receptor agonists, not directly from effects of these drugs alone but from interactions with baroreflex and sympathoneural pathophysiologic mechanisms occurring as part of the disease process.

3. VALSALVA MANEUVER

A particular pattern of beat-to-beat blood pressure responses to the Valsalva maneuver can detect sympathetic neurocirculatory failure *(30)*. Because of deficient reflexive, sympathetically mediated cardiovascular stimulation in response to decreased cardiac filling during Phase II of the maneuver the blood pressure decreases progressively, and during Phase IV, the pressure fails to exceed the baseline value (Fig. 1).

In our series thus far, extending over 8 years, all patients with unequivocal PD and orthostatic hypotension (and who have been able to perform a technically adequate Valsalva maneuver) have shown this abnormal pattern, regardless of levodopa/carbidopa treatment. In contrast, only about one fourth of patients with unequivocal PD lacking orthostatic hypotension have shown the abnormal pattern. Failure of reflexive sympathetically mediated cardiovascular stimulation in response to acutely decreased venous return to the heart therefore seems to characterize orthostatic hypotension in PD.

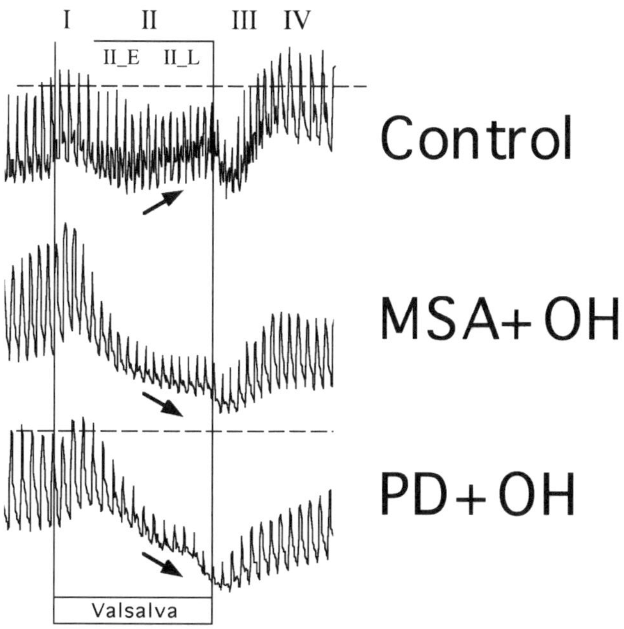

Fig. 1. Blood pressure associated with the Valsalva maneuver in a control patient, a patient with MSA and orthostatic hypotension (OH) (MSA + OH) and a patient with PD and orthostatic hypotension (PD + OH). Note that in the late portion of Phase II (II_L), blood pressure fails to increase and in Phase IV the blood pressure fails to "overshoot" the baseline value in the patients with MSA + OH or PD + OH. This pattern characterizes sympathetic neurocirculatory failure.

4. PLASMA NOREPINEPHRINE

Concentrations of norepinephrine in antecubital venous plasma provide a means—albeit indirect—to detect sympathetic denervation in the body overall. Thus, patients with orthostatic hypotension from pure autonomic failure have low plasma norepinephrine levels during supine rest *(31,32)*.

Previous work has noted that patients with PD and orthostatic hypotension have lower plasma norepinephrine concentrations than do patients without orthostatic hypotension *(21,33)*. Our results agree: patients with PD lacking orthostatic hypotension have a mean plasma norepinephrine level about 50% greater than do patients with PD and orthostatic hypotension (2.3 versus 1.4 nmol/L, $p = 0.005$).

In patients with PD and orthostatic hypotension, plasma norepinephrine levels, although significantly lower than in patients without orthostatic hypotension, are not particularly low for healthy people of similar age and are clearly higher than in patients with pure autonomic failure. Partial loss of sympathetic fibers possibly leads to augmented traffic in the remaining fibers, resulting in increased proportionate release of norepinephrine from the reduced vesicular stores. Moreover, because denervation would produce concurrent decreases in both release and reuptake of norepinephrine, plasma norepinephrine levels might fail to detect a real decrease in norepinephrine release.

5. BAROREFLEX FAILURE IN PD

Normally, plasma norepinephrine levels approximately double within 5 minutes of standing from the supine position *(34)*. Among patients who have PD without orthostatic hypotension, most have an increase in plasma norepinephrine levels of 60% or more during orthostasis, whereas in patients who have PD with orthostatic hypotension, most have an orthostatic increment less than 60%. The finding that orthostatic hypotension in PD is almost always associated with failure to increase norepinephrine levels appropriately during orthostasis is consistent with decreased baroreflex-sympathoneural function.

Studies have disagreed about whether baroreflex-sympathoneural gain changes as a function of aging *(35–49)*. Some of this inconsistency seems to have resulted from the different types of measures used—direct indices (e.g., peroneal muscle sympathetic activity) or indirect indices (e.g., limb vascular resistance). When both direct and indirect measurements have been applied in the same subjects, cardiopulmonary baroreflex control of sympathetic outflow, assessed by exposure of subjects to lower body negative pressure, has been found to be augmented, not impaired, with age in healthy humans; meanwhile, reflexive limb vasoconstriction is attenuated *(41)*. The ability to inhibit sympathetic outflow in response to increased cardiac filling from head-down tilt also does not decrease with normal human aging *(44)*. Regulation of sympathetic outflow by arterial baroreceptors, measured by sympathetic microneurography after injection of vasoactive drugs, remains approximately unchanged *(45)*, even with lower body negative pressure applied concurrently to keep central venous pressure constant *(42)*.

In contrast, studies have consistently found that baroreflex-cardiovagal gain decreases with normal human aging *(36,45,46,50)*. Relatively few studies have reviewed baroreflex-cardiovagal gain in PD *(51)*, and none to our knowledge has stratified patients regarding the occurrence of orthostatic hypotension. We have estimated baroreflex-cardiovagal gain from the slope of the relationship between interbeat interval and systolic blood pressure during Phase II of the Valsalva maneuver. Nearly all patients with PD and orthostatic hypotension have a baroreflex-cardiovagal gain less than 2 ms/mmHg. The mean value, less than 1 ms/mmHg, is far below the average value of about 6 ms/mmHg in age-matched control subjects. (Normal values in response to a fall in blood pressure can be somewhat less than those in response to an increase in blood pressure [*45*].) In contrast, among patients with PD lacking orthostatic hypotension, only about half have a baroreflex-cardiovagal gain less than 2 ms/mmHg, with a mean value of 3.2 ms/mmHg. Thus, in PD lacking orthostatic hypotension, baroreflex-cardiovagal gain is statistically decreased from normal, but in PD with orthostatic hypotension, baroreflex-cardiovagal gain is virtually always low.

In our series currently, 21 of 22 patients with PD and orthostatic hypotension have had both a supine plasma norepinephrine level less than 2 nmol/L and baroreflex-cardiovagal gain less than 2 ms/mmHg, whereas only 6 of 15 patients with PD lacking orthostatic hypotension have had both these findings ($p = 0.0002$). The combination of low baroreflex-cardiovagal gain and relatively low plasma norepinephrine levels therefore seems to characterize PD with orthostatic hypotension. Alternatively, of 10 patients with PD and either a plasma norepinephrine level less than 2 nmol/L or baroreflex-cardiovagal gain less than 2 ms/mmHg, but not both, only 1 patient has had orthostatic hypotension. This finding leads to the proposal that a combination of baroreflex-cardiovagal failure and at least some loss of sympathetic nerves may be required for orthostatic hypotension to become manifest in PD. It should be noted that baroreflex failure itself is not thought to produce orthostatic hypotension *(52,53)*.

6. CARDIAC SYMPATHETIC DENERVATION IN PD

More than 20 recent studies have agreed on the remarkable finding that virtually all patients with PD have loss of sympathetic innervation of the heart, as indicated by low myocardial concentrations of radioactivity after injection of the sympathoneural imaging agents, ^{123}I-MIBG *(16–19,54–59* and 6-[^{18}F]fluorodopamine *(14,60,61)*, as well as by neurochemical assessments during right heart catheterization *(61)*.

In patients with PD who lack orthostatic hypotension, about half have had a loss of 6-[^{18}F]fluorodopamine-derived radioactivity diffusely in the left ventricular myocardium, and slightly fewer than half have had loss localized to the lateral or inferior walls, with relative preservation in the septum or anterior wall. Only a very small minority have had entirely normal cardiac 6-[^{18}F]fluorodopamine-derived radioactivity (Fig. 2). Thus, virtually all patients with PD have evidence of at least some loss

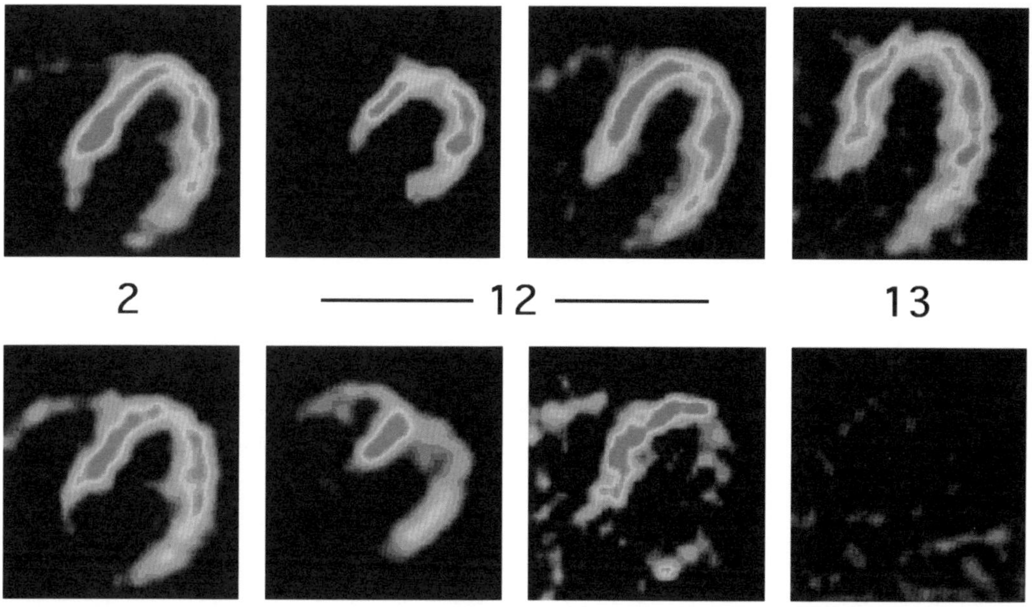

Fig. 2. Cardiac positron emission tomography scans in patients with PD lacking orthostatic hypotension. Top row shows ^{13}N-ammonia perfusion scans and bottom row shows 6-[^{18}F]fluorodopamine sympathoneural scans. Of 27 patients, 13 had markedly decreased 6-[^{18}F]fluorodopamine-derived radioactivity throughout the left ventricular myocardium, 12 localized decreases in the lateral or inferior walls with relatively more radioactivity in the interventricular septum, and only 2 normal 6-[^{18}F]fluorodopamine-derived radioactivity.

of cardiac sympathetic innervation, which agrees with the many studies from European and Japanese centers that have used ^{123}I-MIBG for cardiac sympathetic neuroimaging.

The extent of loss of sympathetic innervation in PD seems to vary among organs. Normal tissue concentrations of 6-[^{18}F]fluorodopamine-derived radioactivity have been noted in the liver, spleen, salivary glands, and nasopharyngeal mucosa, but there have been decreased concentrations in the thyroid gland and renal cortex *(14)*.

A case report noted markedly decreased cutaneous vasoconstrictor responses, indicated by laser-Doppler flowmetry, in a patient with autonomic failure and uncomplicated PD *(62)*. Many studies about cutaneous sympathetic function in PD have relied on measurements of skin humidity or electrical conductance as indices of sweat production; results have been variable *(63–69)*. However, thermoregulatory, gustatory, and emotional sweating depend on sympathetic cholinergic innervation, not sympathetic noradrenergic innervation. Patients with PD and orthostatic hypotension have intact sympathetic cholinergic innervation, as measured by the quantitative sudomotor axon reflex test, despite sympathetic neurocirculatory failure *(70)*.

7. ABSENCE OF POSTGANGLIONIC LESION IN MSA

Perhaps as remarkable as the finding that virtually all patients with PD and orthostatic hypotension have cardiac sympathetic denervation is the indication that all patients with MSA, with or without orthostatic hypotension, have intact cardiac sympathetic innervation, as measured by sympathetic neuroimaging *(16,54,55,71)*, and normal or even increased rates of entry of norepinephrine and other catechols into coronary sinus plasma *(61)*.

Validation of the approach in diagnosing PD differentially from MSA, based on the occurrence of cardiac sympathetic denervation in the former but not the latter, requires a standard, such as postmortem pathology, that unequivocally distinguishes these diseases *(72)*. Two recent studies have provided this important evidence *(73,74)*. All patients with autonomic failure, central neurodegeneration, and decreased cardiac ^{123}I-MIBG-derived radioactivity submitted to postmortem study have had nigrostriatal Lewy bodies, pathognomonic of PD, and absent tyrosine hydroxylase staining in the heart, indicating sympathetic noradrenergic denervation. All patients with normal cardiac ^{123}I-MIBG-derived radioactivity have had an absence of nigrostriatal Lewy bodies, glial cytoplasmic inclusions thought to be characteristic of MSA, and normal myocardial tyrosine hydroxylase staining.

8. DENERVATION SUPERSENSITIVITY IN PD

Clinical and preclinical studies of chronic autonomic failure have consistently noted increased blood pressure or vasoconstrictor responses to exogenously administered adrenoceptor agonists in PD with orthostatic hypotension. This type of finding would be consistent with "denervation supersensitivity," as described classically by Cannon *(75)*. Some of this supersensitivity may result from increased expression of α- or β-adrenoceptors or altered intracellular signalling after receptor occupation *(76–80)*. Moreover, cardiac sympathetic denervation supersensitivity may predispose to the development of arrhythmias *(81)*.

Augmented cardiovascular responsiveness to adrenoceptor agonists can have other explanations, such as decreased baroreflex buffering of sympathetic outflows, which as noted seems to characterize PD with orthostatic hypotension. Structural adaptations of vascular walls with increases in wall:lumen ratios occur commonly in hypertension, and supine hypertension often seems to attend orthostatic hypotension in patients with autonomic failure *(82)*. Hence, although studies of patients with PD have noted augmented pressor responses to exogenously administered norepinephrine, and the augmentation is seen mainly or exclusively in patients with PD and orthostatic hypotension *(20,21)*, the results do not necessarily lead to the conclusion that PD with orthostatic hypotension features denervation supersensitivity.

9. CONCLUSIONS AND FUTURE TRENDS

A combination of loss of sympathetic nerves and baroreflex failure can explain orthostatic hypotension in PD and the worsening of orthostatic symptoms during treatment with levodopa/carbidopa or dopamine receptor agonists. Cardiac sympathetic denervation characterizes most patients with PD and virtually all patients with PD and orthostatic hypotension. This evidence contrasts with normal cardiac sympathetic innervation in MSA.

The functional consequences of cardiac sympathetic denervation in PD, relationship between central dopaminergic and peripheral noradrenergic pathologies, and basis for cardioselective sympathetic denervation in PD without orthostatic hypotension remain unknown.

REFERENCES

1. Magalhaes M, Wenning GK, Daniel SE, Quinn NP. Autonomic dysfunction in pathologically confirmed multiple system atrophy and idiopathic Parkinson's disease—a retrospective comparison. Acta Neurol Scand 1995;91:98–102.
2. Martignoni E, Pacchetti C, Godi L, Micieli G, Nappi G. Autonomic disorders in Parkinson's disease. J Neural Transm Suppl 1995;45:11–19.
3. Wenning GK, Scherfler C, Granata R, et al. Time course of symptomatic orthostatic hypotension and urinary incontinence in patients with postmortem confirmed parkinsonian syndromes: a clinicopathological study. J Neurol Neurosurg Psychiatry 1999;67:620–623.
4. Senard JM, Rai S, Lapeyre-Mestre M, et al. Prevalence of orthostatic hypotension in Parkinson's disease. J Neurol Neurosurg Psychiatry 1997;63:584–589.
5. Senard JM, Brefel-Courbon C, Rascol O, Montastruc JL. Orthostatic hypotension in patients with Parkinson's disease: pathophysiology and management. Drugs Aging 2001;18:495–505.
6. Aminoff MJ, Wilcox CS. Control of blood pressure in Parkinsonism. Proc R Soc Med 1972;65:944–946.
7. Appenzeller O, Goss JE. Autonomic deficits in Parkinson's syndrome. Arch Neurol 1971;24:50–57.

8. Birkmayer W, Birkmayer G, Lechner H, Riederer P. DL-3,4-threo-DOPS in Parkinson's disease: effects on orthostatic hypotension and dizziness. J Neural Transm 1983;58:305–313.
9. Bloem BR. Postural instability in Parkinson's disease. Clin Neurol Neurosurg 1992;94:S41–S45.
10. Micieli G, Martignoni E, Cavallini A, et al. Postprandial and orthostatic hypotension in Parkinson's disease. Neurology 1987;37:386–393.
11. Mathias CJ. Cardiovascular autonomic dysfunction in parkinsonian patients. Clin Neurosci 1998;5:153–166.
12. Cardiovascular disorders in Parkinson disease are underrated. Fortschr Neurol Psychiatr 1999;67:A8–A9.
13. Hoehn MM. Levodopa-induced postural hypotension. Treatment with fludrocortisone. Arch Neurol 1975;32:50–51.
14. Goldstein DS, Holmes C, Dendi R, et al. Orthostatic hypotension from sympathetic denervation in Parkinson's disease. Neurology 2002;58:1247–1255.
15. Shy GM, Drager GA. A neurological syndrome associated with orthostatic hypotension. Arch Neurol 1960;3:511–527.
16. Braune S, Reinhardt M, Schnitzer R, et al. Cardiac uptake of [123I]MIBG separates Parkinson's disease from multiple system atrophy. Neurology 1999;53:1020–1025.
17. Satoh A, Serita T, Seto M, et al. Loss of 123I-MIBG uptake by the heart in Parkinson's disease: assessment of cardiac sympathetic denervation and diagnostic value. J Nucl Med 1999;40:371–375.
18. Takatsu H, Nishida H, Matsuo H, et al. Cardiac sympathetic denervation from the early stage of Parkinson's disease: Clinical and experimental studies with radiolabeled MIBG J Nucl Med 2000;41:71–77.
19. Yoshita M, Hayashi M, Hirai S. Decreased myocardial accumulation of 123I-meta-iodobenzyl guanidine in Parkinson's disease. Nucl Med Commun 1998;19:137–142.
20. Niimi Y, Ieda T, Hirayama M, et al. Clinical and physiological characteristics of autonomic failure with Parkinson's disease. Clin Auton Res 1999;9:139–144.
21. Senard JM, Valet P, Durrieu G, et al. Adrenergic supersensitivity in parkinsonians with orthostatic hypotension. Eur J Clin Invest 1990;20:613–619.
22. Senard JM, Rascol O, Durrieu G, et al. Effects of yohimbine on plasma catecholamine levels in orthostatic hypotension related to Parkinson disease or multiple system atrophy. Clin Neuropharmacol 1993;16:70–76.
23. Tohgi H, Abe T, Yamazaki K, et al. Effects of the catechol-O-methyltransferase inhibitor tolcapone in Parkinson's disease: correlations between concentrations of dopaminergic substances in the plasma and cerebrospinal fluid and clinical improvement. Neurosci Lett 1995;192:165–168.
24. Kaakkola S, Mannisto PT, Nissinen E, et al. The effect of an increased ratio of carbidopa to levodopa on the pharmacokinetics of levodopa. Acta Neurol Scand 1985;72:385–391.
25. Rose S, Jenner P, Marsden CD. The effect of carbidopa on plasma and muscle levels of L-dopa, dopamine and their metabolites following L-dopa administration to rats. Mov Disord 1988;3:117–125.
26. Myllyla VV, Sotaniemi KA, Illi A, et al. Effect of entacapone, a COMT inhibitor, on the pharmacokinetics of levodopa and on cardiovascular responses in patients with Parkinson's disease. Eur J Clin Pharmacol 1993;45:419–423.
27. Yeh BK, McNay JL, Goldberg LI. Attenuation of dopamine renal and mesenteric vasodilation by haloperidol: Evidence for a specific dopamine receptor. J Pharmacol Exp Ther 1969;168:303–309.
28. Lokhandwala MF, Hegde SS. Cardiovascular pharmacology of dopamine receptor agonists. In: Amenta F, ed. Peripheral Dopamine Pathophysiology. CRC Press, Inc., Boca Raton, FL, 1990, pp. 63–77.
29. Durrieu G, Senard JM, Tran MA, et al. Effects of levodopa and bromocriptine on blood pressure and plasma catecholamines in parkinsonians. Clin Neuropharmacol 1991;14:84–90.
30. Goldstein DS, Tack C. Non-invasive detection of sympathetic neurocirculatory failure. Clin Auton Res 2000;10:285–291.
31. Ziegler MG, Lake CR, Kopin IJ. The sympathetic-nervous-system defect in primary orthostatic hypotension. N Engl J Med 1977;296:293–297.
32. Goldstein DS, Polinsky RJ, Garty M, et al. Patterns of plasma levels of catechols in neurogenic orthostatic hypotension. Ann Neurol 1989;26:558–563.
33. Senard JM, Rascol O, Durrieu G, et al. Effects of yohimbine on plasma catecholamine levels in orthostatic hypotension related to Parkinson disease or multiple system atrophy. Clin Neuropharmacol 1993;16:70–76.
34. Lake CR, Ziegler MG, Kopin IJ. Use of plasma norepinephrine for evaluation of sympathetic neuronal function in man. Life Sci 1976;18:1315–1325.
35. Ebert TJ, Morgan BJ, Barney JA, et al. Effects of aging on baroreflex regulation of sympathetic activity in humans. Am J Physiol 1992;263:H798–H803.
36. Matsukawa T, Sugiyama Y, Mano T. Age-related changes in baroreflex control of heart rate and sympathetic nerve activity in healthy humans. J Auton Nerv Syst 1996;60:209–212.
37. Shimada K, Kitazumi T, Sadakane N, et al. Age-related changes of baroreflex function, plasma norepinephrine, and blood pressure. Hypertension 1985;7:113–117.
38. Shimada K, Kitazumi T, Ogura H, et al. Effects of age and blood pressure on the cardiovascular responses to the Valsalva maneuver. J Am Geriatr Soc 1986;34:431–434.
39. Ebert TJ, Morgan BJ, Barney JA, et al. Effects of aging on baroreflex regulation of sympathetic activity in humans. Am J Physiol 1992;263:H798–H803.

40. Matsukawa T, Sugiyama Y, Mano T. Age-related changes in baroreflex control of heart rate and sympathetic nerve activity in healthy humans. J Auton Nerv Syst 1996;60:209–212.
41. Davy KP, Seals DR, Tanaka H. Augmented cardiopulmonary and integrative sympathetic baroreflexes but attenuated peripheral vasoconstriction with age. Hypertension 1998;32:298–304.
42. Davy KP, Tanaka H, Andros EA, et al. Influence of age on arterial baroreflex inhibition of sympathetic nerve activity in healthy adult humans. Am J Physiol 1998;275:H1768–H1772.
43. Matsukawa T, Sugiyama Y, Watanabe T, et al. Baroreflex control of muscle sympathetic nerve activity is attenuated in the elderly. J Auton Nerv Syst 1998;73:182–185.
44. Tanaka H, Davy KP, Seals DR. Cardiopulmonary baroreflex inhibition of sympathetic nerve activity is preserved with age in healthy humans. J Physiol 1999;515:249–254.
45. Rudas L, Crossman AA, Morillo CA, et al. Human sympathetic and vagal baroreflex responses to sequential nitroprusside and phenylephrine. Am J Physiol 1999;276:H1691–H1698.
46. O'Mahony D, Bennett C, Green A, Sinclair AJ. Reduced baroreflex sensitivity in elderly humans is not due to efferent autonomic dysfunction. Clin Sci 2000;98:103–110.
47. Ferrari AU. Modifications of the cardiovascular system with aging. Am J Geriatr Cardiol 2002;11:30–33.
48. Seals DR, Monahan KD, Bell C, et al. The aging cardiovascular system: changes in autonomic function at rest and in response to exercise. Int J Sport Nutr Exerc Metab 2001;11 Suppl:S189–S195.
49. Niimi Y, Iwase S, Fu Q, et al. Effect of aging on muscle sympathetic nerve activity and peripheral venous pressure in humans. Environ Med 2000;44:56–59.
50. Bristow JD, Honour J, Pickering GW, et al. Diminished baroreflex sensitivity in high blood pressure. Circulation 1969;39:48–54.
51. Szili-Torok T, Kalman J, Paprika D, et al. Depressed baroreflex sensitivity in patients with Alzheimer's and Parkinson's disease. Neurobiol Aging 2001;22:435–438.
52. Robertson D, Hollister AS, Biaggioni I, et al. The diagnosis and treatment of baroreflex failure. N Engl J Med 1993;329:1449–1455.
53. Robertson D, Hollister AS, Biaggioni I. Arterial baroreflex failure in man. Clin Auton Res 1993;3:212.
54. Druschky A, Hilz MJ, Platsch G, et al. Differentiation of Parkinson's disease and multiple system atrophy in early disease stages by means of I-123-MIBG-SPECT. J Neurol Sci 2000;175:3–12.
55. Reinhardt MJ, Jungling FD, Krause TM, Braune S. Scintigraphic differentiation between two forms of primary dysautonomia early after onset of autonomic dysfunction: value of cardiac and pulmonary iodine-123 MIBG uptake. Eur J Nucl Med 2000;27:595–600.
56. Orimo S, Ozawa E, Nakade S, et al. (123)I-metaiodobenzylguanidine myocardial scintigraphy in Parkinson's disease. J Neurol Neurosurg Psychiatry 1999;67:189–194.
57. Ohmura M. Loss of 123I-MIBG uptake by the heart in Parkinson's disease: assessment of cardiac sympathetic denervation and diagnostic value. J Nucl Med 2000;41:1594–1595.
58. Braune S, Reinhardt M, Bathmann J, et al. Impaired cardiac uptake of meta-[123I]iodobenzylguanidine in Parkinson's disease with autonomic failure. Acta Neurol Scand 1998;97:307–314.
59. Satoh A, Serita T, Tsujihata M. Total defect of metaiodobenzylguanidine (MIBG) imaging on heart in Parkinson's disease: assessment of cardiac sympathetic denervation. Nippon Rinsho 1997;55:202–206.
60. Goldstein DS, Holmes C, Cannon RO, III, et al. Sympathetic cardioneuropathy in dysautonomias. N Engl J Med 1997;336:696–702.
61. Goldstein DS, Holmes C, Li ST, et al. Cardiac sympathetic denervation in Parkinson disease. Ann Intern Med 2000;133:338–347.
62. Baron R, Feldmann R, Lindner V. Small fibre function in primary autonomic failure. J Neurol 1993;241:87–91.
63. De Marinis M, Stocchi F, Gregori B, Accornero N. Sympathetic skin response and cardiovascular autonomic function tests in Parkinson's disease and multiple system atrophy with autonomic failure. Mov Disord 2000;15:1215–1220.
64. Haapaniemi TH, Korpelainen JT, Tolonen U, et al. Suppressed sympathetic skin response in Parkinson disease. Clin Auton Res 2000;10:337–342.
65. Choi BO, Bang OY, Sohn YH, Sunwoo IN. Sympathetic skin response and cardiovascular autonomic function tests in Parkinson's disease. Yonsei Med J 1998;39:439–445.
66. Braune HJ, Korchounov AM, Schipper HI. Autonomic dysfunction in Parkinson's disease assessed by sympathetic skin response: a prospective clinical and neurophysiological trial on 50 patients. Acta Neurol Scand 1997;95:293–297.
67. Denislic M, Meh D. Sympathetic skin response in parkinsonian patients. Electromyogr Clin Neurophysiol 1996;36:231–235.
68. Hirashima F, Yokota T, Hayashi M. Sympathetic skin response in Parkinson's disease. Acta Neurol Scand 1996;93:127–132.
69. Wang SJ, Fuh JL, Shan DE, et al. Sympathetic skin response and R-R interval variation in Parkinson's disease. Mov Disord 1993;8:151–157.
70. Sharabi Y, Li ST, Dendi R, Holmes C, Goldstein DS. Neurotransmitter specificity of sympathetic denervation in Parkinson's disease. Neurology 2003;60:1036–1039.

71. Yoshita M, Hayashi M, Hirai S. Iodine 123-labeled meta-iodobenzylguanidine myocardial scintigraphy in the cases of idiopathic Parkinson's disease, multiple system atrophy, and progressive supranuclear palsy. Rinsho Shinkeigaku 1997;37:476–482.
72. Goldstein DS. Cardiac sympathetic neuroimaging to distinguish multiple system atrophy from Parkinson disease. Clin Auton Res 2001;11:341–342.
73. Orimo S, Ozawa E, Oka T, et al. Different histopathology accounting for a decrease in myocardial MIBG uptake in PD and MSA. Neurology 2001;57:1140–1141.
74. Orimo S, Oka T, Miura H, et al. Sympathetic cardiac denervation in Parkinson's disease and pure autonomic failure but not in multiple system atrophy. J Neurol Neurosurg Psychiatry 2002;73:776–777.
75. Cannon WB. A law of denervation. Am J Med Sci 1939;198:737–750.
76. Davies B, Sudera D, Sagnella G, et al. Increased numbers of alpha receptors in sympathetic denervation supersensitivity in man. J Clin Invest 1982;69:779–784.
77. Kurvers H, Daemen M, Slaaf D, et al. Partial peripheral neuropathy and denervation induced adrenoceptor supersensitivity. Functional studies in an experimental model. Acta Orthop Belg 1998;64:64–70.
78. Vatner DE, Lavallee M, Amano J, et al. Mechanisms of supersensitivity to sympathomimetic amines in the chronically denervated heart of the conscious dog. Circ Res 1985;57:55–64.
79. Warner MR, Wisler PL, Hodges TD, et al. Mechanisms of denervation supersensitivity in regionally denervated canine hearts. Am J Physiol 1993;264:H815–H820.
80. Baser SM, Brown RT, Curras MT, et al. Beta-receptor sensitivity in autonomic failure. Neurology 1991;41:1107–1112.
81. Inoue H, Zipes DP. Results of sympathetic denervation in the canine heart: Supersensitivity that may be arrhythmogenic. Circulation 1987;75:877–887.
82. Biaggioni I, Robertson RM. Hypertension in orthostatic hypotension and autonomic dysfunction. Cardiol Clin 2002;20:291–301.

13
Thermoregulatory Dysfunction

Mark S. LeDoux

SUMMARY

Patients with Parkinson's disease (PD) must maintain core body temperature in a narrow range despite fluctuations in both endogenous heat production and environmental conditions. The hypothalamus and peripheral autonomic nervous system are essential neuroanatomical substrates for thermoregulation. In the preoptic/anterior hypothalamus, dopamine excites warm-sensitive neurons and inhibits cold-sensitive neurons. Hypothalamic dopamine deficiency may perturb normal thermoregulatory responses. Several features of both the neuroleptic malignant syndrome (NMS) and the NMS-like syndrome associated with levodopa withdrawal are likely the result of inadequate stimulation of hypothalamic dopamine receptors. In PD, thermoregulatory dysfunction can also manifest as heat and cold intolerance, paroxysmal head and neck hyperhidrosis, and dry skin in the lower extremities. Tests of sudomotor function, such as the sympathetic skin response, quantitative sudomotor axon reflex test, thermoregulatory sweat test, silastic sweat imprint, and quantitative thermoregulatory sweat test, are often abnormal in PD, particularly in its more advanced stages. Therefore, clinicians should be cautious when using thermoregulatory testing to differentiate PD from other neurodegenerative disorders (e.g., multiple system atrophy [MSA]). In early PD, thermoregulatory dysfunction is mostly consistent with central and preganglionic autonomic dysfunction. As PD progresses, an increasing percentage of patients will also show evidence of postganglionic sympathetic abnormalities.

Key Words: Thermoregulation; Parkinson's disease (PD); hypothalamus; exothermic; radiation; conduction; sweat; dopamine; temperature; sudomotor; sympathetic; postganglionic; hyperhidrosis; neuroleptic malignant syndrome; seborrhea; xerosis.

1. INTRODUCTION

1.1. Normal Thermoregulatory Mechanisms

Patients with Parkinson's disease (PD) have cells that need energy to do their work. Energy exists in forms like light, heat, and chemical bonds. Most types of energy can be classified as either kinetic or potential. Thermal (heat) and radiant (light) are two major kinds of kinetic energy. The first law of thermodynamics states that the various types of energy can be changed from one form to another. The process of photosynthesis, for example, converts the kinetic energy of light into the potential energy of covalent bonds. Concentration and charge gradients are other forms of potential energy that are critical to biological systems.

Biological systems continuously require energy for the performance of mechanical work, active transport of molecules and ions, and synthesis of macromolecules. Chemotrophs (e.g., humans) obtain free energy by the oxidation of foods, a process in which adenosine diphosphate (ADP) is converted to adenosine triphosphate (ATP). ATP serves as the principal carrier of free energy in biological systems.

From: *Current Clinical Neurology*
Parkinson's Disease and Nonmotor Dysfunction
Edited by: R. F. Pfeiffer and I. Bodis-Wollner © Humana Press Inc., Totowa, NJ

ATP contains two energy-rich phosphoanhydride bonds, and a large amount of energy is liberated when ATP is hydrolyzed to ADP.

The sequences of reactions required for the production of ATP are exothermic. In exothermic reactions, the products contain less bond energy than the reactants, and the excess energy is usually liberated as heat. On average, one third of the potential energy contained in foods is converted to heat during the process of ATP generation. Heat is also generated in the body during the turnover of cellular macromolecules, such as proteins. Heat production by the body is normally expressed in terms of metabolic rate, which is governed by basal cellular metabolism, muscular activity, thyroid hormones, and levels of circulating epinephrine and norepinephrine. Metabolic rate can be quantified by direct calorimetry, which measures the total quantity of heat liberated from the body during a fixed period of time.

In addition to endogenous production, heat may also be gained from exogenous sources via mechanisms like radiation and conduction. Radiation is the transfer of heat by electromagnetic radiation. When environmental temperatures are greater than body temperatures, a thermal gradient is present, and heat can be transferred to humans by radiation. Conduction is heat exchange between objects that are in contact with one another. For instance, a person can gain heat by conduction while sitting on asphalt pavement on a scorching summer day.

Homeotherms, like humans, must maintain core body temperature in a narrow range, despite fluctuations in environmental conditions and endogenous heat production. Humans have a variety of mechanisms for heat loss that can be used to prevent core temperature elevations. The vast majority of heat in humans is generated by deep tissues (e.g., brain, liver, heart, and skeletal muscles). For effective elimination, this heat must be first transferred to the skin, then from the skin to the surroundings. A robust microvascular network is present in the dermis and subdermal connective tissues. Draining veins from skin capillaries are directly connected to a venous plexus located in the lower dermis and subdermal connective tissue. In the hands, feet, and ears, muscular arteriovenous anastomoses directly link small arteries to this venous plexus. When necessary, blood flow to the skin venous plexus can increase to one fourth of cardiac output.

At an ambient temperature of 22°C, most heat is lost from the skin surface by radiation and conduction. Conduction of heat to the air layer surrounding the body is greatly augmented by convection. Heat from the skin that is conducted to the surrounding air is carried away by convection air currents.

Evaporation is the final major mechanism for heat loss and becomes critical when environmental temperatures exceed body temperature. Evaporation of 1 g of water removes 0.58 kcal of heat from the body. Most of this water is derived from sweat, but insensible losses from the lungs, upper airways, and skin average 50 mL per hour. During strenuous physical activity in a hot environment, sweat secretion can exceed 1600 mL per hour. Urination, defecation, and respiration only account for 2 to 3% of heat loss in normal circumstances.

1.2. Neuroanatomical Substrates of Thermoregulation

An array of autonomic, behavioral, endocrine, and somatic thermoregulatory responses is involved in the maintenance of core temperature within a narrow range. Mechanisms activated by heat include sweating, cutaneous vasodilatation, and movement to a cooler environment. Mechanisms catalyzed by cold include vasoconstriction, piloerection, movement to a warmer environment, shivering, and possibly, increased output of thyroxine. The hypothalamus has a central role in these thermoregulatory responses.

The anterior/preoptic hypothalamus contains both warm- and cold-sensitive neurons. Warm-sensitive neurons outnumber cold-sensitive neurons by a 3:1 ratio. Increased core temperatures are associated with increased firing rates of warm-sensitive neurons, whereas cold-sensitive neurons increase their firing rates when core temperatures fall *(1)*. Although much less significant in the maintenance of core temperature, temperature sensors are also present in the skin and deep visceral tissues. In the skin, there are ten times more cold receptors than heat receptors. Afferent pathways for thermal receptors in the skin begin in the dorsal roots and ascend predominantly in the spinothalamic tract. Thermal receptors in deep tissues, such as the abdominal viscera, may course through the vagus and splanchnic nerves before entering the central nervous system. Both skin and deep thermal receptor pathways terminate in the preoptic/anterior and posterior hypothalamic areas. The posterior hypothalamus integrates signals from the skin, deep tissues, and preoptic/anterior hypothalamus. Integrated signals are compared with the setpoint for core temperature. The posterior hypothalamus then triggers autonomic responses appropriate for temperature correction. Lesion and stimulation studies highlight the complex and interrelated roles of the preoptic/anterior and posterior hypothalamus. Stimulation of the preoptic/anterior hypothalamic area produces cutaneous vasodilatation and sweating, whereas stimulation of the posterior hypothalamus causes vasoconstriction and shivering. In comparison, lesions of the preoptic/anterior hypothalamus result in hyperthermia and impair the normal responses to environmental heat (i.e., sweating and cutaneous vasodilatation). Lesions of the posterior hypothalamus lead to hypothermia in cold environments because heat conservation and generation mechanisms are impaired.

The intermediolateral and intermediomedial cell columns of spinal segments T1 to L3 of the spinal cord are the origin of preganglionic sympathetic outflow. These preganglionic neurons receive first- and higher-order control from cell groups in the hypothalamus and brainstem, including the rostral ventrolateral medulla, rostral ventromedial medulla, caudal raphe nuclei, A5 noradrenergic cell group, lateral and posterior hypothalamus, and periaqueductal gray and preoptic area *(2)*. The axons of preganglionic neurons form the white rami communicantes that pass to the sympathetic trunk. Preganglionic axons may synapse with postganglionic neurons in the sympathetic ganglia and rejoin the spinal nerves as gray rami communicantes. Preganglionic axons may also ascend or descend the sympathetic trunk before making synapses on postganglionic neurons. Other preganglionic fibers course through the sympathetic ganglia and form the splanchnic nerves that synapse in the prevertebral ganglia. Acetylcholine is the neurotransmitter released at preganglionic synapses on postganglionic neurons. It is also released by the postganglionic sympathetic innervation of sweat glands, whereas norepinephrine is released by the vast majority of postganglionic nerves that innervate blood vessels. Other neurotransmitters, particularly peptides, may be released in combination with either acetylcholine or norepinephrine.

1.3. Dopamine Effects on Thermoregulation

The potential role of dopamine in the modulation of neuronal activity in the preoptic/anterior hypothalamus has been studied in a variety of model systems. When directly injected into the preoptic/anterior hypothalamus of rats, the dopamine agonist, apomorphine, causes hypothermia. In contrast, local injections of dopaminergic antagonists like haloperidol cause hyperthermia *(3)*. An in vitro study by Scott and Boulant *(4)* detailed the effects of dopamine on individual hypothalamic neurons; single-unit activity was recorded from the preoptic/anterior hypothalamic area in rat tissue slices. Dopamine excited 41% of warm-sensitive neurons and inhibited 100% of the cold-sensitive neurons. Dopamine also decreased the thermosensitivity of the cold-sensitive neurons. Hasegawa and colleagues *(5)* used in vivo microdialysis to monitor the levels of dopamine and its metabolites in the preoptic/anterior hypothalamus of exercising rats. The levels of the dopamine metabolites 3,4-dihydroxyphenylacetic acid and homovanillic acid increased during exercise. In aggregate, these experimental findings indicate that dopaminergic innervation of the preoptic/anterior hypothalamus is involved in heat-loss mechanisms. More recent work suggests that dopamine D1/D5 and D2 receptors may be independent factors in thermoregulatory mechanisms *(6,7)*.

2. TESTING THERMOREGULATORY MECHANISMS

2.1. Core and Skin Temperature

Human core temperatures undergo circadian fluctuations of up to 0.6°C. Core temperature is lowest during sleep and, in most people, reaches its nadir at about 6:00 AM. Core temperature is highest in the evenings and rises with physical activity. In women, core temperature rises during ovulation.

Esophageal and bladder temperature-sensing devices may be superior to rectal probes for highly accurate measures of core temperature *(8)*. However, rectal temperatures are reliable enough for most routine clinical applications and more easily acquired in the outpatient setting. Oral temperatures are typically 0.5°C below rectal temperatures and are relatively unstable during long-term recordings. Axillary temperatures are not dependable, and tympanic membrane temperature measurements may be compromised by cerumen, narrow external auditory canals, and tympanic membrane defects from previous trauma *(9)*.

Contrary to core temperature, skin temperature may vary greatly from one body surface area to another and is highly reliant on both environmental temperature and the body's need to dissipate heat. Skin temperature patterns can be analyzed in two ways: infrared pyrometry and infrared telethermograhy. Pyrometry is the measurement of radiation emitted from an object. Pyrometers work without making contact with the object of interest. An infrared pyrometer can be used to document skin temperatures at several standard sites (e.g., forearm, thenar pad, hypothenar pad, distal pads of each finger, thigh, anterior leg, dorsum of the foot, and each toe pad) on each half of the body. Alternatively, infrared telethermography provides a more sophisticated color-coded digital representation of body-surface temperatures. High-resolution digital images of the trunk, face, extremities, palmar surfaces of the hands, and plantar surfaces of the feet can be obtained in minutes. Side-to-side differences of more than 1°C are considered clinically significant.

2.2. *Sudomotor Function*

2.2.1. *Sympathetic Skin Response*

The sympathetic skin response (SSR) has also been called the somatosympathetic response because the afferent component of its neural pathway is mediated predominantly by types 2 and 3 myelinated fibers. Although a variety of stimuli can be used to elicit the SSR, many laboratories provide a shock stimulus to the supraorbital or sural nerves. The efferent component of the SSR is mediated by the type B and C sympathetic innervation of sweat glands. Using the standard electrophysiological equipment typically used in nerve conduction studies, potentials are acquired from all four palmar and plantar surfaces. On the hand, the cathode is placed over the second palmar interspace and anode is over the pulp of the middle finger. On the foot, the cathode is placed over the second plantar interspace and the anode is on the pulp of the second toe. Because the SSR is sensitive to a variety of environmental factors, the patient should be relaxed, the room should be very quiet and dimly lit, and the test should be performed before other potentially painful neurophysiological studies (e.g., needle electromyography). Voltage is recorded for 10 seconds. In a study by Knevzevic and Bajada *(10)*, the average latency to onset of the palmar and plantar responses was 1.5 and 2.1 milliseconds, respectively. In normals, an early negative potential is followed by positive, then late long-duration negative potentials.

The SSR diminishes with age, and the plantar SSR may be absent in elderly subjects. The SSR also habituates; repeat studies should be performed at intervals of at least 30 seconds. The SSR is widely used in clinical neurology, and SSR abnormalities have been described in numerous diseases of both the central and peripheral nervous systems. Unfortunately, this test suffers from poor sensitivity and specificity in routine clinical application.

2.2.2. *Quantitative Sudomotor Axon Reflex Test*

The quantitative sudomotor axon reflex test (QSART) depends on the integrity of postganglionic sympathetic sudomotor axons and sweat glands. The stimulus for the QSART is iontophoretically applied acetylcholine *(11)*. Acetylcholine activates the terminals of postganglionic sympathetic axons, and the impulse is transmitted antidromically to a branch point and then orthodromically to activate sweat glands. The QSART requires a multicompartment sweat cell; one compartment serves as the stimulus compartment for delivery of acetylcholine and another for evaporation of sweat by nitrogen gas. An intervening compartment blocks the diffusion of sweat between the stimulus and evaporation compartments. Recordings are typically performed from multiple sites, such as the medial forearm, proximal leg, distal leg, and dorsum of the foot. The latency, duration, and amplitude of the response are recorded. The QSART is both sensitive and reproducible.

The QSART is usually normal in purely central and preganglionic disorders, but it is frequently abnormal in axonal neuropathies, as in diabetes. In early diabetic axonal neuropathy, only distal sites (e.g., dorsum of the foot) may show QSART abnormalities. As distal axonal neuropathies progress in severity, postganglionic failure may be detected at more proximal sites.

2.2.3. *Thermoregulatory Sweat Test*

The thermoregulatory sweat test (TST) provides a global assessment of the sympathetic sudomotor pathway *(12,13)*. A normal TST requires the integrity of high-order centers in the hypothalamus and brainstem, intermediolateral cell columns, white rami communicantes, sympathetic ganglia, postganglionic neurons, and sweat glands. To perform the TST, an indicator powder (one part alizarin red, two parts corn starch, one part sodium carbonate) is first applied to the unclothed body surface. The powder is light orange when dry and purple when wet. The subject is then enclosed in a chamber at 45 to 50°C with a relative humidity of 35 to 40%. Oral temperature is continuously monitored throughout the procedure and should not exceed 38.5°C. Under these conditions, a heating time of 30 to 45 minutes is required to elicit a maximal sweat response. A digital camera is used to photograph the body and provide a permanent record of sweating patterns. An image analysis program can then be used to determine the percentage of anterior body surface anhidrosis (%TST).

When used in combination with the QSART, the TST can determine whether an abnormality is preganglionic or postganglionic in most circumstances. However, it is important to note that the transsynaptic effects of longstanding preganglionic lesions can impair postganglionic sympathetic sudomotor function *(12,14)*. The TST may be used to evaluate sudomotor dysfunction in a variety of neurological diseases, including hypothalamic structural lesions, spinal cord pathology (e.g., vitamin B_{12} deficiency, syrinx, traumatic myelopathy, multiple sclerosis), neurodegenerative disorders, such as multiple system atrophy (MSA), and disorders of the peripheral nervous system (e.g., diabetes, amyloidosis, and other small-fiber neuropathies). In patients with compensatory regional hyperhidrosis, the TST can be used to demonstrate anhidrosis in other body regions.

2.2.4. *Silastic Sweat Imprint Test*

The silastic sweat imprint test (SSIT) directly measures the sweat gland response to a muscarinic agent, pilocarpine. Denervated glands fail to respond. In many laboratories, acetylcholine is used in place of pilocarpine, although sweating in response to acetylcholine reflects the stimulation of both muscarinic and nicotinic receptors. After intradermal injection of pilocarpine, sweat imprints are formed by the secretion of active sweat glands into a plastic (Silastic) imprint. Following removal, the indentations in the Silastic material can be examined with a microscope, photographed in either digital or analog format, and analyzed with a variety of morphometric software packages. The test can determine sweat gland density, sweat droplet size, and sweat volume per area. Denervated sweat glands lose their sudomotor response to pilocarpine.

The SSIT is sensitive, reproducible, and complements the QSART. The QSART detects postganglionic sudomotor dysfunction among a population of sympathetic axons and sweat glands. In contrast, the SSIT method provides quantitative information about individual sweat glands. The QSART may be more sensitive than the SSIT method for detection of early autonomic neuropathy.

2.2.5. *Quantitative Thermoregulatory Sweat Test*

Subjects are acclimatized to a room with stable temperature (40°C) and humidity (40%) for 30 minutes *(15)*. Local sweat rates are measured using the ventilated capsule method. Plastic capsules are attached to two skin-recording areas (forearm and thigh) and connected to plastic tubing. Low-humidity air is passed at a constant flow rate through the capsule, and changes in relative humidity are measured using capacitance hygrometry. Resting sweat rates and the frequency of sweat expulsions are measured for 10 minutes from the two recording sites. Thyrotropin-releasing hormone (TRH) is then infused while the resting sweat rates and frequency of sweat expulsions are measured for another 10 minutes. Control subjects show significant increases in sweat rates and number of sweat expulsions during infusion of TRH.

2.3. Skin Blood Flow

Laser Doppler flow meters can be used to measure skin blood flow before, during, and after autonomic maneuvers *(16)*. Modern laser Doppler flow meters provide real-time assessment of perfusion in very small volumes of tissue (1 mm^3). Changes in blood flow are measured in response to perturbations intended to increase or decrease sympathetic innervation of the cutaneous vasculature. Measurements are frequently acquired from the finger and toe pads because sympathetic activity in these areas is limited to vasoconstriction. Simultaneous continuous noninvasive measurements of blood pressure and laser Doppler perfusion from the forearm allow for calculation of cutaneous vascular resistance in response to both sympathetic vasoconstrictor (deep inspiration and foot immersion in cold water) and vasodilator (postischemic reactive hyperemia and heating of the body) responses *(17)*.

3. CLINICAL MANIFESTATIONS OF THERMOREGULATORY DYSFUNCTION IN PD

3.1. Heat and Cold Intolerance

Heat and cold intolerance are both difficult to define and fairly common in the elderly population. A person with heat intolerance may feel unusually hot and dizzy after vigorous activity or on a torrid summer day. Other manifestations of heat intolerance may include flushing, malaise, and generalized weakness. Cold intolerance is seemingly a more common complaint noted on review of systems. However, cold intolerance is usually interpreted by patients to mean an inability to keep their hands and feet warm, particularly in cold weather. A more significant manifestation of cold intolerance would be difficulty maintaining core temperature with associated weakness and dulling of consciousness in chilly environments. One report suggests that Parkinsonian patients may have an increased susceptibility to hypothermia *(18)*. A comprehensive autonomic symptom survey in PD analyzed the relative frequency (1 day/week to 7 days/week) of subjective heat and cold intolerance in patients who had PD in comparison to age-matched controls *(19)*. On average, cold intolerance was more common in the PD group, but this result did not reach statistical significance. In contrast, no differences were found between patients with PD and age-matched controls in heat intolerance.

3.2. Paroxysmal Hyperhidrosis and Other Sweating Abnormalities

Sweating (i.e., sudomotor) abnormalities were included in early descriptions of PD prior to the availability of levodopa *(20,21)*. More recently, patients have reported that sweating abnormalities may antedate their initial diagnosis of PD. Ray Kennedy, for example, a renowned soccer player in England during the 1970s, exhibited "unprovoked bouts of perspiration accompanying feelings of heat" before his PD was diagnosed and then treated with levodopa *(22)*. Most studies indicate that sweating abnormalities increase in severity with declining motor function in PD. Both hypohidrosis and hyperhidrosis have been described in PD. Hypohidrosis is most common in the lower extremities; hyperhidrosis, if present, tends to occur in the upper trunk, neck, and face. Head and neck hyperhidrosis could be a compensatory response to impaired sweating in other body regions *(23)*. However, in some patients with PD, profuse sweating may seemingly involve the entire body surface.

Hyperhidrosis may occur on a paroxysmal basis with the paroxysms being triggered by "off" periods. Sage and Mark *(24)* described copious sweating during "off" periods in four patients with advanced PD. Plasma levodopa concentration was measured in one of their patients and correlated with clinical signs. Drenching sweats started just before the noted decline in plasma levodopa levels and continued into the motor "off" period for about 1 hour.

Dry skin (i.e., xerosis), especially in the lower extremities, is a common complaint among patients with PD. Manifestations may include redness, dry scaling, pruritus, and fine crackling. Dry skin is likely a manifestation of appendicular sudomotor dysfunction in PD.

3.3. *Levodopa and/or Dopamine Agonist-Withdrawal Neuroleptic Malignant-Like Syndrome*

The NMS most commonly occurs 4–14 days after therapy initiation with a neuroleptic; approximately 90% of NMS cases occur within 10 days of neuroleptic initiation. Although the clinical spectrum of NMS is broad, certain features are necessary to make a diagnosis: hyperthermia (>38°C), muscular rigidity, delirium, and autonomic dysfunction. Autonomic features may include hypertension, hypotension, tachycardia, diaphoresis, sialorrhea, and incontinence. Rhabdomyolysis with elevated creatinine kinase is present in many cases; renal failure may result. An NMS-like syndrome may occur after the withdrawal of levodopa and/or dopamine agonists. Concomitant use of either lithium or anticholinergics increases the risk of both NMS and NMS-like syndromes.

In patients with PD, an NMS-like syndrome may occur during "off" periods *(25),* following reduction in levodopa or dopamine agonist therapy *(26,27),* and even during the premenstrual period, despite the lack of levodopa withdrawal *(28).* The average age was 72 years, and mean disease duration was 9.5 years in a recent series of 11 patients with PD who developed an NMS-like syndrome after sudden discontinuation of levodopa therapy *(29).* In this series, the NMS-like syndrome appeared at a mean latency of 93 hours after stopping levodopa.

The first and most important component of treating the NMS-like syndrome in patients who have PD, is immediate reinstitution of therapy with levodopa and/or a dopamine agonist. Patients with an NMS-like syndrome must be closely monitored in an intensive care unit. A nasogastric feeding tube should be inserted if the patient is delirious and unable to take medications orally. If available, apomorphine can be administered until a feeding tube can be used or in patients with upper gastrointestinal dysfunction (e.g., anatomical obstruction and recent laparotomy). The serum creatinine kinase and urine myoglobin should be checked for evidence of muscle necrosis. Urine output should be monitored with an indwelling catheter. It is important to correct volume depletion and hypotension with intravenous fluids. Methods to reduce body temperature include cooling blankets and oral or rectal acetaminophen. Benzodiazepines can be can be used to calm the agitated patient. Dantrolene has been used in patients with NMS to reduce rigidity and lessen the severity of rhabdomyolysis. Forced diuresis with a mannitol drip can prevent renal failure in patients with laboratory evidence of rhabdomyolysis. Clinical outcomes are good in the majority of patients who receive proper intensive medical management.

3.4. *Seborrhea and Seborrheic Dermatitis*

Seborrheic dermatitis is a red, scaly, itchy rash that most commonly occurs in areas that have the highest concentration of sebaceous glands, such as the nose, eyebrows, eyelids, behind the ears, and middle of the chest. Seborrhea is oiliness of the skin, particularly of the face and scalp, without associated redness or scaly rash. Seborrhea and seborrheic dermatitis are more common in PD than in age-matched controls. The etiology and pathophysiology of seborrhea and seborrheic dermatitis are poorly understood. A variety of factors, including androgens, lipophilic *Malassezia* yeast, and dysfunction of the central and peripheral nervous systems, may contribute to the development of seborrheic dermatitis.

The pathophysiology of seborrheic dermatitis is peripherally related to thermoregulation in PD. The sebaceous glands secrete sebum, an oily substance that helps prevent sweat loss from the skin and thus contributes to thermoregulation. Sebum is a component of the hydrolipid system that is partly responsible for the skin's barrier function. The hydrolipid system consists of sweat, sebum, and other moisturizing factors (e.g., urea). Sebum helps keep the skin pliable and crack-free and prevents the hair from becoming brittle and split. In essence, sebum "waterproofs" the skin and hair.

Table 1
Tests of Sudomotor Function in Parkinson's Disease

Name	Technique	Pathway (s) analyzed	Findings in Parkinson's disease	References
Sympathetic skin response (SSR)	Record palmar and plantar current change in response to shock stimulus	Types 2 and 3 mechano-receptor afferents and sympathetic efferents	Incidence of absent or diminished responses that increase with increasing disease severity	*(38,41,42)*
Quantitative sudomotor axon reflex test (QSART)	Measure sweat volume and latency of response to iontophoresis of acetylcholine	Postganglionic sympathetic innervation of sweat glands	Mildly abnormal, in general, and degree of abnormality increases with disease severity	*(37,55)*
Thermoregulatory sweat test (TST)	Apply indicator powder to whole body prior to whole-body heating	Central and peripheral sudomotor pathways	Patchy or mainly lower extremity anhidrosis or hypohidrosis in the majority of patients	*(23,35–37, 43)*
Silastic sweat imprint test (SSIT)	Obtain imprints of sweat droplets after iontophoresis of pilocarpine or acetylcholine	Postganglionic sympathetic innervation of sweat glands	Mean total volume and sweat droplet density lower in PD	*(41,42)*
Quantitative thermo-regulatory sweat test (QTST)	Measure resting sweat rate and frequency of sweat expulsions before and after infusion of TRH	Central and peripheral sudomotor pathways, including hypothalamic control centers	Absent response to TRH in early PD	*(40)*

TRH, thyrotropin-releasing hormone.

The development of seborrhea and seborrheic dermatitis is somehow related to dopamine deficiency. For example, seborrheic dermatitis is quite common in patients with neuroleptic-induced Parkinsonism *(30)*. Anecdotal evidence suggests that improvement in parkinsonian motor dysfunction shown with levodopa and/or dopamine agonists may be associated with corresponding improvement in seborrheic dermatitis. Finally, quantitative methods have been used to prove that levodopa and the dopamine agonist, bromocriptine, reduce sebum production in patients with PD *(31–33)*.

Cutaneous vascular instability, particularly on the face, may occur in up to one third of patients with PD and may coexist with seborrheic dermatitis *(34)*. Interestingly, there is an anatomical overlap among hyperhidrosis, seborrhea, and cutaneous vascular instability in patients with PD. Cranial hyperhidrosis and cutaneous vascular instability are possibly associated with the development of seborrheic dermatitis.

4. THERMOREGULATORY TEST ABNORMALITIES IN PD

Sudomotor and other thermoregulatory test abnormalities are present in many patients with PD (*see* Table 1). In early PD, test abnormalities are mostly consistent with central and preganglionic autonomic dysfunction. In more advanced PD, an increasing percentage of patients will additionally show evidence of postganglionic sympathetic abnormalities. As in most other neuropathies, the postganglionic sympathetic neuropathy in PD initially becomes manifest in the longest axons (i.e., those to the distal lower extremities). Given that idiopathic PD is most appropriately classified as a neurodegenerative syndrome with variable and broad expressivity, it is not surprising that even within a particular

Hoehn and Yahr (H & Y) stage, sudomotor testing will be normal in some patients and yet strikingly abnormal in others. Therefore, thermoregulatory testing may not be particularly useful for diagnosing PD in an individual patient but may supply information important for the clinical management of a patient already diagnosed with PD based on standard clinical criteria.

The TST was used in two early studies of autonomic dysfunction in PD. Appenzeller and Goss *(23)* reported a normal TST in 8 of 18 patients with PD; the remaining patients had almost complete anhidrosis on the trunk and limbs with hyperhidrosis on the face. The authors suggested that the facial hyperhidrosis was a compensatory response to anhidrosis elsewhere on the body. In the same year, Aminoff and Wilcox described patchy impairment of the TST in 4 of 11 patients with PD *(35)*.

In 1986, Goetz and colleagues published their studies of autonomic function in 31 patients with PD *(36)*. Average patient age, disease duration, and H & Y stage were 61 years, 123 months, and 3.1, respectively. Findings were compared to those of 10 age-matched controls. Skin temperature after heat stress, measured while patients were off medication, was lower in the PD group than in controls. Off-medication head and neck sweating, as indicated with TST, was significantly greater in the PD group. In contrast, there were no differences in skin temperature and sweating between the control group and patients with PD on medication, thereby showing a substantial role for dopaminergic neurotransmission in thermoregulation. A study of 35 carefully selected PD patients with the TST at the Mayo Clinic revealed a mean anterior hypohidrosis of about 40% *(37)*. Of these 35 patients, 50% had H & Y stage III disease, approximately 30% had stage IV disease, no one had stage V disease, and the remainder had either stage I or II disease.

Quantitative measures of sweating using instrumentation that generates continuous dependent variables (evaporimetry and capacitance hygrometry) also show that patients with PD sweat more in the head and neck region than age-matched normal subjects. Patients who have PD also tend to exhibit lower extremity hypohidrosis, particularly as their disease progresses. Also consistent with distal sympathetic dysfunction, foot temperature may be colder in patients with PD than in controls *(38)*. Turkka and Myllylä *(39)* found that sweating in the upper body parts was greater in patients with PD than in controls both before and after heating. Upper body relative hyperhidrosis also ascended with increasing disease severity. Patients who had PD sweated less on the foot than the control subjects after a 5-minute heating stimulus.

In early PD, sweating abnormalities are both less frequent and less severe. For example, Kihara and coworkers *(40)* measured local sweat rates on the forearm and thigh in 10 patients with early PD (H & Y stages I and II) and found that forearm sweat rates were virtually identical to control values. In distinction, the control group had a higher average thigh sweat rate than the PD group, but this difference did not reach statistical significance. A quantitative thermoregulatory sweat test (QTST) was included in the same study, and it was found that patients with early PD failed to increase local sweat rates with TRH infusion. This result is intriguing and suggests the need for additional testing with a larger cohort of patients to establish the reproducibility, sensitivity, and specificity of the QTST as a marker of early PD.

Several groups have demonstrated SSR abnormalities in PD *(38,41,42)*. Because the SSR is mediated by both central and peripheral autonomic pathways, it can be loosely interpreted as a general measure of sudomotor integrity. The incidence of abnormal SSRs increases and response amplitudes decrease with rising H & Y stages and United Parkinson's Disease Rating Scale scores. In PD, therapy with levodopa or dopamine agonists has no significant effect on the SSR *(38,42)*. SSR abnormalities are more pronounced on limbs with greater motor dysfunction (e.g., tremor, rigidity) than on their contralateral, less impaired, counterparts *(38)*.

Asymmetrical thermoregulatory test abnormalities in patients with asymmetrical motor signs have been reported by some *(38,42)* but not all investigators *(36,39)*. De Marinis et al. *(43)* reported both asymmetrical sweating and facial telethermography in patients who had PD. In their study, facial cutaneous dilatation was induced by sublingual administration of nitroglycerin. Facial telethermography was performed at baseline and at 15 and 30 minutes after nitroglycerin administration. Both sweating and cutaneous facial dilatation were reduced in patients with PD. Decreased heat elimination and sweating were more pronounced on the hemibody (arms and legs) with greater motor dysfunction. As initially described by Gowers *(20)*, excessive head and neck sweating in patients with PD may only involve the parkinsonian side of the body. Therefore, asymmetrical head and neck sweating in PD may be a compensatory response to asymmetrical hypohidrosis elsewhere. Asymmetric autonomic dysfunction has also been described in patients with strokes and other focal structural abnormalities of the central nervous system *(44–46)*. Lesions of the hypothalamus are associated with contralateral hyperhidrosis *(45,46)*. It is possible that dopaminergic projections to the preoptic/anterior hypothalamus and/or the posterior hypothalamus are defective ipsilateral to the side of the brain with greater dopaminergic cell loss. Alternatively, the activities of cortical-hypothalamic projections that contribute to thermoregulation are distorted by defective signaling within cortical-basal ganglia loops.

Postganglionic sympathetic innervation of sweat glands, as measured by the QSART and SSIT, may show abnormalities in PD, particularly in more advanced stages of the disease. In the study of 35 patients with PD from the Mayo Clinic cited previously, the QSART was 37% abnormal at the forearm and 40% abnormal at the foot *(37)*. However, the QSART abnormalities were mild in most patients who had PD. In two studies, SSITs were used to show the decreased total sweat volume and sweat droplet density in patients with PD in comparison to age-matched controls *(41,42)*. In the report by Mano and colleagues, the average sweat volume per gland was 0.0143 mm^3 in patients with PD (1, H & Y stage I; 11, H & Y stage II; 11, H & Y stage III; 11, H & Y stage IV; 0, H & Y stage V) and 0.0327 mm^3 in controls *(41)*. Mean total sweat volume was 3.6 mm^3 per cm^2 in PD patients and 11.9 mm^3 per cm^2 in controls.

5. PATHOLOGICAL BASES FOR THERMOREGULATORY DYSFUNCTION IN PD

The thermoregulatory test abnormalities and clinical manifestations of thermoregulatory dysfunction in PD suggest the presence of widespread neural pathology that encompasses both preganglionic neurons and sympathetic ganglion cells as well as higher-order autonomic centers in the brainstem and hypothalamus. Postmortem pathological findings provide the anatomical basis for specific sudomotor and other thermoregulatory findings in PD. Because neuronal loss occurs at sites where Lewy bodies are numerous, Lewy bodies have been used as a marker for neuronal degeneration in PD. All comprehensive pathological studies have shown that Lewy bodies are not limited to the substantia nigra, pars compacta. Clearly, PD is not a disease restricted to midbrain dopamine neurons. In fact, the earliest pathological descriptions of PD noted the presence of Lewy bodies within an important component of the central autonomic nervous system—the dorsal motor nucleus of the vagus nerve *(47)*. Den Hartog Jager and Bethlem *(48)* emphasized the widespread distribution of Lewy bodies in their seminal pathological study of PD, being detected in the sympathetic ganglia in five of six PD cases. In the central nervous system, there were several Lewy bodies in the locus ceruleus, hypothalamus, and brainstem. In four cases, Lewy bodies were found in the lateral horns of the spinal cord. Den Hartog Jager and Bethlem stated, "…we believe that every investigation into the pathogenesis of idiopathic paralysis agitans will have to make allowance for this widespread neuronal degeneration."

Subsequent postmortem pathological studies corroborated and expanded on previous findings in PD. Rajput and Rozdilsky *(49)* examined the brains from six patients with PD, one with MSA, and one control. Lewy bodies in sympathetic ganglia were seen in five of the PD cases; using nonstereological methods, associated ganglion cell loss was present in three of these cases. Intermediolateral cell column Lewy bodies were prominent in the MSA case but were detected in only one of the six PD cases. In sympathetic ganglia from PD, Lewy bodies are certainly a symbol of neurodegeneration, not a trivial consequence of aging. Forno and Norville *(50)* examined the stellate ganglia from 9 patients with PD, 9 patients with Parkinsonism without nigral Lewy bodies, and 17 controls. Stellate ganglia Lewy bodies were limited to the PD cases. In a more recent study, Lewy bodies in the paravertebral sympathetic ganglia were found in 28 of 30 PD cases, but in only 5 of 60 non-Parkinsonian controls over age 60 years *(51)*.

Although less severe than that noted in MSA cases *(52)*, neuronal loss within the intermediolateral cell column of the spinal cord has been well-documented in PD, despite a relative paucity of Lewy bodies *(53)*. In a study of 25 PD and 25 control cases, there was a 31% relative reduction of neurons within the intermediolateral cell column at the second thoracic segment in the PD cases. A more striking 63% reduction in neurons was seen at the ninth thoracic segment.

In addition to the substantia nigra, locus ceruleus, and dorsal motor nucleus of the vagus *(49)*, a report by Langston and Forno *(54)* indicates that Lewy bodies are also consistently found in the hypothalamus. In their study of 30 PD brains, at least 2 Lewy bodies were identified in each hypothalamus. More than 60 Lewy bodies were detected in 6 of the brains. Lewy bodies were concentrated in the tuberomamillary, lateral, and posterior hypothalamic nuclei. Degeneration in the posterior hypothalamus could explain some of the thermoregulatory abnormalities in PD. It is noteworthy that shivering, which is controlled by the posterior hypothalamus, was shown to be severely impaired in one patient who had PD and was exposed to experimental lowering of body temperature *(18)*.

6. THERMOREGULATORY TESTING TO DIFFERENTIATE PD FROM OTHER NEURODEGENERATIVE DISORDERS

In an individual patient, testing of thermoregulatory function or even autonomic function generally may not distinguish patients with PD from those with other neurodegenerative disorders, such as MSA *(55)*, progressive supranuclear palsy (PSP), the Guamanian Parkinsonism-amyotrophic lateral sclerosis (ALS)-dementia complex, and cortical-basal ganglionic degeneration. Nevertheless, when coupled with a careful history and physical examination, magnetic resonance imaging, and additional neurophysiological studies (e.g., electronystagmography, electromyography), tests of thermoregulatory function, particularly sudomotor function, can assist PD diagnosis and, in a very high percentage of cases, allow for accurate differentiation of PD from other, less common, disease processes.

Delineation of MSA from PD is a major diagnostic dilemma for both general neurologists and specialists in movement disorders. Because first-rate facilities for testing autonomic function are not available at many medical centers, neurologists at these sites rely heavily on clinical clues to differentiate PD with autonomic dysfunction from MSA, such as: (1) good response to carbidopa/levodopa, (2) presence of a resting tremor, (3) asymmetry of motor signs, (4) absence of significant anterocollis, (5) absence of upper motor neuron signs, and (6) absence of the "cold hands sign" *(56)*. Unfortunately, even highly skilled clinicians have difficulty distinguishing some cases of PD from MSA. When available, thermoregulatory testing may provide additional evidence supporting one diagnosis or the other. These tests range from simple bedside tests to complex overnight studies. Index-finger temperature can be measured in the clinic with a routine digital thermometer. In one study, mean (± standard deviation) index finger skin temperatures were 29.5 ± 3.9°C in 9 patients with MSA, 32.6 ± 0.9°C in 10 patients with PD, and 32.2 ± 1.1°C in 10 age-matched control subjects. Values from five of the MSA patients were within the range of patients with PD and controls. On average, patients with MSA are more likely than those with PD to exhibit severe abnormalities on thermoregulatory tests, e.g., QSART and TST, that are commonly performed in specialized autonomic function laboratories *(37,57,58)*. Specifically, in one study, mean anterior anhidrosis was nearly 90% in a group of 75 patients with MSA undergoing the TST *(37)*. The SSR can be performed in most neurology clinics with standard electromyography equipment and is also more likely to be absent or markedly diminished in MSA than in PD *(58,59)*. Contrasting to PD, TRH may enhance sweating in MSA *(15,40)*. Finally, long-term measurement of core temperature with a rectal probe has shown that the normal nocturnal fall in core temperature is blunted in MSA patients *(60)*. Certainly, a patient is unlikely to have idiopathic PD if not treated with levodopa or a dopamine agonist and with minimal or absent resting tremor, mild symmetric rigidity, cold digits, absent SSRs, and marked anhidrosis as documented with a QSART.

To prevent potential diagnostic confusion, it is important to recognize that thermoregulatory testing may also be abnormal in other, less typical, neurodegenerative disorders, e.g., PSP and the Guamanian

Parkinsonism-ALS-dementia complex. Low and colleagues at the Mayo Clinic examined autonomic function in 16 Guamanian Parkinsonism-ALS-dementia complex patients *(61)*. Deficits in postganglionic sudomotor function (i.e., QSART) were greater in the Guamanian Parkinsonism-ALS-dementia complex patients than in non-Guamanian PD, but less severe than that seen in MSA. In a series of 12 PSP patients with moderate to advanced disease, average anterior anhidrosis on the TST and percent abnormality on the QSART were slightly more than that found in a group of 35 patients who had PD of H & Y stages I–IV *(37)*. It is doubtful that thermoregulatory testing would be very useful in distinguishing early PSP from early PD.

7. TREATMENT OF THERMOREGULATORY DYSFUNCTION IN PD

7.1. Cold Intolerance

Patients with cold intolerance should be informed of several common sense approaches in dealing with cold weather conditions. Most importantly, they must wear warm socks, mittens, or gloves, and the head should be covered with a wool hat or cap. In windy conditions, the head, neck, and upper chest should be protected with a hood and scarf, windbreaker jacket, or other suitable apparel. If walking through snow, it is important to wear waterproof shoes to keep the feet dry. Cigarette smoking should be avoided, as smoking can impair circulation in the hands and feet. Finally, patients should be encouraged to wear several layers of clothing; one or more layers can be easily peeled off indoors.

7.2. Heat Intolerance

Anticholinergics (e.g., benztropine and trihexyphenidyl) and other medications with anticholinergic effects, such as diphenhydramine and tricyclic antidepressants, should be avoided in patients with heat intolerance. These patients should be instructed to limit physical activity in hot or humid environments and make a special effort to keep well-hydrated during warmer months. For example, they should not mow their lawn during the early afternoon of a hot summer day. Outdoor activities should be limited to the early morning and late afternoon or evening. A wide-brimmed hat limits exposure to direct sunlight, and loose lightweight clothing allows convection to occur. Patients taking diuretics should be particularly cautious in hot environments.

7.3. Hyperhidrosis

Because head and neck hyperhidrosis may be an appropriate thermoregulatory compensatory response to appendicular sudomotor dysfunction, it should not be specifically treated. However, patients can carry a handkerchief to wipe sweat from their foreheads and avoid wearing shirts with a tight collar. Episodic hyperhidrosis that occurs at the onset of motor "off" periods may improve with adjustments in dopaminergic therapy, such as addition of a dopamine agonist *(24)*, closer spacing of levodopa dosing, and use of a catechol-*O*-methyltransferase inhibitor.

7.4. Dry Skin (Xerosis)

Emollients containing either 40% urea (Carmol 40®) or 12% ammonium lactate (Lac-Hydrin®) are effective for xerosis. In one study, clinical improvement occurred in less time with the 40% urea cream than with the 12% ammonium lactate cream *(62)*. Both Carmol 40® and Lac-Hydrin® are available as either a lotion or a cream. These medications should be thoroughly rubbed into affected areas twice daily. A positive clinical response may require a range of several days to a week or more of applications.

7.5. Seborrheic Dermatitis

Low-potency topical corticosteroids (e.g., 1% hydrocortisone cream) are frequently used to treat seborrheic dermatitis and usually decrease erythema and flaking. Unfortunately, the benefits of corticosteroids are often transient with recurrence of seborrheic dermatitis within days after discontinuation of topical corticosteroid application. The antimycotic, ketoconazole, is more efficient than topical corticosteroids to treat seborrheic dermatitis and greatly increases the time to recurrence *(63)*. Ketoconazole is available in both topical cream and shampoo forms. Ketoconazole cream (2%) should be applied to affected areas twice daily for 4 weeks or until clinical clearing. Oral antimycotics, e.g., terbinafine, can be used with substantial efficacy in the more severe cases of seborrheic dermatitis *(64)*.

REFERENCES

1. Kelso SR, Perlmutter MN, Boulant JA. Thermosensitive single-unit activity of in vitro hypothalamic slices. Am J Physiol 1982;242:R77–R84.
2. Smith JE, Jansen AS, Gilbey MP, Loewy AD. CNS cell groups projecting to sympathetic outflow of tail artery: neural circuits involved in heat loss in the rat. Brain Res 1998;786:153–164.
3. Lin MT, Chandra A, Tsay BL, Chern YF. Hypothalamic and striatal dopamine receptor activation inhibits heat production in the rat. Am J Physiol 1982;242:R471–R481.
4. Scott IM, Boulant JA. Dopamine effects on thermosensitive neurons in hypothalamic tissue slices. Brain Res 1984;306:157–163.
5. Hasegawa H, Yazawa T, Yasumatsu M, Otokawa M, Aihara Y. Alteration in dopamine metabolism in the thermoregulatory center of exercising rats. Neurosci Lett 2000;289:161–164.
6. Salmi P. Independent roles of dopamine D1 and D2/3 receptors in rat thermoregulation. Brain Res 1998;781:188–193.
7. Perachon S, Betancur C, Pilon C, et al. Role of dopamine D3 receptors in thermoregulation: a reappraisal. Neuroreport 2000;11:221–225.
8. Lefrant JY, Muller L, De La Coussaye JE, et al. Temperature measurement in intensive care patients: comparison of urinary bladder, oesophageal, rectal, axillary, and inguinal methods versus pulmonary artery core method. Intensive Care Med 2003;29:414–418.
9. Fulbrook P. Core body temperature measurement: a comparison of axilla, tympanic membrane and pulmonary artery blood temperature. Intensive Crit Care Nurs 1997;13:266–272.
10. Knezevic W, Bajada S. Peripheral autonomic surface potential. A quantitative technique for recording sympathetic conduction in man. J Neurol Sci 1985;67:239–251.
11. Low PA, Opfer-Gehrking TL, Kihara M. In vivo studies on receptor pharmacology of the human eccrine sweat gland. Clin Auton Res 1992;2:29–34.
12. Cohen J, Low P, Fealey R, et al. Somatic and autonomic function in progressive autonomic failure and multiple system atrophy. Ann Neurol 1987;22:692–699.
13. Fealey RD, Low PA, Thomas JE. Thermoregulatory sweating abnormalities in diabetes mellitus. Mayo Clin Proc 1989;64:617–628.
14. Faden AI, Chan P, Mendoza E. Progressive isolated segmental anhidrosis. Arch Neurol 1982;39:172–175.
15. Kihara M, Sugenoya J, Takahashi A. The assessment of sudomotor dysfunction in multiple system atrophy. Clin Auton Res 1991;1:297–302.
16. Bornmyr S, Castenfors J, Svensson H, et al. Detection of autonomic sympathetic dysfunction in diabetic patients. A study using laser Doppler imaging. Diabetes Care 1999;22:593–597.
17. Stanton AW, Levick JR, Mortimer PS. Assessment of noninvasive tests of cutaneous vascular control in the forearm using a laser Doppler meter and a Finapres blood pressure monitor. Clin Auton Res 1995;5:37–47.
18. Gubbay SS, Barwick DD. Two cases of accidental hypothermia in Parkinson's disease with unusual EEG findings. J Neurol Neurosurg Psychiatry 1966;29:459–466.
19. Siddiqui MF, Rast S, Lynn MJ, et al. Autonomic dysfunction in Parkinson's disease: a comprehensive symptom survey. Parkinsonism Relat Disord 2002;8:277–284.
20. Gowers WR. A Manual of Diseases of the Nervous System. Blakiston, Philadelphia, PA, 1888.
21. Charcot JM. Maladies de Système Nerveux, vol. 1. Battaille, Paris, France, 1892.
22. Lees AJ. When did Ray Kennedy's Parkinson's disease begin? Mov Disord 1992;7:110–116.
23. Appenzeller O, Goss JE. Autonomic deficits in Parkinson's disease. Arch Neurol 1971;24:50–57.
24. Sage JI, Mark MH. Drenching sweats as an off phenomenon in Parkinson's disease: treatment and relation to plasma levodopa profile. Ann Neurol 1995;37:120–122.
25. Pfeiffer RF, Sucha EL. "On-Off"-induced lethal hyperthermia. Mov Disord 1989;4:338–341.
26. Keyser DL, Rodnitzky RL. Neuroleptic malignant syndrome in Parkinson's disease after withdrawal or alteration of dopaminergic therapy. Arch Intern Med 1991;151:794–796.
27. Gordon PH, Frucht SJ. Neuroleptic malignant syndrome in advanced Parkinson's disease. Mov Disord 2001;16:960–962.
28. Mizuta E, Yamasaki S, Nakatake M, Kuno S. Neuroleptic malignant syndrome in a parkinsonian woman during the premenstrual period. Neurology 1993;43:1048–1049.
29. Serrano-Duenas M. Neuroleptic malignant syndrome-like, or –dopaminergic malignant syndrome–due to levodopa therapy withdrawal. Clinical features in 11 patients. Parkinsonism Relat Disord 2003;9:175–178.

30. Binder RL, Jonelis FJ. Seborrheic dermatitis in neuroleptic-induced Parkinsonism. Arch Dermatol 1983;119:473–475.
31. Burton JL, Shuster S. Effect of L-dopa on seborrhoea of Parkinsonism. Lancet 1970;2:19–20.
32. Streifler M, Avrami E, Rabey JM. L-dopa and the secretion of sebum in Parkinsonian patients. Eur Neurol 1980;19:43–48.
33. Villares JC, Carlini EA. Sebum secretion in idiopathic Parkinson's disease: effect of anticholinergic and dopaminergic drugs. Acta Neurol Scand 1989;80:57–63.
34. Fischer M, Gemende I, Marsch WC, Fischer PA. Skin function and skin disorders in Parkinson's disease. J Neural Transm 2001;108:205–213.
35. Aminoff MJ, Wilcox CS. Assessment of autonomic function in patients with a Parkinsonian syndrome. Br Med J 1971;4:80–84.
36. Goetz CG, Lutge W, Tanner CM. Autonomic dysfunction in Parkinson's disease. Neurology 1986;36:73–75.
37. Sandroni P, Ahlskog JE, Fealey RD, Low PA. Autonomic involvement in extrapyramidal and cerebellar disorders. Clin Auton Res 1991;1:147–155.
38. Haapaniemi TH, Korpelainen JT, Tolonen U, et al. Suppressed sympathetic skin response in Parkinson disease. Clin Auton Res 2000;10:337–342.
39. Turkka JT, Myllylä VV. Sweating dysfunction in Parkinson's disease. Eur Neurol 1987;26:1–7.
40. Kihara M, Kihara Y, Tukamoto T, et al. Assessment of sudomotor dysfunction in early Parkinson's disease. Eur Neurol 1993;33:363–365.
41. Mano Y, Nakamuro T, Takayanagi T, Mayer RF. Sweat function in Parkinson's disease. J Neurol 1994;241:573–576.
42. Hirashima F, Yokota T, Hayashi M. Sympathetic skin response in Parkinson's disease. Acta Neurol Scand 1996;93:127–132.
43. De Marinis M, Stocchi F, Testa SR, et al. Alterations of thermoregulation in Parkinson's disease. Funct Neurol 1991;6:279–283.
44. Korpelainen JT, Sotaniemi KA, Myllylä VV. Autonomic nervous system disorders in stroke. Clin Auton Res 1999;9:325–333.
45. Ueno M, Tokunaga Y, Terachi S, et al. Asymmetric sweating in a child with multiple sclerosis. Pediatr Neurol 2000;23:74–76.
46. Smith CD. A hypothalamic stroke producing recurrent hemihyperhidrosis. Neurology 2001;56:1394–1396.
47. Lewy FH. Paralysis agitans. I. Pathologische Anatomie. In: Lewandowsky M, ed. Handbuch der Neurologie, vol. 3. Springer, Berlin, 1912, pp. 920–933.
48. Den Hartog Jager WA, Bethlem J. The distribution of Lewy bodies in the central and autonomic nervous systems in idiopathic paralysis agitans. J Neurol Neurosurg Psychiatry 1960;23:283–290.
49. Rajput AH, Rozdilsky B. Dysautonomia in Parkinsonism: a clinicopathological study. J Neurol Neurosurg Psychiatry 1976;39:1092–1100.
50. Forno LS, Norville RL. Ultrastructure of Lewy bodies in stellate ganglia. Acta Neuropathol 1976;34:183–197.
51. Wakabayashi K, Takahashi H. Neuropathology of autonomic nervous system in Parkinson's disease. Eur Neurol 1997;38(Suppl 2):2–7.
52. Wenning GK, Tison F, Ben Shlomo Y, et al. Multiple system atrophy: a review of 203 pathologically proven cases. Mov Disord 1997;12:133–147.
53. Wakabayashi K, Takahashi H. The intermediolateral nucleus and Clarke's column in Parkinson's disease. Acta Neuropathol 1997;94:287–289.
54. Langston JW, Forno LS. Hypothalamus in Parkinson's disease. Ann Neurol 1978;3:129–133.
55. Riley DE, Chelimsky TC. Autonomic nervous system testing may not distinguish multiple system atrophy from Parkinson's disease. J Neurol Neurosurg Psychiatry 2003;74:56–60.
56. Klein C, Brown R, Wenning G, Quinn N. The "cold hands sign" in multiple system atrophy. Mov Disord 1997;12:514–518.
57. Low PA. Composite autonomic scoring scale for laboratory quantification of generalized autonomic failure. Mayo Clin Proc 1993;68:748–752.
58. Bordet R, Benhadjali J, Destee A, et al. Sympathetic skin response and R-R interval variability in multiple system atrophy and idiopathic Parkinson's disease. Mov Disord 1996;11:268–272.
59. De Marinis M, Stocchi F, Gregori B, Accornero N. Sympathetic skin response and cardiovascular autonomic function tests in Parkinson's disease and multiple system atrophy with autonomic failure. Mov Disord 2000;15:1215–1220.
60. Pierangeli G, Provini F, Maltoni P, et al. Nocturnal body core temperature falls in Parkinson's disease but not in multiple-system atrophy. Mov Disord 2001;16:226–232.
61. Low PA, Ahlskog JE, Petersen RC, et al. Autonomic failure in Guamanian neurodegenerative disease. Neurology 1997;49:1031–1034.
62. Ademola J, Frazier C, Kim SJ, et al. Clinical evaluation of 40% urea and 12% ammonium lactate in the treatment of xerosis. Am J Clin Dermatol 2002;3:217–222.
63. Faergemann J. Management of seborrheic dermatitis and pityriasis versicolor. Am J Clin Dermatol 2000;1:75–80.
64. Scaparro E, Quadri G, Virno G, et al. Evaluation of the efficacy and tolerability of oral terbinafine (Daskil) in patients with seborrheic dermatitis. A multicentre., randomized, investigator-blinded, placebo-controlled trial. Br J Dermatol 2001;144:854–857.

14
Respiratory Dysfunction

Holly A. Shill

SUMMARY

Pulmonary complications remain a primary cause of morbidity and mortality in Parkinson's disease (PD). Obstructive and restrictive airway deficits are related to disordered motor control of the respiratory musculature. Although this may sometimes lead to overt symptoms, such as stridor and respiratory failure, it more commonly results in silent aspiration and atelectasis, predisposing patients to pneumonia. Anti-Parkinson medications may produce pulmonary side effects (e.g., pleuropulmonary fibrosis associated with ergot-based dopamine agonists). Finally, motor fluctuations in patients with advanced PD may affect the respiratory system. Recognizing these pulmonary complications will assist the clinician in appropriately managing the disease and potentially reducing the impact of the abnormal respiratory system on the overall health of the patient with PD.

Key Words: Parkinson's disease; upper airway obstruction; restrictive abnormality; stridor; pleuropulmonary fibrosis; respiratory dyskinesia; hypophonia.

1. INTRODUCTION

In 1817, James Parkinson described a man who spoke "with such a low voice and indistinct articulation, as hardly to be understood but by those who were constantly with him. He fetched his breath rather hard" *(1)*. Thus, involvement of the airway and respiratory apparatus has been appreciated since the original description of the shaking palsy. In the early reports on morbidity and mortality in Parkinson's disease (PD), pneumonia was a common cause of early death *(2)*. More recently, reports indicate that, although patient lifespan is improving with optimal medical management, pulmonary complications remain the most frequent cause of death *(3–6)*. Clinician attention to these prevalent complications is therefore paramount. Many of the clinical aspects of respiratory dysfunction in PD discussed in this chapter are, in actuality, related to underlying Parkinsonian motor dysfunction in some manner, but they are often evaluated and treated by non-neurologists and consequently remain appropriate subjects for consideration and discussion under the rubric of nonmotor dysfunction in PD.

2. HYPOPHONIA

Dysarthria with hypophonia, owing to bradykinesia and rigidity of the vocal cords, is common and can be considered a cardinal sign of PD *(7)*. Its severity can be graded both in terms of subjective perception of difficulties by the patient and objective findings on clinical examination. More than 70% of patients experience problems with speech, and 30% find the difficulty to be the most debilitating aspect of their disease *(8,9)*. Patients are often reluctant to speak in front of others, talk on the telephone, or go out socially because they fear the difficulty in being understood.

From: *Current Clinical Neurology*
Parkinson's Disease and Nonmotor Dysfunction
Edited by: R. F. Pfeiffer and I. Bodis-Wollner © Humana Press Inc., Totowa, NJ

Strategies to improve vocal quality have been quite broad. Neurologists generally approach the problem by manipulating dopaminergic medications, and speech ability typically responds to this to a certain extent. Simple speech therapy has been used, as well as more specific therapies designed to circumvent the abnormal basal ganglia circuitry in PD. A therapy program, termed the Lee Silverman Voice Treatment, focuses on "think loud, think shout" and may change the neural control of speech to a more "reflex" production of speech *(10)*. A second method, the Pitch Limiting Voice Treatment, may improve speech without the straining associated with the previous method *(11)*. Although otolaryngologists have used permanent therapies to augment voice, such as laryngoplasty and alloplastic or autologous vocal cord injections, evidence for their efficacy in PD is limited. Percutaneous collagen injection into the vocal cords may offer a more tolerable, albeit nonpermanent, option for patients *(12,13)*. Neurosurgical approaches, e.g., pallidotomy and deep-brain stimulation of the thalamus and subthalamic nucleus, are beneficial for many PD symptoms and signs, yet are typically less helpful for hypophonia. In fact, bilateral therapies and unilateral gamma knife therapy may have an unacceptable adverse effect on speech *(14–17)*. Therefore, patients should be appropriately counseled regarding expectations with these surgical therapies and their potential effect on voice.

3. OBSTRUCTIVE COMPLICATIONS

In initial reports, a lower airway obstructive defect, similar to chronic obstructive pulmonary disease, was thought to be the prominent ventilatory abnormality in PD *(18,19)*. If symptomatic, this is manifest clinically as wheezing and decreased expiratory flow rate. However, with a combination of improved medical therapies, better patient characterization, and control for obstructive risk factors (e.g., smoking), this entity is now known to be less common than previously thought.

Attention has subsequently shifted to upper airway obstruction, manifest clinically as stridor. There are two typical obstructive patterns of the upper airway associated with PD *(20)*. Type A, termed "respiratory flutter," shows an oscillatory pattern on a flow-volume loop with a frequency similar to tremor. This pattern results from vibration of the vocal cords and supraglottic structures, rather than diaphragmatic oscillations. Type B has irregular and abrupt changes in airflow, sometimes with intermittent complete obstructions and may be owing to both upper airway obstruction and poor control of the ventilatory pump. Both patterns are believed to be the consequence of poor basal ganglia control of the striated muscles of the ventilatory system. In an early study of 21 patients with PD, 12 had a type A pattern and 6 a type B pattern. One third of patients met respiratory criteria for upper airway obstruction (UAO). Only four patients had respiratory symptoms. Patients with airway obstruction had more advanced PD, as measured by Hoehn and Yahr staging. Many of the patients in this study were smokers, and PD medications were not controlled, which necessitates caution in interpreting this study. In a second, similarly performed study of 31 nonsmoking, respiratory symptom-free patients with advanced PD, a type A pattern was present in 4 and a type B pattern in 16; 9 displayed UAO *(21)*. Patients in this study were on levodopa treatment. This suggests that even asymptomatic, medically managed patients may have subclinical evidence of UAO.

Based on these early studies, UAO has been generally considered to be relatively asymptomatic and present primarily in more advanced and sedentary patients who have PD. Consequently, it has received little clinical attention. However, it is important to recognize its presence, because it may have significant relevance in patient management. Stridor may be a presenting symptom of PD and respond to levodopa *(22)*. Stridor and respiratory failure may also result from abruptly stopping dopaminergic medication *(23–25)*. Such reports have fueled further study into the effects of medication on respiratory function. Both levodopa and dopamine agonists may improve ventilatory parameters, particularly UAO *(26–28)*. Patients undergoing spirometry show a much higher prevalence of UAO while off levodopa therapy in comparison to during therapy *(29,30)*. In patients with the combination of poor upper airway control and sensitivity to dopaminergic medications, withdrawal of oral medications near the time of surgery might contribute to the higher frequency of aspiration pneumonias and longer hospital stays seen in surgical patients with PD *(31)*. Thus, this "asymptomatic" abnormality, coupled with an impaired cough reflex *(32)*, might be more relevant from a clinical standpoint than previously thought.

Careful attention to the manipulation of PD medications is important pertaining to the upper airway. Every attempt should be made to continue PD medications through any type of procedure or surgery *(33)*. In the outpatient setting, doses should be changed gradually in an effort to reduce these types of respiratory complications.

Finally, upper airway obstruction and central hypoventilation are associated with the Parkinsonism-plus syndrome—multiple system atrophy (MSA; *34,35*). Autonomic insufficiency, clinically manifest as impotence, incontinence, and orthostatic hypotension, eventually develops in most individuals with MSA. MSA is characterized by poor response to PD medications. Stridor occurring in the MSA setting is generally also not responsive to PD medications and is a poor prognostic sign *(36)*. Patients should be counseled appropriately after developing this sign because of its poor prognosis, and tracheostomy should be considered.

4. RESTRICTIVE ABNORMALITIES

Restrictive abnormalities of the pulmonary apparatus in PD have also been recognized. Chest-wall muscles may develop bradykinesia and cocontraction with a consequent increase in chest-wall compliance *(29)*. The intercostal and scalene muscles may also develop a tremor pattern, which contributes to decreased coordinated activity of the respiratory pump *(37)*. Furthermore, in individuals with PD, repetitive muscle activity results in early fatigue *(38)*. This result may, in turn, lead to apparent weakness of the chest-wall muscles during normal respiration, similar to what is indicated in primary neuromuscular disorders, and manifest in pulmonary function testing as a restrictive abnormality *(39,40)*. Postural and arthritic changes from longstanding disease may also mechanically restrict ventilation *(30,41)*. Restrictive changes may further adversely affect the overall clinical state by reducing vital capacity, leading to symptoms of fatigue. Additionally, poor expansion of the lungs leads to atelectasis, which predisposes to pneumonia. Restrictive abnormalities are less responsive to dopaminergic therapy, but may be affected by pulmonary rehabilitation (*see* the Exercise and Ventilation section).

Medical therapy for PD may also produce restrictive abnormalities in the lung tissue itself. All of the ergot dopamine agonists have been reported to cause pleuropulmonary fibrosis *(42,43)*. This phenomenon appears to be specific to the ergot dopamine agonists and has not been found with newer, nonergot agents, such as pramipexole and ropinirole. Clinical symptoms of pleuropulmonary fibrosis include dyspnea, pleuritic pain, and nonproductive cough; pulmonary infiltrates and pleural effusions appear on chest radiographs. The sedimentation rate may be elevated, and pleural fluid may show inflammatory cells with a predominance of eosinophils. Although initially believed to be present in 2–5% of patients on these agents, this condition is now known to be exceedingly rare *(44,45)*. Discontinuing the offending dopamine agonist usually reverses the abnormalities. The pathophysiology for this entity is poorly understood, but it may reflect serotonergic activation that triggers an inflammatory response *(46)*. More recently, a link between this response and prior exposure to asbestos was postulated *(47)*.

5. FLUCTUATIONS

Although levodopa therapy improves respiratory and motor function, development of levodopa-induced dyskinesias may also affect ventilation. Patients with respiratory dyskinesias may complain of dyspnea and chest pain shortly after levodopa administration *(48)*. Serial pulmonary function testing demonstrates the appearance of rapid shallow breathing and a decline in pulmonary functions in conjunction with the clinical onset of limb and orofacial dykinesias that are typical of peak-dose levodopa-induced dyskinesias *(49)*. Because complaints of acute chest pain and shortness of breath in this older population might result in an extensive evaluation for cardiac and pulmonary disorders, this side effect of treatment should be considered early in the differential diagnosis. Generally, the dyskinesias subside with reduced dopaminergic medication.

Additionally, in more advanced patients, the wearing-off phenomena between levodopa doses may induce acute pulmonary complaints. Dystonia of the laryngeal muscles, causing stridor, is an example *(50)*. Chest-wall tightness with shortness of breath and anxiety, superficially resembling a panic attack, may also occur *(51)*. In part, this may be a psychological reaction to the sudden appearance of chest-wall rigidity, causing an acute restrictive condition. These types of wearing-off phenomena are treated similarly to other motor fluctuations *(52)*. Generally, the strategy is to smooth the levodopa response by providing appropriate dose overlap or initiating longer-acting therapies that reduce abrupt withdrawal symptoms.

Although it might be anticipated that these kinds of nonmotor symptoms are rare complications of long-term therapy, it is becoming apparent that they are more common and debilitating than previously realized. In a survey of a group of patients who had PD with motor fluctuations, 40% complained of dyspnea, 21% had stridor as a wearing-off symptom, and 8% had intermittent coughing *(53)*. All of these respiratory symptoms were linked to the patient's motor state; the correlation with PD fluctuations suggests they are a part of the primary pathophysiology in PD.

6. EXERCISE AND VENTILATION

Defective motor control of ventilatory muscles is the primary contributor to the obstructive and restrictive changes found in PD. However, patients who have PD may also have trouble regulating breathing when walking because they are not able to effectively synchronize breathing with locomotion *(54)*. This may lead to decreased exercise tolerance and also could contribute to the fatigue that many patients experience *(53)*. Patients who exercise regularly seem to maintain better respiratory status *(55)*, and those undergoing a formal pulmonary rehabilitation program may experience improvement in ventilatory function *(56,57)*. Thus, patients complaining of fatigue and poor exercise tolerance should be considered for these nonpharmacological interventions.

7. SUMMARY

PD affects the ventilatory system at all levels. Laryngeal involvement brings forth hypophonia, which possibly responds to both medical treatment and nonpharmacological therapies. Upper airway involvement may generally present clinically as stridor or subclincally as silent aspiration and responds well to dopaminergic therapy. Restrictive impairment can perhaps manifest as fatigue and predispose to atelectasis and pneumonia. Motor fluctuations in PD may also present as pulmonary symptoms and are addressed by appropriate adjustment of dopaminergic medications. Dopamine agonists can potentially induce pleuropulmonary fibrosis. Finally, attention to the respiratory tract may improve exercise capacity and reduce fatigue. Awareness of all the pulmonary complications can help to reduce morbidity and mortality in PD.

REFERENCES

1. Parkinson J. An Essay on the Shaking Palsy. Sherwood, Nealy and Jones, London, 1817.
2. Hoehn MM, Yahr MD. Parkinsonism: onset, progression and mortality. Neurology 1967;17:427–442.
3. Mosewich RK, Rajput AH, Shuaib A, et al. Pulmonary embolism: an under-recognized yet frequent cause of death in Parkinsonism. Mov Disord 1994;9:350–352.
4. Nakashima K, Maeda M, Tabata M, et al. Prognosis of Parkinson's Disease in Japan. Tottori University Parkinson's Disease Epidemiology (TUPDE) Study Group Eur Neurol 1997;38:60–63.
5. Morgante L, Salemi G, Meneghini F, et al. Parkinson disease survival: a population-based study. Arch Neurol 2000;57:507–512.
6. Beyer MK, Herlofsen K, Arsland D, Larsen JP. Causes of death in a community-based study of Parkinson's disease. Acta Neurol Scand 2001;103:7–11.
7. Baker KK, Ramig LO, Luschei ES, Smith ME. Thyroarytenoid muscle activity associated with hypophonia in Parkinson disease and aging. Neurology 1998;51:1592–1598.
8. Logemann JA, Fisher HB, Boshes B, Blonsky ER. Frequency and cooccurrence of vocal tract dysfunction in the speech of a large sample of Parkinson patients. J Speech Hear Disord 1978;43:47–57.

9. Hartelius L, Svensson P. Speech and swallowing symptoms associated with Parkinson's disease and multiple sclerosis: a survey. Folia Phon Log 1994;46:9–17.
10. Liotti M, Ramig LO, Vogel D, et al. Hypophonia in Parkinson's disease. Neural correlates of voice treatment revealed by PET. Neurology 2003;60:432–440.
11. Swart BJM, Willemse SC, Maassen BAM, Horstink MWIM. Improvement of voicing in patients with Parkinson's disease by speech therapy. Neurology 2003;60:498–500.
12. Berke GS, Gerratt B, Kreiman J, Jackson K. Treatment of Parkinson hypophonia with percutaneous collagen augmentation. Laryngoscope 1999;1098:1295–1299.
13. Kim SH, Kearney JJ, Atkins JP. Percutaneous collagen augmentation for treatment of parkinsonian hypophonia. Otolaryngol Head Neck Surg 2002;126:653–656.
14. Jankovic J, Cardoso F, Grossman RG, Hamilton WJ. Outcome after stereotactic thalamotomy for parkinsonian, essential, and other types of tremor. Neurosurgery 1995;37:680–687.
15. Lang AE, Duff J, Saint-Cyr JA, et al. Posteroventral medial pallidotomy in Parkinson's disease. J Neurol 1999;246(Suppl 2):28–41.
16. Okun MS, Stover NP, Subramanian T, et al. Complications of gamma knife surgery for Parkinson's disease. Arch Neurol 2001;58:1995–2002.
17. Romito LM, Scerrati M, Contarin MF, et al. Long-term follow up of subthalamic nucleus stimulation in Parkinson's disease. Neurology 2002;58:15.
18. Neu HC, Connolly JJ, Jr., Schwertley FW, et al. Obstructive respiratory dysfunction in parkinsonian patients. Am Rev Respir Dis 1967;95:33–47.
19. Obenour WH, Stevens PM, Cohen AA, McCutchen JJ. The causes of abnormal pulmonary function in Parkinson's disease. Am Rev Respir Dis 1972;105:382–387.
20. Vincken WG, Gauthier SG, Dollfuss RE, et al. Involvement of upper-airway muscles in extrapyramidal disorders. A cause of airflow limitation. N Engl J Med 1984;311:438–442.
21. Hovestadt A, Bogaard JM, Meerwaldt JD, et al. Pulmonary function in Parkinson's disease. J Neurol Neurosurg Psychiatry 1989;52:329–333.
22. Read D, Young A. Stridor and Parkinsonism. Postgrad Med J 1983;59:520–521.
23. Fink ME, Klebanoff LM, Lennihan L, Fahn S. Acute respiratory failure during drug manipulation in patients with Parkinson's disease. Neurology 1989;39:348.
24. Riley DE, Grossman G, Martin L. Acute respiratory failure from dopamine agonist withdrawal. Neurology 1992;42:1843–1844.
25. Easdown LJ, Tessler MJ, Minuk J. Upper airway involvement in Parkinson's disease resulting in postoperative respiratory failure. Can J Anaesth 1995;42:344–347.
26. Langer H, Woolf CR. Changes in pulmonary function Parkinson's syndrome after treatment with L-dopa. Am Rev Respir Dis 1971;104:440–442.
27. de Bruin PF, de Bruin VM, Lees AJ, Pride NB. Effects of treatment on airway dynamics and respiratory muscle strength in Parkinson's disease. Am Rev Respir Dis 1993;148:1576–1580.
28. Herer B, Arnulf I, Housset B. Effects of levodopa on pulmonary function in Parkinson's disease. Chest 2001;119:387–393.
29. Izquierdo-Alonso JL, Jimenez-Jimenez FJ, Cabrera-Valdivia F, Mansilla-Lesmes M. Airway dysfunction in patients with Parkinson's disease. Lung 1994;172:47–55.
30. Sabate M, Gonzalez I, Ruperez F, Rodriguez M. Obstructive and restrictive pulmonary dysfunctions in Parkinson's disease. J Neurol Sci 1996;138:114–119.
31. Pepper PV, Goldstein MK. Postoperative complications in Parkinson's disease. J Am Geriatr Soc 1999;47:967–972.
32. Fontana GA, Pantaleo T, Lavorini F, et al. Defective motor control of coughing in Parkinson's disease. Am J Respir Crit Care Med 1998;158:458–464.
33. Galvez-Jimenez N, Lang AE. Perioperative problems in Parkinson's disease and their management: apomorphine with rectal domperidone. Can J Neurol Sci 1996;23:198–203.
34. Chester CS, Gottfried SB, Cameron DI, Strohl KP. Pathophysiological findings in a patient with Shy-Drager and alveolar hypoventilation syndromes. Chest 1988;94:212–214.
35. Apps MCP, Scheaff PC, Ingram DA, et al. Respiration and sleep in Parkinson's disease. J Neurol Neurosurg Psychiatry 1985;48:1240–1245.
36. Silber MH, Levine S. Stridor and death in multiple system atrophy. Mov Disord 2000;15:699–704.
37. Estenne M, Hubert M, De Troyer A. Respiratory-muscle involvement in Parkinson's disease. N Engl J Med 1984;311:1516–1517.
38. Schwab RD, England AC, Peterson E. Akinesia, in Parkinson's disease. Neurology 1959;9:65–72.
39. Nugent CA, Harris HW, Cohn J, et al. Dyspnea as a symptom in Parkinson's syndrome. Am Rev Tuberc 1958;78:682–691.
40. Tzelepis GE, McCool FD, Friedman JH, Hoppin FG, Jr. Respiratory muscle dysfunction in Parkinson's disease. Am Rev Respir Dis 1988;138:266–271.
41. Sabate M, Rodriguez M, Mendez E, et al. Obstructive and restrictive pulmonary dysfunction increases disability in Parkinson disease. Arch Phys Med Rehabil 1996;77:29–34.

42. Bhatt MH, Keenan SP, Fleetham JA, Calne DB. Pleuropulmonary disease associated with dopamine agonist therapy. Ann Neurol 1991;30:613–616.
43. Geminiani G, Fetoni V, Genitrini S, et al. Cabergoline in Parkinson's disease complicated by motor fluctuations. Mov Disord 1996;11:495–500.
44. McElvaney NG, Wilcox PG, Churg A, Fleetham JA. Pleuropulmonary disease during bromocriptine treatment of Parkinson's disease. Arch Intern Med 1988;148:2231–2236.
45. Todman DH, Oliver WA, Edwards RL. Pleuropulmonary fibrosis due to bromocriptine treatment for Parkinson's disease. Clin Exp Neurol 1990;27:79–82.
46. LeWitt PA, Calne DB. Pleuropulmonary changes during long-term bromocriptine treatment for Parkinson's disease. Lancet 1981;1:44–45.
47. Hillerdal G, Lee J, Blomkvist A, et al. Pleural disease during treatment with bromocriptine in patients previously exposed to asbestos. Eur Respir J 1997;10:2711–2715.
48. Weiner WJ, Goetz CG, Nausieda PA, Klawans HL. Respiratory dyskinesias: extrapyramidal dysfunction and dyspnea. Ann Intern Med 1978;88:327–331.
49. Zupnick HM, Brown LK, Miller A, Moros DA. Respiratory dysfunction due to L-dopa therapy for Parkinsonism, diagnosis using serial pulmonary function tests and respiratory inductive plethysmography. Am J Med 1990;89:109–114.
50. Corbin DO, Williams AC. Stridor during dystonic phases of Parkinson's disease. J Neurol Neurosurg Psychiatry 1987;50:821–822.
51. Hartman DE. Stridor during dystonia phases of Parkinson's disease. J Neurol Neurosurg Psychiatry 1988;51:161.
52. Vazquez A, Jimenez-Jimenez FJ, Garcia-Ruiz P, Garcia-Urra D. "Panic attacks" in Parkinson's disease. A long-term complication of levodopa therapy. Acta Neurol Scand 1993;87:14–18.
53. Stacy M. Pharmacotherapy for advanced Parkinson's disease. Pharmacotherapy 2000;20:8S–16S.
54. Witjas T, Kaphan E, Azulay JP, et al. Nonmotor fluctuations in Parkinson's Disease. Neurology 2002;59:408–413.
55. Canning CG, Alison JA, Allen NE, Groeller H. Parkinson's disease: an investigation of exercise capacity, respiratory function, and gait. Arch Phys Med Rehabil 1997;78:199–207.
56. Bergen JL, Toole T, Elliott RG, et al. Aerobic exercise intervention improves aerobic capacity and movement initiation in Parkinson's disease patients. Neurorehabilitation 2002;17:161–168.
57. Koseoglu F, Inan L, Ozel S, et al. The effects of a pulmonary rehabilitation program on pulmonary function tests and exercise tolerance in patients with Parkinson's disease. Funct Neurol 1997;12:319–325.

III Sleep-Related Dysfunction in Parkinson's Disease

15
Insomnia

Maria L. Moro-de-Casillas and David E. Riley

SUMMARY

Insomnia is the most common sleep disturbance in Parkinson's disease (PD), affecting 40–90% of patients. Insomnia usually takes the form of frequent nocturnal awakenings ("sleep fragmentation"). There are numerous factors contribute to insomnia in PD, including the persistence or recurrence of PD symptoms (especially tremor and immobility) during light stages of sleep, effects of medications used to treat PD on sleep, depression, restless legs syndrome, and nocturia. Identification and minimization of such factors is the first step in proper management. General sleep hygiene principles are outlined. Avoidance of regular hypnotic therapy is encouraged, but recommendations regarding the use of hypnotic drugs in selected cases are provided.

Key Words: Insomnia; sleep fragmentation; restless legs syndrome; sleep hygiene; hypnotics.

1. INTRODUCTION

The International Classification of Sleep Disorders defines insomnia as "difficulty in initiating and/or maintaining sleep" *(1)*. However, several definitions exist; there is no clear consensus in this matter. The core elements of insomnia are an inadequate quantity or quality of sleep *(2,3)* with both nocturnal and daytime consequences *(4)*. Traditionally, insomnia has been subgrouped into sleep-onset insomnia, sleep-maintaining insomnia, and insomnia with early morning awakening. However, there is extensive overlap, and most insomniacs fit into more than one subgroup *(2,5)*.

There are many consequences of insomnia in a patient's daily life. Aside from the obvious complications of daytime fatigue and somnolence, insomniacs have an increased incidence of psychiatric disorders, such as depression and anxiety, increased use of over-the-counter medications and alcohol, and a higher incidence of accidents and unemployment, among others *(2,4)*. The economic impact of insomnia in our society is enormous: an estimate of the total direct annual cost of insomnia in the United States placed it above $13 billion *(4)*. Insomnia is the most commonly reported sleep problem in the United States and in industrialized nations worldwide *(6–9)*. Bixler and colleagues *(7)* reported an overall prevalence of insomnia of 42% in a sample of 1006 subjects ages 18–80. Women are 1.3 times more likely to report insomnia symptoms than men *(4,10)* The elderly (>65 years old) have a prevalence rate of sleep difficulty 1.5 times higher than that of adults younger than 65 *(4,10)*. In a study of the prevalence of insomnia in an older population (ages 53–97), Schubert et al. *(11)* found that almost half (49%) of the population reported at least one insomnia trait (difficulty getting to sleep, difficulty returning to sleep after waking up, or repeated awakenings) occurring at least five times per month.

Against this background, it is difficult to determine the contribution of superimposed illness to the problem of insomnia in affected patients. Nevertheless, insomnia has been associated with many medical conditions, e.g., neurodegenerative disorders like Parkinson's disease (PD; *12,13*). Nonmotor manifestations of PD, including sleep disorders, have a major impact on the quality of life of patients

From: *Current Clinical Neurology*
Parkinson's Disease and Nonmotor Dysfunction
Edited by: R. F. Pfeiffer and I. Bodis-Wollner © Humana Press Inc., Totowa, NJ

and their families *(14)*. In the investigations of Karlsen et al., the two most important nonmotor complaints associated with poor quality of life in patients with PD were depression and insomnia *(15,16)*.

2. SLEEP PHYSIOLOGY

The definition of sleep is based on both behavioral and physiologic criteria *(17)*. The behavioral criteria are: eye closure, reduced responsiveness to environmental stimuli, decreased or absent movements, and a reversibly unconscious state *(17,18)*. Physiologically, sleep normally proceeds through cycles of five stages. The first four, collectively known as non-rapid eye movement NREM sleep, are numbered consecutively and represent progressively deeper states of somnolence. They account for 75–80% of sleep time in a healthy adult *(17)*. During these phases, electroencephalography displays varying amounts of high-voltage slow activity and delta waves (1–4 Hz) with characteristic sleep spindles (12–14 Hz) and K-complexes during stage II. The fifth stage of sleep is characterized by rapid eye movement (REM), atonia, low-voltage fast brain activity, cardiorespiratory irregularities, and dreaming *(17)*. Sleep cycles last 90–100 minutes, and a normal sleep period has four to six cycles. The duration of REM sleep increases from the first to the last cycle and can persist for as long as 1 hour at the end of the sleep period *(17)*. Interference with the initiation, orderly progression, and completion of normal cycles of sleep result in insomnia.

The sleep cycle is regulated by a variety of neurochemical systems and is the result of active and passive mechanisms. Multiple monoamines, including serotonin, norepinephrine, and histamine, as well as acetylcholine and the neuropeptide hypocretin *(17,19–22)*, appear to be involved in the modulation of the sleep–wake cycle. Recently, interest has re-emerged about the role of dopamine and its systems in the sleep–wake cycle. The most prominent pathways that utilize dopamine include the mesostriatal, mesocortical, and mesolimbic systems *(23)*. Midbrain dopaminergic neurons may have the potential to influence thalamocortical neuronal excitability, and theoretically the sleep–wake state, through connections with the striatum and via extensive collaterals to the thalamus *(23)*. Neural mechanisms closely related to behavioral states have been associated with the modulation of "burst-firing" patterns of dopaminergic neurons *(19)*. REM sleep deprivation may produce a significant increase in striatal dopamine levels, suggesting that sleep deprivation can induce plasticity in the mesostriatal dopamine system *(19,24,25)*. Dopamine activity is itself under the influence of a circadian rhythm *(19,26)*. Perhaps the strongest evidence of the role of dopaminergic systems in the modulation of sleep–wake cycles derives from clinical studies *(19)*. Abnormal sleep and impaired daytime alertness both occur in the majority of patients with PD *(27,28)*. Clinical observations of sleepiness in PD further support the role of dopamine in the sleep–wake cycle *(19)*. The effects of levodopa and dopamine agonists on sleep *(29)* also imply a role of dopaminergic systems in sleep. Therefore, it is not surprising that most patients who have PD experience difficulties with sleep owing to the disease, its treatment, or both *(30,31)*.

3. INSOMNIA IN PD

Sleep disorders are common in patients with PD *(27,32,33)*. Their frequency appears to be higher than that expected from the effects of age alone *(27)*, but not all authors agree *(31)*. Measurements of the prevalence of sleep disorders in PD range from 40% to 98% *(28,31,34,35)*. Sleep disturbances can occur at any stage of PD, but they are more common as the disease progresses, which suggests a direct relation between impaired sleep and disease severity *(35,36)*. However, sleep impairment becomes more typical with advancing age in the absence of PD, and some studies have failed to show a significant association with the stage of PD *(31)*.

Insomnia is the most common sleep complaint in both the general population and in patients who have PD *(14)*. Polysomnographic data in patients with PD have shown: (1) light-fragmented sleep *(37)*, (2) decreased sleep efficiencies *(38)*, (3) increased wakefulness *(38)*, (4) decreased amounts of REM sleep *(38)*, (5) increased REM sleep latencies *(39)*, (6) fragmented REM sleep *(38)*, (7) increased frequency of arousals *(38)*, (8) decreased amounts of sleep spindles *(39,40)*, (9) poorly formed K complexes *(39,40)*, and (10) increased muscle activity in REM sleep (REM without atonia; *38*). Evidently, both the macro- and microstructure of sleep are affected in this group of patients.

The most common form of insomnia in patients with PD is that of frequent nocturnal awakenings, also known as sleep fragmentation *(27,28,39)*. Factor and colleagues *(27)* studied sleep complaints and the effect of sleep on motor symptoms through a survey in 78 patients with PD (median age 67 years old; average disease duration 6.7 years) and 43 elderly controls (median age 63 years old). Sleep initiation problems occurred frequently in both groups with no significant difference between them, but sleep fragmentation was more common in patients who had PD (88.5% in PD versus 74.4% in the control group). In a community-based study, Tandberg et al. *(34)* found that the most common sleep complaints reported by 245 patients with PD were sleep fragmentation and early awakening. In their study, patients with PD indicated sleep disorders significantly more often than patients with diabetes and healthy control subjects, and one third of the patients with PD rated their overall nighttime problem as moderate-to-severe. Another study *(41)* compared 90 patients who had PD to 71 age-matched healthy subjects, showing a high prevalence of sleep disturbances in both groups (81% patients with PD versus 92% controls). There were no differences between the groups regarding the prevalence of disturbances of sleep initiation or maintenance; however, those patients with PD who experienced sleep maintenance difficulties reported a significantly greater number of awakenings.

Kumar and colleagues *(35)* studied the frequency and nature of sleep disturbances in 149 patients with PD and 115 age-matched controls and found that 42% of patients who had PD reported sleep problems when compared to 12% of a healthy control population. Insomnia was reported by 39.6% of patients and 5% of the control group. Within the PD group, those patients with sleep complaints had a longer duration of disease and higher Unified Parkinson's Disease Rating Scale (UPDRS) scores and received higher levodopa doses. They also had longer sleep latencies than those without sleep problems. Nighttime awakenings were significantly associated with rigidity and Hoehn and Yahr (H & Y) scores.

The frequency of sleep initiation difficulties in patients with PD is not as well-established as that of sleep maintenance. Most studies have not observed significant differences between patients with PD and control subjects *(27,34,41)*. However, Kales et al. *(30)* found sleep initiation problems to be a prominent issue in patients who had PD.

Although it has been suggested that sleep deprivation influences dopamine systems *(42)*, data on the effects of sleep deprivation on motor symptoms in patients who have PD are scarce and controversial. Bertolucci et al. *(43)* reported improvement in rigidity, bradykinesia, gait, and posture disturbances lasting 2 weeks after a single night of total sleep deprivation in 12 patients with PD. These results supported the positive effects of REM-sleep deprivation shown in an animal model of PD *(44)*. However, beneficial results are not universal. There were 15 patients with PD who underwent one night of total sleep deprivation, one night of partial sleep deprivation, and one control night of normal sleep. Mean UPDRS motor scores and tapping velocities were not substantially affected by sleep deprivation. Only four patients following PSD showed an improvement in their motor score of greater than 20% when compared to the score after normal sleep *(42)*.

4. CONTRIBUTING FACTORS

The etiology of light and fragmented sleep in PD is multifactorial *(28,32,37,45)*. Treated patients with more advanced disease typically experience wearing-off of medication effect at night, resulting in recurrence of tremor, rigidity, and akinesia, and increased sleep latency. Rigidity and akinesia both contribute to the inability to turn in bed, which has been rated as the most troublesome nocturnal symptom, affecting 65% of 220 patients who had PD in one study *(28)*. Multiple motor symptoms persist during sleep and interfere with its normal physiology *(32,33)*. During light sleep, PD tremor can reappear *(33)*. The effect of sleep on the involuntary movements or dyskinesias in PD and other movement disorders was studied by Fish et al. *(46)*. They reported that involuntary movements or dyskinesias in PD were most likely to occur after awakenings or in stage 1 sleep; these movements were very rare during the deeper phases of sleep. The movements that occurred without awakenings were usually preceded by arousal phenomena and, rarely, by sleep spindles or slow waves.

Repetitive muscle contractions can occur during NREM sleep. Askenasy and colleagues reported that NREM sleep transforms the waking "alternating" parkinsonian tremor into subclinical repetitive muscle contractions. Their amplitude and duration decreased as NREM sleep progressed and disappeared during REM sleep *(47)*. Additional motor abnormalities that are factors to sleep fragmentation include dystonia, which can lead to pain *(28)*, blinking and blepharospasm *(32,33)*, painful leg cramps *(28)*, and fragmentary myoclonus *(45)*.

A common complaint of patients who have PD is frequent urination, and nocturia was the most common form of nighttime disability in a group of 220 patients who had PD *(28)*. In this study, 79% of the patients had to "visit the lavatory" during the night, and one third needed to urinate three or more times. When nocturnal urinary frequency is compounded with the inability to walk without assistance (e.g., as in 35% of these 220 patients; *28*), nocturia can represent a major source of stress and disability in PD. Urinary frequency in PD may be a result of disease-related dysautonomia or age-related urological abnormalities and can increase patients' morbidity, as it exposes them to frequent falls and consequent injuries, including fractures *(45)* and further immobility.

Coexisting psychiatric and medical disorders can also affect sleep in patients with PD. Depression may have an important role in modulating normal sleep architecture, and early-morning awakening with inability to return to sleep is a classic symptom of depression. The high prevalence of depression in PD patients makes it an important consideration in the differential diagnosis of insomnia. (Depression is discussed in detail in an earlier Chapter 1.)

Other sleep disturbances that can contribute to insomnia, namely REM-sleep behavior disorder (Chapter 16) and sleep-related breathing disorders (Chapter 18), are detailed elsewhere in this volume. Other PD nonmotor symptoms discussed elsewhere that may affect the ability to sleep restfully include pain (Chapter 22), anxiety (Chapter 2), and hallucinosis (Chapter 5) *(32,33,45)*.

5. RESTLESS LEGS SYNDROME

Restless legs syndrome (RLS) is characterized by an irresistible urge to move the limbs that (1) becomes evident or is accentuated in the evening and at nighttime (2), occurs when the legs are rested (sitting or lying down) and is relieved by moving the legs or walking, and (3) is accompanied by paresthesias or dysesthesias variously described as creeping, crawling, itching, burning, pulling, aching, restless, tingling, cramping, or other sensations. The onset is unilateral in 40–50% of cases. The legs are almost always involved, but the arms may be affected as well in 25–50%. Most patients also experience periodic limb movements in sleep, and many display similar dyskinesias while awake *(48)*. Symptoms tend to increase with age. RLS may affect as much as 5% of the population and 10% of those over age 65. The main effect on sleep of RLS is sleep-latency insomnia (i.e., delaying the onset of sleep), but RLS may also cause fragmented, nonrestorative sleep and occasionally excessive daytime sleepiness.

Many cases are idiopathic or hereditary. Yet, as with insomnia in general, RLS is a common disorder that is even more typical when associated with a variety of chronic illnesses, including PD. Approximately 20% of patients with PD report symptoms consistent with RLS; in over 70% of cases, the onset of PD preceded or occurred concomitantly with the development of RLS *(49)*. Tan and colleagues *(50)* could not find any patients who had PD with RLS in a survey of 125 consecutive patients, but the same authors reported a prevalence of RLS of only 0.6% in their general population. Some patients with PD clearly relate their RLS symptoms to the development of motor symptoms when the benefit from their medications wears off *(50–52)*. Gunal and colleagues *(53)* identified 5 such instances among 72 consecutive patients who had PD with motor fluctuations.

It is important to identify RLS because of its response to specific treatment. Systematic survey of patients with PD indicates that the majority of affected individuals will not volunteer symptoms of RLS *(49)*. In cases where the symptoms of RLS fluctuate in tandem with motor manifestations of PD, patients may assume that such symptoms are typical of "off" periods, not a distinct experience. Thus, such historical information must be actively and specifically sought to establish the diagnosis of RLS.

6. EFFECTS OF ANTI-PARKINSONIAN TREATMENT

Pharmacological agents used in PD treatment may be a cause of sleep disorders. Anti-Parkinsonian medications alter the sleep–wake cycle *(29,31)*, and dopaminergic medications have prominent effects on both circadian rhythms and sleep–wake modulatory systems *(32)*. The effects of levodopa on sleep are nonspecific. They are exerted through pre- and postsynaptic mechanisms and via interaction with different neurotransmitters *(32)*. Levodopa suppresses REM sleep and delays REM-sleep latency *(29,32,54)*; it has improved daytime vigilance in narcoleptic patients *(55)*. In a questionnaire study, Nausieda et al. *(31)* found that the use and duration of levodopa therapy were associated in patients who had PD with a higher frequency of sleep disruption, and sleep fragmentation was the most common sleep complaint.

Bromocriptine has induced changes in sleep architecture similar to levodopa in patients who had PD, including shorter REM sleep, superficial sleep, and prolongation of REM-sleep latency *(56)*. Pergolide, bromocriptine, and apomorphine produce "biphasic effects" (opposite effects at low and high doses) on sleep architecture in rats *(57)*. At low doses, they decrease wakefulness and increase NREM sleep. In a 71-year-old sleep-deprived patient with PD, pergolide suppressed REM-sleep rebound phenomena *(58)*. The newer nonergoline dopaminergic agonists, ropinirole and pramipexole, also affect sleep physiology. At lower doses, D3 agonists increase NREM and REM sleep and reduce locomotion in rats *(59)*; with higher doses, D2/D3 agonists improve locomotion without major sedation *(59)*. In one study, ropinirole was shown to improve sleep efficiency and total sleep time in five patients with chronic insomnia secondary to RLS *(60)*. The potential clinical effect of dopamine agonists and levodopa to induce "sleep attacks" is reviewed in Chapter 17. Selegiline can suppress REM sleep *(61)*. Puca et al. reported an increase in sleep spindle activity in Parkinsonian patients following administration of amantadine *(62)*.

7. TREATMENT OF INSOMNIA IN PD

7.1. Contributing Factors

The first step in insomnia management in PD is accurate identification of contributing factors. A detailed history provided by the patient and any bedmate or caregiver is crucial. For those with complicated or varying sleep problems, a symptom diary could be useful. In some instances, diagnostic testing with polysomnography might be necessary. Successful treatment of sleep disturbances in patients with PD can postpone their institutionalization, allow the caregiver better sleep, and improve their quality of life *(45)*.

If a specific cause for insomnia is found, it should be treated first *(2)*. Comorbid conditions, such as nocturia, sleep apnea, RLS, anxiety, and depression, should be addressed, as their treatment will likely improve sleep quality. General sleep hygiene rules should be recommended as appropriate to each individual. Some of these instructions include:

1. Reduce excessive time in bed.
2. Increase exercise and physical activity.
3. Curtail caffeine intake.
4. Observe a fixed wake-up time.
5. Avoid naps.
6. Avoid caffeine, alcohol, or heavy meals before bedtime.
7. Limit fluid intake after 5 pm.

8. Use available aids for getting in and out of bed.
9. Make medications, water, and a bathroom or commode chair easily accessible *(2,32,45)*.

Sleep hygiene rules should be instituted only once at a time to enhance compliance. Behavioral therapy (through stimulus control), sleep restriction, sleep hygiene education, and chronotherapy, are important factors in the treatment of insomnia *(32,45,63)*.

7.2. Dopaminergic Medication Adjustment

Insomnia in a Parkinsonian patient should always prompt careful reassessment of dopaminergic therapy *(45)*. Dosage adjustment must be carefully individualized. In some patients, excessive dosages of dopaminergic medications should be avoided at night. Levodopa can have an arousal effect, potentiate wakefulness, and enhance sleep fragmentation *(45)*. Alternatively, increased doses of dopaminergic medications may significantly improve sleep by improving motor symptoms, specifically tremor and akinesia. Activity and immobility during sleep was recorded by a wrist monitor in 84 patients with PD and 83 age- and sex-matched normal controls *(64)*. In mild-to-moderate disease, levodopa or dopamine agonists were disruptive to sleep by their effects on sleep regulation. However, in more severe PD forms, the drugs had beneficial effects on nocturnal disability *(64)*. The influence on sleep of other medications, e.g., anticholinergics, selegiline, and amantadine, should also be considered.

7.3. Sedatives/Hypnotics

Use of hypnotics is usually not indicated, as the primary role of these medications is to treat acute insomnia, and in chronic insomnia, there is a risk of dependence *(32,45)*. If benzodiazepines are used, the short-acting kinds are preferred; those with a long half-life can produce daytime sedation, dozing, and disturbances in perceptual skills *(2,45)*. Newer, nonbenzodiazepine hypnotic agents have been well-accepted in the treatment of insomnia in the general population. Zolpidem and zaleplon have hypnosedative actions comparable with that of benzodiazepines, but they display specific properties. These agents share a short plasma half-life (zaleplon, 1 hour; zolpidem, 5 hours) and a limited duration of action, and they are less sedating than benzodiazepines *(65)*. A double-blind placebo-controlled trial of zolpidem in 10 patients with PD suggested that it may be helpful for parkinsonian motor symptoms as well as insomnia *(66)*.

Melatonin effects in the treatment of insomnia in the general population is controversial *(2)*. Its use in PD requires further investigation.

7.4. Treatment of Nocturia

Nocturia frequently causes sleep disruption in patients who have PD. Oral anticholinergic agents, such as oxybutynin and tolterodine, may provide sufficient antispasmodic effects on the urinary bladder, and both are available in sustained-release preparations for nighttime dosing. Suchowersky et al. *(67)* found intranasal desmopressin to be a safe and effective tool for nocturnal polyuria in PD.

7.5. Treatment of RLS

Fortunately, RLS shares responsiveness to dopaminergic medication with PD, and dopamine agonists are particularly appropriate in the management of RLS because of levodopa's greater tendency to produce augmentation *(68)*. Other effective agents in treatment include gabapentin, clonazepam, and opiates.

7.6. Deep-Brain Stimulation Surgery

Sleep architecture in PD may improve with subthalamic nucleus (STN) stimulation *(69)*, or pallidotomy *(70)*. In 10 insomniac patients with PD on dopaminergic therapy, STN improved nighttime akinesia by 60%, suppressed axial dystonia, and increased total sleep time by 47% and sleep efficiency by 36%. It also decreased the duration of wakefulness following sleep. Periodic leg movements and motor behavior during REM sleep were not influenced by stimulation *(69)*.

8. CONCLUSION

Insomnia is a common complaint and one of the most important determinants of quality of life in patients with PD. The most typical form of insomnia in patients who have PD is frequent nocturnal awakenings. Insomnia may be a direct complication of PD or its treatment, or it may be a byproduct of other complications like depression, nocturia and RLS. Proper management of insomnia involves the identification and treatment of contributing factors, careful assessment of the regimen of anti-Parkinsonian medications, institution of effective sleep hygiene measures, and judicious use of hypnotic medication.

REFERENCES

1. American Sleep Disorders Association. The International Classification of Sleep Disorders: Diagnostic and Coding Manual. American Sleep Disorders Association, Rochester, MN, 1997.
2. Hauri PJ. Insomnia. Clin Chest Med 1998;19:157–168.
3. Spielman AJ, Nunes J, Glovinsky PB. Insomnia. Neurol Clin 1996;14:513–543.
4. Walsh J, Ustun TB. Prevalence and Health Consequences of Insomnia. Sleep 1999;22(Suppl 3):S427–S436.
5. Hohagen F, Kappler C, Schramm E, et al. Sleep onset insomnia, sleep maintaining insomnia and insomnia with early morning awakening—temporal stability of subtypes in a longitudinal study on general practice attenders. Sleep 1994;17:551–554.
6. Sateia MJ, Doghramji K, Hauri PJ, Morin CM. Evaluation of chronic insomnia. An American Academy of Sleep Medicine review. Sleep 2000;23:243–308.
7. Bixler EO, Kales A, Soldatos CR, et al. Prevalence of sleep disorders in the Los Angeles metropolitan area. Am J Psychiatry 1979;136:1257–1262.
8. Blais FC, Morin CM, Boisclair A, et al. Insomnia. Prevalence and treatment of patients in general practice [Article in French]. Can Fam Physician 2001;47:759–767.
9. Ohayon MM, Hong SC. Prevalence of insomnia and associated factors in South Korea. J Psychosom Res 2002;53:593–600.
10. Mellinger GD, Balter MB, Uhlenhuth EH. Insomnia and its treatment. Prevalence and correlates. Arch Gen Psychiatry 1985;42:225–232.
11. Schubert CR, Cruickshanks KJ, Dalton DS, et al. Prevalence of sleep problems and quality of life in an older population. Sleep 2002;25:889–893.
12. Aldrich MS. Insomnia in neurological diseases. J Psychosom Res 1993;37(Suppl 1):3–11.
13. Chokroverty S. Sleep and degenerative neurologic disorders. Neurol Clin 1996;14807–826.
14. Larsen JP. Sleep disorders in Parkinson's disease. Adv Neurol 2003;91:329–334.
15. Karlsen KH, Larsen JP, Tandberg E, Maeland JG. Quality of life measurements in patients with Parkinson's disease: A community-based study. Eur J Neurol 1998;5:443–450.
16. Karlsen KH, Larsen JP, Tandberg E, Maeland JG. Influence of clinical and demographic variables on quality of life in patients with Parkinson's disease. J Neurol Neurosurg Psychiatry 1999;66:431–435.
17. Chokroverty S. An overview of sleep. In: Chokroverty S, ed. Sleep Disorders Medicine: Basic Science, Technical Considerations, and Clinical Aspects. Butterworth-Heinemann, Boston, MA, 1999, pp. 7–20.
18. Tobler I. Is sleep fundamentally different between mammalian species? Behav Brain Res 1995;69:35–41.
19. Rye DB, Jankovic J. Emerging views of dopamine in modulating sleep/wake state from an unlikely source: PD. Neurology 2002;58:341–346.
20. Silber MH, Rye DB. Solving the mysteries of narcolepsy: the hypocretin story. Neurology 2001;56:1616–1618.
21. McCarley RW. Sleep neurophysiology: basic mechanisms underlying control of wakefulness and sleep. In: Chrokroverty S, ed. Sleep Disorders Medicine: Basic Science, Technical Considerations, and Clinical Aspects. Butterworth-Heinemann, Boston, MA, 1999, pp. 21–50.
22. Steriade M. Neurophysiologic mechanisms of non-rapid eye movement (resting) sleep. In: Chrokroverty S, ed. Sleep Disorders Medicine: Basic Science, Technical Considerations, and Clinical Aspects. Butterworth-Heinemann, Boston, MA, 1999, pp. 51–62.
23. Freeman A, Ciliax B, Bakay R, et al. Nigrostriatal collaterals to thalamus degenerate in parkinsonian animal models. Ann Neurol 2001;50:321–329.
24. Farber J, Miller JD, Crawford KA, McMillen BA. Dopamine metabolism and receptor sensitivity in rat brain after REM sleep deprivation. Pharmacol Biochem Behav 1983;18:509–513.
25. Ghosh PK, Hrdina PD, Ling GM. Effects of REMS deprivation on striatal dopamine and acetylcholine in rats. Pharmacol Biochem Behav 1976;4:401–405.
26. Smith AD, Olson RJ, Justice JBJ. Quantitative microdialysis of dopamine in the striatum: effect of circadian variation. J Neurosci Methods 1992;44:33–41.
27. Factor SA, McAlarney T, Sanchez-Ramos JR, Weiner WJ. Sleep disorders and sleep effect in Parkinson's disease. Mov Disord 1990;5:280–285.

28. Lees AJ, Blackburn NA, Campbell VL. The nighttime problems of Parkinson's disease. Clin Neuropharmacol 1988;11:512–519.
29. Schafer D, Greulich W. Effects of parkinsonian medication on sleep. J Neurol 2000;247(Suppl 4):24–27.
30. Kales A, Ansel RD, Markham CH, et al. Sleep in patients with Parkinson's disease and normal subjects prior to and following levodopa administration. Clin Pharmacol Ther 1971;12:397–406.
31. Nausieda PA, Weiner WJ, Kaplan LR, et al. Sleep disruption in the course of chronic levodopa therapy: an early feature of the levodopa psychosis. Clin Neuropharmacol 1982;5:183–194.
32. Garcia-Borreguero D, Larrosa O, Bravo M. Parkinson's disease and sleep. Sleep Med Rev 2003;7:115–129.
33. Comella CL. Sleep disturbances in Parkinson's disease. Curr Neurol Neurosci Rep 2003;3:173–180.
34. Tandberg E, Larsen JP, Karlsen K. A community-based study of sleep disorders in patients with Parkinson's disease. Mov Disord 1998;13:895–899.
35. Kumar S, Bhatia M, Behari M. Sleep disorders in Parkinson's disease. Mov Disord 2002;17:775–781.
36. Partinen M. Sleep disorder related to Parkinson's disease. J Neurol 1997;244(4 Suppl 1):S3–S6.
37. Askenasy JJ, Yahr MD. Reversal of sleep disturbance in Parkinson's disease by antiparkinsonian therapy: a preliminary study. Neurology 1985;35:527–532.
38. Hogl BE, Gomez-Arevalo G, Garcia S, et al. A clinical, pharmacologic, and polysomnographic study of sleep benefit in Parkinson's disease. Neurology 1998;50:1332–1339.
39. Poewe W, Hogl B, Parkinson's disease and sleep. Curr Opin Neurol 2000;13:423–426.
40. Friedman A. Sleep pattern in Parkinson's disease. Acta Med Pol 1980;21:193–199.
41. van Hilten JJ, Weggeman M, van der Velde EA, et al. Sleep, excessive daytime sleepiness and fatigue in Parkinson's disease. J Neural Transm Park Dis Dement Sect 1993;5:235–244.
42. Hogl B, Peralta C, Wetter TC, et al. Effect of sleep deprivation on motor performance in patients with Parkinson's disease. Mov Disord 2001;16:616–621.
43. Bertolucci PH, Andrade LA, Lima JG, Carlini EA. Total sleep deprivation and Parkinson disease. Arq Neuropsiquiatr 1987;45:224–230.
44. Andrade LA, Lima JG, Tufik S, et al. Rem sleep deprivation in an experimental model of Parkinson's disease. Arq Neuropsiquiatr 1987;45:217–223.
45. Askenasy JJ. Sleep disturbances in Parkinsonism. J Neural Transm 2003;110:125–150.
46. Fish DR, Sawyers D, Allen PJ, et al. The effect of sleep on the dyskinetic movements of Parkinson's disease, Gilles de la Tourette syndrome, Huntington's disease, and torsion dystonia. Arch Neurol 1991;48:210–214.
47. Askenasy JJ, Yahr MD. Parkinsonian tremor loses its alternating aspect during non-REM sleep and is inhibited by REM sleep. J Neurol Neurosurg Psychiatry 1990;53:749–753.
48. Stiasny K, Oertel WH, Trenkwalder C. Clinical symptomatology and treatment of restless legs syndrome and periodic limb movement disorder. Sleep Med Rev 2002;6:253–265.
49. Ondo WG, Vuong KD, Jankovic J. Exploring the relationship between Parkinson disease and restless legs syndrome. Arch Neurol 2002;59:421–424.
50. Tan EK, Lum SY, Wong MC. Restless legs syndrome in Parkinson's disease. J Neurol Sci 2002;196:33–36.
51. Quinn NP. Classification of fluctuations in patients with Parkinson's disease. Neurology 1998;51(2 Suppl 2):S25–29.
52. Riley DE, Lang AE. The spectrum of levodopa-related fluctuations in Parkinson's disease. Neurology 1993;43:1459–1464.
53. Gunal DI, Nurichalichi K, Tuncer N, et al. The clinical profile of nonmotor fluctuations in Parkinson's disease patients. Can J Neurol Sci 2002;29:61–64.
54. Galarraga E, Corsi-Cabrera M, Sangri M. Reduction in paradoxical sleep after L-dopa administration in rats. Behav Neural Biol 1986;46:249–256.
55. Boivin DB, Montplaisir J. The effects of L-dopa on excessive daytime sleepiness in narcolepsy. Neurology 1991;41:1267–1269.
56. Vardi J, Glaubman H, Rabey J, Streifler M. EEG sleep patterns in Parkinsonian patients treated with bromocryptine and L-dopa: a comparative study. J Neural Transm 1979;45:307–316.
57. Monti JM, Hawkins M, Jantos H, et al. Biphasic effects of dopamine D-2 receptor agonists on sleep and wakefulness in the rat. Psychopharmacology (Berl) 1988;95:395–400.
58. Askenasy JJ, Yahr MD. Suppression of REM rebound by pergolide. J Neural Transm 1984;59:151–159.
59. Uitti RJ, Wszolek ZK. Dopamine agonists, sleep disorders, and driving in Parkinson's disease. Adv Neurol 2003;91:343–349.
60. Estivill E, de la Fuente V. The efficacy of ropinirole in the treatment of chronic insomnia secondary to restless legs syndrome: polysomnography data. [Article in Spanish]. Rev Neurol 1999;29:805–807.
61. Hublin C, Partinen M, Heinonen EH, et al. Selegiline in the treatment of narcolepsy. Neurology 1994;44:2095–2101.
62. Puca FM, Bricolo A, Turella G. Effect of L-dopa or amantadine therapy on sleep spindles in Parkinsonism. Electroencephalogr Clin Neurophysiol 1973;35:327–330.
63. Petit L, Azad N, Byszewski A, et al. Non-pharmacological management of primary and secondary insomnia among older people: review of assessment tools and treatments. Age Ageing 2003;32:19–25.
64. van Hilten B, Hoff JI, Middelkoop HA, et al. Sleep disruption in Parkinson's disease. Assessment by continuous activity monitoring. Arch Neurol 1994;51:922–928.

65. Terzano MG, Rossi M, Palomba V, et al. New drugs for insomnia: comparative tolerability of zopiclone, zolpidem and zaleplon. Drug Saf 2003;26:261–282.
66. Daniele A, Albanese A, Gainotti G, et al. Zolpidem in Parkinson's disease. Lancet 1997;349:1222–1223.
67. Suchowersky O, Furtado S, Rohs G. Beneficial effect of intranasal desmopressin for nocturnal polyuria in Parkinson's disease. Mov Disord 1995;10:337–340.
68. Earley CJ. Clinical practice. Restless legs syndrome. N Engl J Med 2003;348:2103–2109.
69. Arnulf I, Bejjani BP, Garma L, et al. Improvement of sleep architecture in PD with subthalamic nucleus stimulation. Neurology 2000;55:1732–1734.
70. Favre J, Burchiel KJ, Taha JM, Hammerstad J. Outcome of unilateral and bilateral pallidotomy for Parkinson's disease: patient assessment. Neurosurgery 2000;46:344–353.

16
Rapid Eye Movement Sleep Behavior Disorder

Suzanne Stevens and Cynthia Comella

SUMMARY

Rapid eye movement sleep behavior disorder (RBD) is a rapid eye movement (REM) parasomnia in which the normal muscle atonia of REM sleep is absent. The lack of muscle atonia may lead to motor activation and the appearance of dream-related behaviors. Dream content during RBD is vivid and often has aggressive themes, such as being threatened, chased, or attacked. During an episode, both the patient with RBD and their bed partner are at risk for serious injuries (e.g., bruises, lacerations, and bone fractures). Diagnosis of RBD currently requires the presence of established clinical criteria, but polysomnography is recommended to confirm the diagnosis and differentiate it from other sleep disorders, including sleep apnea. Controlled trials are lacking; yet, clonazepam has been effective in treating symptoms in up to 90% of patients with RBD. Other treatment approaches are dopaminergic agonists, antiepileptic agents, α-adrenergic agonists, acetylcholinesterase inhibitors, and melatonin. RBD is frequently associated with synucleinopathies, such as multiple system atrophy, dementia with Lewy bodies, and Parkinson's disease. In these patients, RBD symptoms may precede motor symptoms by months to years. Abnormalities in central dopaminergic mechanisms have been postulated.

Key Words: REM sleep; REM sleep behavior disorder; parasomnia; dreams; polysomnography; clonazepam.

1. INTRODUCTION

Rapid eye movement (REM) sleep typically comprises 15 to 25% of the normal sleep cycle and is the stage in which at least 80% of dreaming occurs. REM sleep is defined electrophysiologically by a desynchronized cortical electroencephalogram (EEG), skeletal muscle atonia, REM, autonomic instability, and pontogenicular (PGO) spikes. REM sleep behavior disorder (RBD) was initially described as a parasomnia by Schenk in 1986 *(1)*. RBD is an abnormal state of REM in which normal REM-associated muscle atonia is absent, enabling the activation of the motor system. Loss of REM-associated muscle atonia may lead to an enactment of dream content. Dream content during RBD episodes often involves aggressive themes of being threatened, chased, or attacked. Hence, the activities observed during RBD may include talking, yelling, clapping, punching, thrashing, kicking, sitting up, falling out of bed, and running. Because of these sometimes violent behaviors, several reports exist of injuries during sleep, including lacerations, ecchymoses, bone fractures, and subdural hematomas. These injuries have been indicated in both patients and bed partners during episodes. The bed partner may be suddenly awakened by being pummeled or choked by the spouse, who exhibits no evidence of hostility during waking hours. The bed partner often seeks refuge by sleeping in another room. Then, the patient awakens in the morning with no recollection of these behaviors, but associated dreams may be recalled.

Idiopathic RBD is diagnosed when no concurrent neurological disease is found; symptomatic RBD is found when additional neurological findings are present. RBD is more common in the

From: *Current Clinical Neurology*
Parkinson's Disease and Nonmotor Dysfunction
Edited by: R. F. Pfeiffer and I. Bodis-Wollner © Humana Press Inc., Totowa, NJ

elderly population, affects men more than women, and is particularly frequent in certain neurodegenerative disorders that have common features of Parkinsonism and pathological findings of synuclein pathology (e.g., idiopathic Parkinson's disease [PD], multiple system atrophy [MSA], and dementia with Lewy bodies [DLB; *2*].)

2. PREVALENCE

The prevalence of RBD in the general population is approximately 0.05%. The male predominance is significant; up to 87% of patients with RBD are men *(3,4)*. Gender predisposition has not yet been explained. The mean age of onset with RBD symptoms is in the age range of 52 to 62 years, but RBD has been reported in patients from 9 to 84 years old. Cross-sectional analysis of large groups of patients with RBD shows that idiopathic RBD is less common than symptomatic RBD. In three large case series, 25 to 43% of patients with RBD were designated as idiopathic, whereas 48 to 75% were classified with symptomatic RBD. The most frequently associated neurological disorders in patients with RBD were neurodegenerative diseases, which comprised 48 to 92% of cases *(3–5)*. Neurodegenerative diseases most often linked with RBD are synucleinopathies, PD, and MSA *(4,6)*, but rare case reports of RBD in progressive supranuclear palsy *(7)* and corticobasalganglionic degeneration (CBD; *8*), both tauopathies, also exist.

RBD frequency in the synucleinopathies has been extensively investigated. In one interview study, 15% of idiopathic patients who had PD were found to have a clinical history meeting the International Classification of Sleep Disorders (ICSD) criteria for RBD. Among the RBD patients, one-third had caused injury to themselves or their caregivers *(9)*. Using polysomnography (PSG) along with clinical history, investigators have shown as many as 58% of patients who had PD tested to have REM sleep without atonia, but 42% of these did not have obvious behavioral abnormalities, suggesting that RBD is a common feature in PD and may be presymptomatic in many *(10)*. In one study that compared clinical features in patients who had PD with RBD to those without, factors related to RBD occurrence in PD included longer duration of PD, more severe disease, and treatment with higher doses of dopaminergic drugs *(11)*.

The prevalence of RBD in MSA has been found to be even greater than that in PD. One study assessing 39 consecutive MSA patients showed that 69% had clinical features consistent with RBD, and 90% were diagnosed with RBD when evaluation included PSG *(12)*. Similarly, in patients with RBD and dementia, these clinical features are highly suggestive of DLB; confirmatory pathological examinations have been performed in some cases *(2,13)*.

One intriguing aspect of the relationship between RBD and these parkinsonian syndromes is the observation that RBD symptoms may precede the onset of parkinsonian symptoms by many years. Schenck reported that in 38% (11/29) of 29 primary RBD male patients, a parkinsonian syndrome developed a mean of 4 years after the clinical diagnosis of RBD and a mean of 13 years after historical symptoms of RBD began *(14)*. This estimate has been confirmed by others *(15)*. In patients with DLB assessed by Boeve et al., 97% developed RBD either before or concurrent with the onset of dementia *(13)*. Similarly, RBD preceded MSA onset of symptoms by at least 1 year in 44% of individuals with MSA *(12)*. Based on these observations, RBD has been theorized to be a harbinger of specific neurodegenerative conditions *(16)*.

3. ETIOLOGY AND PATHOGENESIS

3.1. Anatomy

Anatomic localization and pathophysiological mechanisms underlying RBD remain to be fully elucidated. Jouvet was the first to describe the REM mechanisms in animals *(17,18)*. He also showed that cats lesioned bilaterally in the dorsolateral pontine tegmental region had REM sleep without atonia, which developed into dream enactment behavior in the weeks following lesioning, a phenomenon like that seen in human RBD. In these experiments, lesions of other regions of the brainstem did not result in REM abnormalities. Furthermore, suppression of REM sleep abolished the oneiric behaviors, implying that the abnormality responsible for REM-related motor activation involved the disruption of pathways responsible for the normal components of REM sleep.

Specific anatomic areas suspected to be engaged in the pathogenesis of RBD include the pedunculopontine nucleus (PPN) and lateraldorsal tegmental nucleus (LDT). The PPN is located in the pontomesencephalic tegmentum. Both the PPN and the LDT are cholinergic nuclei with rostral projections to the gigantocellular tegmental field (FTG). Injections of cholinergic agents into the pontine reticular formation enhance the release of acetylcholine in the FTG and induce a REM-like state with EEG desynchronization and the generation of PGO spikes, which implicates that the PPN and LDT may have a pivotal role in the regulation of REM *(19)*. The PPN has also been implicated in the akinesia and gait difficulties in Parkinsonism *(20)*. Although limited work has been done, the PPN has been found in several studies to degenerate in PD with a loss of approximately 50% of the cholinergic neurons *(21,22)*. This finding has led to the hypothesis that a loss of PPN cholinergic neurons may be involved in both selected motor findings in Parkinsonism and RBD development. The pathological findings in a small number of patients with RBD, most with features suggestive of DLB, have included significant neuronal loss in the locus ceruleus. The locus ceruleus has important connections with the PPN and is integrally associated with the control of REM sleep *(23,24)*.

Lai and Siegel have developed a more detailed theory to explain the frequent coexistence of RBD and Parkinsonism *(16)*. In their model, two juxtaposed areas of the brainstem undergo degeneration: the rostroventral midbrain (RVMD) and the ventral mesopontine junction (VMPJ). The RVMD includes the substantia nigra, among other nuclei, and projects to the basal ganglia and basal forebrain. The VMPJ consists of the caudal part of the ventral tegmental area, retrorubral nucleus, and ventral mesencephalic field (among others) and projects to the pontine inhibitory area, locus ceruleus, and nucleus magnocellularis. Lesions in the VMPJ area in animals produce increased phasic and tonic muscle activity during REM sleep. RVMD lesions in animals produce transient Parkinsonism and sleep fragmentation, a sleep disturbance that affects many patients who have PD *(25)*. Lai and Siegel hypothesize that neuronal degeneration occurs simultaneously in both brainstem areas in Parkinsonism. In those patients whose initial symptoms consist of RBD, degeneration may begin in the VMPJ and later involve the adjacent areas of the RVMD. Conversely, Parkinsonism symptoms preceding RBD may implicate the onset of neurodegeneration in the RVMD with subsequent involvement of the VMPJ, thus providing evidence of an anatomic link between Parkinsonism and RBD *(16)*.

3.2. Neuroimaging and Neurophysiology

In symptomatic RBD, magnetic resonance imaging has demonstrated lacunar infarcts in the dorsal pontomesencephalic area in some patients, suggesting that abnormalities in this area may underlie RBD *(26)*. However, in primary RBD, MRI findings do not differ from age-matched controls, and proton magnetic resonance spectroscopy (1H-MRS) does not indicate mesopontine neuronal loss or 1H-MRS-detectable metabolic disturbances *(27)*. However, multiple studies have shown alterations in the dopaminergic system in patients with primary RBD. Using [^{11}C] dihydrotetrabenazine (DTBZ) positron emission tomography (PET) scans, Albin et al. showed a marked reduction in dopaminergic innervation in the caudate nucleus and the anterior and posterior putamen in patients with RBD *(28)*. With the same methodology and the addition of $^{[123I]}$iodobenzovesamicol to measure the density of thalamic cholinergic terminals, Gilman et al. demonstrated an inverse correlation between dopaminergic innervation and the severity of muscle atonia loss in patients who had MSA with RBD. Changes in thalamic cholinergic terminals did not correlate with the severity of REM atonia loss but instead correlated with the severity of sleep apnea in these patients *(29)*.

Single-photon emission-computerized tomography (SPECT) scans using radio-labeled *N*-(3-iodopropene-2-yl)-2β-carbomethoxy-3β-(4-chlorophenyl) tropane demonstrated that in patients with subclinical RBD and clinically manifest idiopathic RBD, there is a progressive reduction in dopamine transporter binding when compared to age matched controls; the reduction is not as profound as that seen in PD *(30,31)*. Studies with DTBZ, a ligand that binds to the VMAT2 receptor and reflects the number of dopamine-producing neurons, show that patients with idiopathic RBD have a reduced density of striatal DTBZ binding, indicating loss of dopaminergic neurons in the substantia nigra and that the degree of loss correlates with the severity of RBD symptoms *(28)*. Together, SPECT and PET scans support the hypothesis that dopaminergic dysfunction may be a primary factor in the pathogenesis of RBD.

4. REM SLEEP BEHAVIOR DISORDER AND HALLUCINATIONS

The recent association of RBD with the occurrence of dopaminergic medication-induced hallucinations in PD suggests that the disorders may be related and that both are manifestations of disordered REM sleep. Comella et al. reported that patients who had PD with hallucinations had reduced nocturnal REM sleep when compared to a similarly treated group without hallucinations *(32)*. Arnulf et al. found that hallucinating patients with PD all demonstrated RBD, and REM intrusions into delusions and hallucinations coincided with REM intrusions into wakefulness *(33)*. Using a similar paradigm, Nomura et al. showed that hallucinating patients had more sleep fragmentation, and 71% had REM sleep without atonia versus only 25% of nonhallucinating patients *(34)*. They also demonstrated that visual hallucinations coincided with periods of REM, and the dream content of the sleep-onset REM periods during the multiple sleep latency test closely resembled the content of their daytime hallucinations. Both hallucinations and RBD symptoms improved with administration of clonazepam, an accepted, although unproven, treatment for RBD. An 8-year longitudinal study in 80 patients who had PD showed that the presence of RBD in PD predicted the later development of hallucinations *(35)*. Overall, these studies suggest that REM sleep disruption may have a pivotal influence, not only in the development of RBD, but also in the pathophysiology of drug-induced hallucinations in PD.

5. CLINICAL PRESENTATION

Individuals with RBD often seek medical evaluation only at the urging of their bed partner, who describes the most prominent clinical feature of RBD—acting out dreams. The history from the bed partner is typically the following: during sleep, the patient often punches, kicks, or vocalizes. Although the patient often attacks the bed partner, the patient is actually responding to dream content occurring during REM sleep, which creates an internal environment to which the patient is actually reacting. If the patient is awakened during an episode, the patient is frequently coherent and has recollection of a vivid dream, commonly involving themes of being chased or having to protect oneself against an attacker. However, the dream content may be mundane as well, such as sitting and having a conversation. This content often matches the physical activity or verbalizations made by the patient. Given that REM sleep occurs more in the later half of the night, history often places the timing of these events to the second half of the night. Yet, they may occur at any time throughout the night.

Case presentation: A 70-year-old man presented with violent behaviors during the night that had begun 8 years previously. He had been unaware of these behaviors, but his wife found these events to be very disturbing. As a result of these nocturnal behaviors, the patient intermittently had injured his wife, and on more than one occasion had awakened to find himself on the floor with bruises and abrasions. He provided three examples of such episodes: (1) He was dreaming of a dog biting and attacking him. In defense, he kicked at the dog, but in actuality was kicking his wife. When awakened by his wife, he was immediately coherent and recalled the content of the dream. (2) He dreamed he knocked a cake platter on the floor and broke it, when he actually had knocked the lamp off of his nightstand table and broken it. (3) He dreamed he was being chased by unknown assailants and was hiding behind a door in a barn. He actually had gotten out of bed, and while running behind a closet, collided with the doorknob and incurred a contusion around his eye.

Two years after his presentation to our sleep disorders clinic, and 7 years after the onset of RBD he developed a resting tremor, cogwheel rigidity, mild bradykinesia, and masked face, consistent with idiopathic Parkinson's disease.

Table 1
Criteria for Diagnosing REM Sleep Behavior Disorder in the International Classification of Sleep Disorders

The minimal diagnostic criteria are B plus C:

A. The patient has a complaint of violent or injurious behavior during sleep.
B. Limb or body movement is associated with dream mentation.
C. At least one of the following occurs:
   1. Harmful or potentially harmful sleep behaviors
   2. Dreams appear to be "acted out."
   3. Sleep behaviors disrupt sleep continuity
D. Polysomnographic monitoring demonstrates at least one of the following:
   1. Excessive augmentation of chin electromyography (EMG) tone
   2. Excessive chin or limb phasic EMG twitching, irrespective of chin EMG activity and one or more of the following clinical features during REM sleep:
      a. Excessive limb or body jerking
      b. Complex, vigorous, or violent behaviors
      c. Absence of epileptic activity in association with the disorder
E. The symptoms are not associated with mental disorders but may be associated with neurologic disorders
F. Other sleep disorders (e.g., sleep terrors or sleepwalking) can be present but are not the cause of the behavior

6. DIAGNOSIS

The ICSD codifies the diagnostic criteria for RBD (Table 1; *36*). PSG is not required for diagnosis of RBD by these criteria, but it is thought to be the gold standard to establish the diagnosis. REM without atonia is not sufficient to confirm diagnosis and must be accompanied by motor activation or vocalization to definitively diagnose RBD *(37)*. Inter-rater reliability for scoring REM sleep in PD has been shown to be high *(38)*. There is little data about the night-to-night variability of RBD, and false-negative studies certainly may be encountered, particularly with a single-night study. If there is a coexisting primary sleep disorder, such as obstructive sleep apnea (OSA) or periodic limb movement disorder (PLMD), the sleep disruption resulting from these disorders may trigger RBD episodes, necessitating treatment of these primary sleep disorders, which may improve coexistent RBD.

The differential diagnosis of a patient presenting with the history of acting out dreams includes sleepwalking and sleep terrors. These are non-REM parasomnias, which often occur during slow-wave sleep and are classified as arousal disorders by the ICSD. Additional diagnostic possibilities are seizure, rhythmic movement disorder, dissociative disorders, and malingering. As mentioned previously, movements associated with other primary sleep disorders, such as arousals associated with obstructive sleep apnea, arm and leg movements associated with periodic limb movement disorder, or seizure, can be ruled out by overnight PSG. These disorders may be the primary cause of motor activity during sleep, or a precipitating factor for RBD.

Eisensehr et al. conducted a retrospective analysis of PSG data while investigating the utility of specialized interviews for detecting RBD *(39)* and found that the specialized interviews had a low sensitivity of 33% for RBD patients with PD but a high specificity of 90%. In contrast, the sensitivity was 100% and specificity was 99.6% in non-PD subjects. They concluded that PSG was required to diagnose RBD in patients with PD, whereas interviews were sufficient for patients without PD. Gagnon et al. prospectively studied 33 subjects with PD and 16 control subjects, who each underwent a structured clinical interview followed by PSG. Of the PD patients 11 (33%) had RBD by PSG, but only half of these were detected by history. Only 1 of the 16 control subjects had RBD by PSG *(10)*.

Clinical interview alone does not appear to be sufficient to diagnose RBD in patients with PD. PSG should be performed to rule out other primary sleep disorders, such as OSA and PLMD, as well as to

Table 2
Medications Reported to Improve REM Sleep Behavior Disorder

Benzodiazepines
Clonazepam
Triazolam
Dopaminergic medications
Carbidopa/levodopa
Antiepileptic medications
Carbamazepine
Gabapentin
α Adrenergic agonists
Clonidine
Acetylcholinesterase inhibitors
Donepezil *(41)*
Others
Melatonin *(42)*

look for epileptiform activity on the EEG. Capturing an RBD episode during PSG validates the diagnosis. Even if there is no confirmation of an RBD episode, REM without atonia may be seen, and the disorders already mentioned can be eliminated if the study is normal.

7. TREATMENT

7.1. *Pharmacological Treatment*

Clonazepam has been shown to be effective in up to 90% of patients who tolerate this medication *(3–5)*, but no controlled clinical trials have been conducted to date. However, in some patients, the long half-life and sedating side effects of clonazepam may result in daytime sleepiness, confusion, or falls, and may worsen underlying OSA *(40)*. There are reports of triazolam improving RBD, but no evidence of other benzodiazepines as yet, although those with a shorter half-life than clonazepam could potentially have less troublesome daytime side effects. The efficacy of clonazepam may be a result of a serotonergic property not shared by other benzodiazepines. Studies in idiopathic RBD have shown that clonazepam decreases the visible motor activities of RBD occurring during sleep, but REM without atonia persists, as measured by EMG. This may indicate the presence of two different systems—one responsible for the actual motor activity of acting out of dreams and the other responsible for REM without atonia—as opposed to these being on a continuum of disease severity. Other medications used to treat RBD are listed in Table 2. Clonidine may be effective through its REM suppression effect. Fluoxetine and tricyclic antidepressants have been indicated to worsen RBD, despite that these classes of medications may also have a REM suppressing influence in some patients. Successful treatment of RBD with levodopa has been reported in patients who have PD. Melatonin has been reported to improve RBD in both idiopathic and symptomatic cases. PSG in some RBD patients treated with melatonin has shown restoration of REM without atonia. No large-scale, randomized studies comparing these various therapies currently exist that would assist in clinical decision-making regarding RBD treatment.

7.2. *Nonpharmacological Treatment*

Safety of the sleeping environment is of the utmost importance in this disorder. Given the severity of injuries that have been reported, securing the environment must be reinforced to patients with this disorder. This may include removing any potentially injurious furniture or other items from the area around the bed, or putting pillows or a mattress on the floor beside the bed if the patient falls out of the bed routinely.

Case presentation (continued): The patient was initially treated with 0.5 mg clonazepam at bedtime, which was subsequently titrated to 3 mg at bedtime without significant improvement. Carbidopa/levodopa was initiated, given his parkinsonian symptoms, but the patient discontinued this medication because of gastrointestinal upset. Clonidine was then tried and titrated up to 0.8 mg at bedtime, with dramatic improvement in the patient's presenting complaint of acting out his dreams.

8. CONCLUSION

RBD is present in many patients with PD and may be owing to the degenerative changes occurring with PD in brainstem structures crucial for generating REM sleep. Patients who have PD with hallucinations appear to have RBD more often than those without hallucinations, offering support to the theory that hallucinations are caused by a REM abnormality. Injury risk with this disorder is high, particularly because the elderly population is at higher risk for developing RBD. PSG should be performed to rule out other causes for motor activity during sleep. When tolerated, clonazepam treatment is highly effective. Patient safety can be improved by securing the sleeping environment to minimize the risk of injury in this disorder.

REFERENCES

1. Schenck CH, Bundlie SR, Ettinger MG, Mahowald MW. Chronic behavioral disorders of human REM sleep: a new category of parasomnia. Sleep 1986;9:293–308.
2. Boeve BF, Silber MH, Parisi JE, et al. Synucleinopathy pathology and REM sleep behavior disorder plus dementia or Parkinsonism. Neurology 2003;61:40–45.
3. Olson EJ, Boeve BF, Silber MH. Rapid eye movement sleep behavior disorder: demographic, clinical and laboratory findings in 93 cases. Brain 2000;123:331–339.
4. Schenck CH, Hurwitz TD, Mahowald MS. REM sleep behavior disorder: an update on a series of 96 patients and a review of the world literature. J Sleep Res 1993;2:224–231.
5. Sforza E, Krieger J, Petiau C. REM sleep behavior disorder: clinical and physiopathological findings. Sleep Med Rev 1997;1:57–69.
6. Boeve BF, Silber MH, Ferman TJ, et al. Association of REM sleep behavior disorder and neurodegenerative disease may reflect an underlying synuclienopathy. Mov Disord 2001;16:622–630.
7. Pajera J, Caminero A, Masa J, Dobato J. A first case of progressive supranuclear palsy and pre-clinical REM sleep behavior disorder presenting as inhibition of speech during wakefulness and somniloquy with phasic muscle twitching during REM sleep. Neurologia 1996;11:304–306.
8. Kimura K, Tachibana N, Toshihiko A, et al. Subclinical REM sleep behavior disorder in a patient with corticobasal degeneration. Sleep 1997;20:891.
9. Comella CL, Nardine TM, Diederich NJ. Sleep-related violence, injury, and REM sleep behavior disorder in Parkinson's disease. Neurology 1998;51:526–529.
10. Gagnon JF, Bedard MA, Fantini ML, et al. REM sleep behavior disorder and REM sleep without atonia in Parkinson's disease. Neurology 2002;59:585–589.
11. Wetter TC, Trenkwalder C, Gershanik O, Hogl B. Polysomnographic measures in Parkinson's disease: a comparison between patients with and without REM sleep disturbances. Wien Klin Wochenschr 2001;113:249–253.
12. Plazzi G, Corsini R, Provini F, et al. REM sleep behavior disorders in multiple system atrophy. Neurology 1997;48:1094–1097.
13. Boeve BF, Silber MH, Ferman TJ, et al. REM sleep behavior disorder and degenerative dementia: an association likely reflecting Lewy Body disease. Neurology 1998;51:363–370.
14. Schenck CH, Bundlie SR, Mahowald MW. Delayed emergence of a parkinsonian disorder in 38% of 29 older men initially diagnosed with idiopathic rapid eye movement sleep behavior disorder. Neurology 1996;46:388–393.
15. Tan A, Salgado M, Fahn S. Rapid eye movement sleep behavior disorder preceding Parkinson's disease with therapeutic response to levodopa. Mov Disord 1996;11:214–216.
16. Lai YY, Siegel JM. Physiological and anatomical link between Parkinson-like disease and REM sleep behavior disorder. Mol Neurobiol 2003;27:137–152.
17. Jouvet M. Paradoxical sleep—A study of its nature and mechanisms. Prog Brain Research 1965;18:867–870.
18. Jouvet M. Paradoxical sleep mechanisms. Sleep 1994;17:S77–S83.
19. Scarnati E, Florio T. The pedunculopontine nucleus and related structures. Adv Neurol 1997;74:97–110.

20. Pahapill PA, Lozano AM. The pedunculopontine nucleus and Parkinson's disease. Brain 2000;123:1767–1783.
21. Hirsch EC, Graybiel AM, Duyckaerts C, Javoy-Agid F. Neuronal loss in the pedunculopontine tegmental nucleus in Parkinson disease and in progressive supranuclear palsy. Proc Natl Acad Sci USA 1987;84:5976–5980.
22. Gai WP, Halliday GM, Blumbergs PC, et al. Substance P-containing neurons in the mesopontine tegmentum are severely affected in Parkinson's disease. Brain 1991;114:2253–2267.
23. Turner RS, D'Amato CJ, Chervin RD, Blaivas M. The pathology of REM sleep behavior disorder with comorbid Lewy body dementia. Neurology 2000;55:1730–1732.
24. Uchiyama M, Isse K, Tanaka K, et al. Incidental Lewy body disease in a patient with REM sleep behavior disorder. Neurology 1995;45:709–712.
25. Factor SA, McAlarney T, Sanchez-Ramos JR, Weiner WJ. Sleep disorders and sleep effect in Parkinson's disease. Mov Disord 1990;5:280–285.
26. Culebras A, Moore JT. Magnetic resonance findings in REM sleep behavior disorder. Neurology 1989;39:1519–1523.
27. Irazano A, Santamaria J, Pujol J, et al. Brainstem proton magnetic resonance spectroscopy in idiopathic REM sleep behavior disorder. Sleep 2002;25:867–870.
28. Albin RL, Koeppe A, Chervin RD, et al. Decreased striatal dopaminergic innervation in REM sleep behavior disorder. Neurology 2000;55:1410–1412.
29. Gilman S, Koeppe A, Chervin RD, et al. REM sleep behavior disorder is related to striatal monoaminergic deficit in MSA. Neurology 2003;61:29–34.
30. Eisensehr I, Linke R, Noachtar S, et al. Reduced striatal dopamine transporters in idiopathic rapid eye movement sleep behavior disorder: comparison with Parkinson's disease and controls. Brain 2000;123:1155–1160.
31. Eisensehr I, Linke R, Tatsch K, et al. Increased muscle activity during rapid eye movement sleep correlates with decrease of striatal presynaptic dopamine transporters. IPT and IBZM SPECT imaging in subclinical and clinically manifest idiopathic REM sleep behavior disorder, Parkinson's disease, and controls. Sleep 2003;26:507–512.
32. Comella CL, Tanner CM, Ristanovic RK. Polysomnographic sleep measures in Parkinson's disease patients with treatment-induced hallucinations. Ann Neurol 1993;34:710–714.
33. Arnulf I, Bonnet AM, Damier P, et al. Hallucinations, REM sleep and Parkinson's disease. Neurology 2000;55:281–288.
34. Nomura T, Inoue Y, Mitani H, et al. Visual hallucinations as REM sleep behavior disorder in patients with Parkinson's disease. Mov Disord 2003;18:812–817.
35. Onofrj M, Thomas A, D'Andreamatteo G, et al. Incidence of RBD and hallucination in patients affected by Parkinson's disease: 8-year follow-up. Neurol Sci 2002;23(Suppl 2):S91–S94.
36. American Sleep Disorders Association. The International Classification of Sleep Disorders. Diagnostic and Coding Manual (Revised). American Sleep Disorders Association, Rochester, MN, 1997.
37. Lapierre O, Montplaisir J. Polysomnographic features of REM sleep behavior disorder: development of a scoring method. Neurology 1992;42(Suppl 6):44–51.
38. Bliwise DL, Williams ML, Irbe D, et al. Inter-rater reliability for identification of REM sleep in Parkinson's disease. Sleep 2000;23:671–676.
39. Eisensehr I, v Lindeiner H, Jager M, Noachtar S. REM sleep behavior disorder in sleep-disordered patients with versus without Parkinson's disease: is there a need for polysomnography? J Neurol Sci 2001;186:7–11.
40. Woods JH, Winger G. Current benzodiazepine issues. Psychopharmacology 1995;118:107–115.
41. Ringman JM, Simmons JH. Treatment of REM sleep behavior disorder with donepezil: a report of three cases. Neurology 2000;55:870–871.
42. Boeve BF, Silber MH, Ferman TJ. Melatonin for treatment of REM sleep behavior disorder in neurologic disorders: results in 14 patients. Sleep Med 2003;4:281–284.

17

Excessive Daytime Sleepiness

David E. Hardesty, Daryl Victor, and Steven J. Frucht

SUMMARY

Excessive daytime sleepiness (EDS) is common in patients with Parkinson's disease (PD) and can lead to serious medical consequences, including depression, cognitive impairment, and death or injury from sleep-related accidents. It can also have a deleterious impact on social functions such as work and marriage. To successfully prevent or remedy such negative outcomes, it is important to periodically screen PD patients for EDS. The Epworth Sleepiness Scale (ESS), which can be completed in about 5 minutes, is a reasonable screening tool when used in conjunction with a focused history. When EDS is present, assessment of safety is a priority, and recommendations should be clearly stated to the patient. Next, an underlying cause of EDS can often be identified. Obstructive sleep apnea (OSA) is a common and treatable cause of EDS in the general population. Patients with PD are also at increased risk for other sleep disorders that cause EDS, such as rapid eye movement (REM), sleep behavioral disorder, and insomnia. PD symptoms can directly cause EDS by dramatically reducing sleep quality. PD treatment can cause EDS directly, or cause hallucinations and dyskinesias that similarly interfere with sleep. Furthermore, medications that reduce these side effects also cause somnolence. Finally, the underlying pathophysiology of PD also appears to directly cause EDS. Polysomnography may be needed to clarify the etiology of EDS, but often history and physical examination can lead to correct diagnosis and specific treatment. When no cause can be found, or treatment is unsuccessful, it may be appropriate to treat patients with wakefulness-promoting agents. Our goal is to provide the clinician with a rational, flexible, and cost-effective approach to evaluate and manage EDS in patients with PD. Sleep attacks and driving are additional issues that we discuss at the end of this chapter

Key Words: Parkinson's disease (PD); excessive daytime sleepiness (EDS); somnolence; hypersomnolence; Epworth Sleepiness Scale; polysomnography, sleep attacks.

1. INTRODUCTION

Sleepiness, or somnolence, describes the state in which there is "an inclination to sleep" *(1)*, referring either to the subjective experience of impending sleep or to an objective and often measurable increased propensity to fall asleep. Definitions of excessive daytime sleepiness (EDS) vary *(2,3)*. Clinically, we define EDS as an increased propensity to fall asleep (with or without subjective sleepiness) that is having a significant impact or posing significant threat to the quality of life of the patient. Standardized tools, such as the Epworth Sleepiness Scale (ESS), provide quantitative estimates of EDS that can assist in making this clinical determination.

EDS is common. In the general population of older adults (55–84 years old), 15% report EDS that interferes with daily activities at least several days a week, and 4% report falling asleep while driving. Although problematic, this is less than the 20% of younger adults (18- to 54-year-olds) who report falling asleep while driving, a statistic that is somewhat surprising. *(4)*. EDS is even more common in neurological disorders, including narcolepsy, multiple sclerosis, dementia, and Parkinson's disease

From: *Current Clinical Neurology*
Parkinson's Disease and Nonmotor Dysfunction
Edited by: R. F. Pfeiffer and I. Bodis-Wollner © Humana Press Inc., Totowa, NJ

(PD). Moderate-to-severe sleepiness is seen in 15.5% of patients with PD compared to 1% of healthy elderly controls and 4% of diabetics *(5)*. Once EDS develops in patients with PD, it often persists, and as many as 6% of patients with PD develop EDS each year *(6)*.

2. MECHANISMS

Primary EDS in PD is the result of damage and adaptation of various critical neurotransmitter systems that modulate sleep and wakefulness, including the dopaminergic system. States of dopamine (DA) deficiency and excess can both cause EDS, depending on the circuitry being modulated. Rats with selectively damaged nigrostriatal pathways develop hypersomnolence *(7)*. Non-human primate models of PD can develop hypersomnolence that reverses with treatment of levodopa and bupropion *(8)*. Medications that deplete or block DA also commonly cause sedation. *(9)*. Furthermore, studies using specific DA reuptake inhibitors have shown that blockade of DA reuptake and/or stimulation of DA release in specific brain regions may mediate the wakefulness-promoting effect of central nervous system stimulants *(10)*. It might seem paradoxical, then, that drugs that increase dopaminergic activity also cause somnolence. However, this side effect is well established, *(11,12)* and may be mediated by agonist activity at the D2 receptor *(10,13)*.

Further complicating the matter, extra-striatal pathology in PD may also contribute to EDS. This point is supported by clinical studies that have found that EDS does *not* correlate with motor scores *(9,14–16)*. Abnormal wakefulness in PD may be the result of pathology in the dorsal raphe nucleus, the locus ceruleus, or the pedunculopontine nucleus, which promotes thalamocortical arousal and REM sleep *(9,17)*.

In summary, the mechanisms that underlie primary and medication-induced EDS in PD are complex. It is important for the clinician to be aware that both PD and the medications used to treat it may cause somnolence, often through mechanisms that are not currently well defined.

3. EVALUATION OF EDS

3.1. History

For various reasons, even patients with severe EDS often neglect to bring it to their physicians' attention. Furthermore, some patients without subjective drowsiness fall asleep inappropriately. As a result, all PD patients should be periodically screened for symptoms of EDS, particularly after medication adjustments. Probably the best approach is to ask the patient directly about EDS, and to supplement this focused history by asking the patient to complete the ESS, as discussed in Subheading 3.3. We often ask "Is being tired or sleepy ever a problem for you?"; "Do you fall asleep in inappropriate situations?"; or "Do others notice that you fall asleep easily?" Spouses or caregivers often provide critical details, and should be invited to participate in the interview whenever possible.

Subjective sleepiness in the absence of an increased propensity to fall asleep may be more consistent with mental fatigue, defined as the "sensation of boredom and lassitude owing to absence of stimulation, monotony, or lack of interest in one's surroundings," and characterized by a lack of energy or motivation. *(3)*. In such circumstances, exploring medical and psychiatric conditions, particularly depression, is warranted. Alternatively, an increased propensity to fall asleep with or without the sensation of sleepiness is more consistent with EDS.

Once EDS is found, the clinician should assess safety and make appropriate recommendations, including (but not limited to) driving restrictions. In the United States particularly, the entire assessment and plan should be clearly documented for legal protection. To determine the etiology of the EDS, the time course over which it developed may provide useful clues. It is not uncommon for sleepiness to emerge with the initiation or escalation of DA agonists or levodopa *(18,19)*. When this association is clear and the patient is being treated with a DA agonist, it is reasonable to reduce the dose, switch to a different DA agonist, or eliminate the drug altogether. When somnolence does occur with levodopa, it usually resolves shortly after the dose is taken, and it rarely limits treatment. Higher doses of levodopa were actually associated with *decreased* somnolence in a fairly large prospective study *(16)*.

Subacute or acute development of EDS in the absence of medication change suggests encephalopathy, and this should focus the history on likely etiologies, such as falls (subdural hematoma), infection, and dehydration.

Sleep hygiene should also be assessed early on, and when markedly abnormal, may be the sole etiology for EDS. In such circumstances, it is appropriate to normalize sleep hygiene before embarking on further work-up, provided close follow-up can be achieved. Assessment of sleep hygiene can also reveal an underlying insomnia.

We next determine if excessive sleep time (hypersomnolence) is present. In some individuals, this presents as increased sleep requirement despite relatively normal sleep times. In the presence of hypersomnia, the clinician must consider a sleep-related breathing disorder (SRBD; *see* Chapter 18). Witnessed apneas, snoring, and large neck size are clearly established risk factors. Other clues to the diagnosis include hypertension, congestive heart failure, hypothyroidism, impotence, morning headaches, recent weight gain, and increased alcohol consumption. Stridorous breathing, which occurs commonly in multiple system atrophy (MSA), may also manifest as a change in snoring pattern, and such patients should be followed very closely. Medications and alcohol can also cause hypersomnolence. Other sleep disorders that cause hypersomnolence include REM sleep behavior disorder (RBD; *see* Chapter 16) and periodic limb movements of sleep (PLMS). Often in these disorders the patient is unaware of problems during sleep, and the history must be obtained from a bed partner. When hypersomnolence is absent, the aforementioned causes of EDS are still in the differential diagnosis, but are less likely. The remainder of the history should focus on the problems listed in Table1 or other issues that seem to be relevant.

3.2. *Physical Exam and Ancillary Tests*

A focused physical exam may be helpful in evaluating patients with EDS. Obesity is a tip-off for a SRBD, although 10% of those afflicted have a normal body mass index. A large-neck circumference and craniofacial abnormalities (e.g., micrognathia) also suggests the diagnosis. Lethargy indicates an underlying encephalopathy. Focal neurological findings may warrant neuroimaging to rule out other neurological processes, such as subdural hematoma or mass. Laboratory tests for EDS should be considered, particularly when the onset is subacute or acute. Thyroid function tests, complete blood count, serum electrolytes and glucose, erythrocyte sedimentation rate, ammonia, and liver function tests may be appropriate to screen for medical etiologies. An iron profile and renal function should be ordered in patients with restless legs syndrome (RLS)/PLMS. When a narcolepsy phenotype is present *with* cataplexy, blood can be sent to determine whether or not the human leukocyte antigen HLA DQB1*0602 is present. The absence of HLA DQB1*0602 dramatically decreases the likelihood of narcolepsy in such individuals *(3)*. The narcolepsy phenotype without cataplexy is common in PD, and HLA testing is rarely necessary.

3.3. *Sleep Testing*

There are several tests available to quantify sleepiness and diagnose sleep disorders. We briefly discuss four of them here: the ESS, polysomnography (PSG), the Multiple Sleep Latency Test (MSLT), and the Maintenance of Wakefulness Test (MWT). The ESS is a quick and useful questionnaire that quantifies an individual's propensity to fall asleep *(20)*. The respondent is asked to rate the chance of dozing in eight situations on a 4-point scale, where 0 represents a situation in which the respondent "would never doze," and 3 represents a "high chance of dozing." The cumulative score ranges from 0 to 24. Normal range for individuals aged 22 to 59 years without sleep disorders (by screening questionnaires) is from 0 to 10 (mean = 2.8 +/– 3.8 standard deviation; *21*). The ESS is easy to use, low in cost, and reliably detects patients with a severely increased propensity to fall asleep.

Table 1 Excessive Daytime Sleepiness

Cause of EDS common to general population
Poor sleep hygiene
Sleep-related breathing disorder
RLS
PLMS
Narcolepsy
Insomnia
Circadian rhythm disturbance
Use of certain medications, alcohol, illicit drugs
PD-specific causes of EDS
Use of medications to treat PD
Virtually any medication can cause EDS, including MAOIs. DA agonists are particularly problematic.
Sleep disorders
RBD
Owing to symptoms of PD or "Wearing Off"
Tremor, rigidity (inability to turn in bed, shoulder pain), dystonia, nocturia, central pain, sweating, etc.
Because of PD treatment/overdose effects
Nightmares, hallucinations, dyskinesias.
Other
DID dyskinesias/dystonia
akathsia
Directly owing to underlying pathology of PD

[a]RLS/PLMs may be more common in PD.

[b]A narcolepsy phenotype without cataplexy also occurs in PD, which often resolves with medication adjustment.

[c]See Chapter 15.

EDS, excessive daytime sleepiness; RLS, restless legs syndrome; PLMS, periodic limb movements of sleep; PD, Parkinson's disease; MAOIs, monoamine oxidase inhibitors; DA, dopamine; RBD, rapid eye movement behavior disorder; DID, drug-induced dyskinesias.

Both narcoleptics and subjects with obstructive sleep apnea have higher average scores on the ESS, and scores decrease with effective interventions. The ESS has several weaknesses that should be acknowledged. It is dependent on the subject's recollection of sleepiness in the recent past, which may be inaccurate. Furthermore, the respondent may have to estimate the likelihood of falling asleep in situations not regularly experienced. Even with accurate reporting, the ESS is only sensitive in detecting marked somnolence *(22)*. However, it is still a useful tool, and helps greatly to supplement the history as a screen for EDS.

Overnight PSG is the diagnostic test of choice for the evaluation of most sleep disorders. While the patient sleeps, simultaneous recordings are obtained from electroencephalogram, submental electromyogram (EMG), electro-oculogram (EOG), electrocardiographic tracings, limb movement (via anterior tibial EMG), body position, oxygen saturation, respiratory effort and airflow. Other monitoring devices used in conjunction with PSG include infrared videorecorders, microphones (to capture snoring), and esophageal pH probes. In the patient who has PD with EDS, PSG may identify treatable disorders that are not obvious by history. Most of the disorders discussed in this chapter can be diagnosed by PSG. The sensitivity of PSG for each disorder varies, and the test may miss the diagnosis in a patient with intermittent events *(21)*. The test is further limited by cost and availability of resources. Some patients also find it difficult to sleep in the sleep laboratory setting. Regardless, the test can provide extremely valuable information and is critical to the diagnosis of many sleep disorders. Repeat PSG may be necessary to monitor response to treatment.

We recommend PSG for the evaluation of suspected SRBD, PLMS, RBD (if there is a need to substantiate the diagnosis), and for significant EDS of unknown etiology that does not improve with routine measures. When sleep apnea is suspected, but PSG is not available, portable monitoring with oximetry may be the next best option, but this method is much less sensitive. When nocturnal stridor is suspected, PSG should be ordered urgently.

The MSLT quantifies sleepiness and is utilized primarily in the diagnosis of narcolepsy. The test should be performed the day after overnight PSG to ensure adequate pretest sleep. During five 20-minute sessions that are spread out at 2-hour intervals, the patient tries to fall asleep in a dark, comfortable room while being monitored in the sleep laboratory. The combination of REM sleep and reduced sleep latency suggests narcolepsy *(21)*. However, similar results can occur with sleep deprivation and various medications, and is not uncommon in PD, which limits the usefulness of this test in PD.

The MWT is similar to the MSLT, but the subject is asked to remain awake, not sleep, and is placed in a somewhat less soporific situation (a dimly lit room, sitting supported by pillows). This test is not commonly used in clinical practice, and results may not predict behavior in daily life *(21)*.

4. CAUSES AND MANAGEMENT OF EDS

4.1. Common or Important Causes of EDS in All Patients

4.1.1. Poor Sleep Hygiene

Poor sleep hygiene can result from insufficient time for sleep, poor sleep environment, poor sleep habits, caffeine, alcohol, or use of prescribed or over-the-counter medications. Normalizing sleep requires patient education, and although this can be time consuming, it is often critical to success. When good sleep hygiene is accomplished, the patient associates easily achieved sleep with a regular sleep location and time. Simple recommendations include establishing regular times for waking up and going to bed, regular exercise (but not for several hours prior to sleep), and avoidance of caffeine, alcohol, and lying in bed when not sleepy.

4.1.2. Sleep-Related Breathing Disorders

Obstructive sleep apnea (OSA), central sleep apnea, and upper airway resistance syndrome are common in the general population, particularly among men. They are important to identify because they are treatable and can otherwise have adverse systemic health consequences. Moderate to severe OSA occurs in approximately 20% of patients who have PD with EDS *(16)*. SRBDs are discussed in detail in Chapter 18, and are mentioned only briefly here. History and physical examination, as previously discussed, determine the risk factors for OSA. Definitive diagnosis is made by PSG.

Conservative treatment consists of weight loss, the use of a lateral sleep position, and avoidance of sedatives and alcohol *(23)*. When treatment is necessary, continuous positive airway pressure (CPAP) is the preferred treatment. If CPAP is not tolerated and OSA is not severe, dental appliances are a reasonable alternative. Otherwise, surgery may be the best option. Treatment of sleep apnea has been shown to improve quality of life, mood, alertness, and the risk of automobile accidents. CPAP has been shown to improve hypertension and cardiac ejection fraction in patients with congestive heart failure *(23)*.

4.1.3. Restless Legs Syndrome and Periodic Limb Movements of Sleep

RLS leads to sleep loss and fragmentation and is often associated with EDS. RLS has a prevalence in the normal adult population of between 2.5% and 15% *(24)*. It is not yet clear if PD increases risk for RLS, and most estimates place the prevalence near the upper border of this range. In RLS, uncomfortable sensations manifest in the legs, particularly at night, and are alleviated by pacing. Differentiating RLS from "off" sensory phenomena may be difficult, if not impossible to do. The presence of a family history of RLS and/or symptoms that predated levodopa-induced fluctuations suggests that RLS may be present. Once RLS is suspected, consider potential etiologies and order appropriate lab tests (*see* Subheading 3.2). Medications that frequently precipitate RLS include antidepressants (tricyclic antidepressants [TCAs], monoamine oxidase inhibitors [MAOIs], selective serotonin reuptake inhibitors, and venlafaxine), lithium, antihistamines, and antipsychotics. When feasible, these medications should be adjusted, switched with alternative therapies, or discontinued. Iron replacement therapy may help patients who have an iron deficiency *(24),* although the effect of iron replacement for RLS in PD is not clear. Pharmacotherapy with DA agonists is often an effective treatment for RLS. However, in PD, RLS often presents in a patient already on a DA agonist, or in a patient who cannot tolerate them, particularly at night. Alternative treatments include opiates, benzodiazepines, gabapentin, and carbamazepine *(25.)* Rebound and augmentation may occur with any treatment, and symptoms may need to be treated during the waking hours.

PLMS is an associated disorder in which involuntary leg movements lasting 4 to 5 seconds occur during sleep. Movements occur at regular intervals of about 20 seconds, and can be unilateral or bilateral. Very often, RLS coexists with PLMS. When PLMS is present without RLS, the clinician should reconsider the possibility of a SRBD or medication-induced PLMS *(26).* PSG will quantify the severity of PLMS, and also helps to negate the possibility of an underlying SRBD, although it is not necessary prior to treatment in all cases. PLMS typically responds to the same pharmacological interventions as RLS *(27).* However, anticonvulsants vary in their effect. For instance, carbamazepine helps RLS but not PLMS, and lamotrigine and valproate are more potent at controlling PLMS.

4.1.4. Narcolepsy

Symptoms of narcolepsy usually begin before middle age, although it is not uncommon for the diagnosis to be missed for decades. Therefore, narcolepsy should be considered in a patient with PD when symptoms of the disorder presented early in life. Narcolepsy is characterized by EDS and/or an irresistible urge to sleep, cataplexy, hypnagogic and/or hypnopompic hallucinations, and sleep paralysis, although it is rare for patients to have all symptoms. Narcolepsy can be familial, and is often associated with deficient levels of hypocretin.

Although narcolepsy is not particularly common, patients with PD often develop a narcolepsy-like syndrome. Out of 54 consecutive PD patients with EDS treated with levodopa, 50% had pathological sleepiness and 39% had early onset REM sleep (determined by MSLT) that is typical of narcolepsy *(16).* However, such patients have normal levels of cerebrospinal fluid (CSF) hypocretin-1 *(28).* Furthermore, patients with PD do not usually have cataplexy. This presentation in PD is often associated with dopaminergic medications, particularly DA agonists, and medication adjustment usually alleviates symptoms. Otherwise, patients can be treated with wakefulness-promoting agents.

When cataplexy is present, narcolepsy should be considered. HLA-DQB1*0602 is present in 93% of narcolepsy patients with cataplexy versus 17% of controls *(29).* Therefore, it is reasonable to send blood for the presence of this antigen in these patients. When absent, it effectively rules out narcolepsy. However, if present, the diagnosis remains uncertain. Measurement of CSF hypocretin-1 levels in such rare cases may be reasonable. Narcolepsy is usually treated with wakefulness-promoting agents, such as modafinil or methylphenidate.*(30)* Cataplexy may be treated with γ-hydroxy-butyrate (GHB) or norepinephrine reuptake inhibitors such as venlafaxine.

4.1.5. Circadian Rhythm Disorders

Disruptions of circadian rhythm represent another treatable form of EDS. Diagnosis should be considered when a patient has a long history of going to sleep at an unusually early or late hour. Light therapy or melatonin may provide significant relief.

4.1.6. Insomnia

Insomnia is particularly problematic in PD, can be very difficult to treat, and may result in EDS. Chapter 15 discusses this in detail.

4.2 PD Specific Causes of EDS

4.2.1. REM Sleep Behavior Disorder

RBD was discussed in detail in the preceding chapter, so it is only mentioned briefly here. RBD is characterized by the loss of normal muscle paralysis during REM sleep, which leads to the enactment of dreams *(31)*. It is seen with a variety of neurological conditions, including PD, and it frequently causes EDS *(32)*. In fact, Olson found that 63% of all patients with RBD had complaints of EDS. Clonazepam is generally an effective treatment. Because RBD is often associated with other sleep disorders, PSG may be required when EDS does not resolve with treatment.

4.2.2. Nightmares, Vivid Dreams, and Hallucinations

Hallucinations and psychosis in PD frequently disrupt sleep and cause EDS. Medications are the usual culprit, although encephalopathy must also be considered. Management of these symptoms are discussed in detail in Chapter 5. Unfortunately, both quetiapine and clozapine also frequently cause EDS. Promoting wakefulness in the morning hours with caffeine, modafinil, or stimulants is sometimes needed, although hallucinations may worsen.

4.2.3. Dyskinesias

When severe, dyskinesias can prevent sleep and cause EDS. They often occur late in the day as the doses of dopaminergic medication accumulate, particularly with extended-release levodopa. In such cases, lowering the overall dose, avoiding nighttime doses, and switching to regular carbidopa/levodopa may resolve the issue. Later doses of entacapone may also be stopped. Amantadine may help reduce dyskinesia severity, but can lead to other complications with sleep. Diphasic dyskinesias can also develop at night, and often respond well to a nighttime dose of an extended-release carbidopa/levodopa.

4.2.4. "Off" Phenomena and Insufficient Treatment of PD Symptoms

Motor and sensory symptoms can interfere with sleep when anti-Parkinsonian agents are no longer sufficient or when wearing off occurs at night. Tremor, inability to turn in bed, pain, sweating, and dystonia often lead to sleep fragmentation. Extended-release levodopa preparations given at bedtime can help alleviate these problems. Anti-cholinergic agents, when tolerable, can reduce frequent awakenings from nocturia and dystonia.

5. "SLEEP ATTACKS" AND DRIVING

In 1999, Frucht and colleagues described eight patients taking pramipexole who had sudden episodes of sleep while driving. Since then, there have been numerous reports of "sleep attacks" with ergot and non-ergot DA agonists, as well as levodopa *(11,12,18)*, sometimes occurring without warning. EEG in one such patient documented a normal background of wakefulness despite a sleep latency of less than 1 minute *(33)*. Sleep episodes may be more common in men and in patients with dysautonomia *(34,35)*.

So how common are "sleep attacks," and can they be predicted? The Canadian Movement Disorder Group *surveyed* 420 nondemented PD patients who continued to drive, and found that of those with EDS (remarkably, 51%), 16 (3.8%) reported sudden-onset sleep episodes while driving *(36)*. Three reported no warning. Unfortunately, data was not collected from a control group. An ESS score greater than 7 predicted 75% of sleep episodes, but this score is well within the normal range, and therefore lacks specificity. A score of 1 on the Inappropriate Sleep Composite Score, which was introduced in this study, had a sensitivity of 52% and a specificity of 82%. Of note, the Canadian Movement Disorder Group did *not* find an increased risk of sleep-related accidents or excessive sleepiness in those taking DA agonists. One problem with the study is that PD patients (with EDS) may not recognize when they have fallen asleep, and in fact do so less often than patients with other sleep disorders (primary hypersomnia and sleep apnea), even with longer nap times during MSLT *(37)*. Furthermore, patients who misperceive falling asleep tend to have lower ESS scores, which underscores the need for a different screening instrument for detecting "sleep attacks."

Regardless of EDS, driving is impaired in PD, in part because of slower reaction times *(38)*. Patients with PD also have an increased frequency of collisions during driving simulation *(39)*. Furthermore, neurologists, unlike driving instructors and psychiatrists, may overestimate the ability of patients with PD to drive *(40)*.

How, then, does one decide on a driving recommendation? Unfortunately, there are no guidelines to determine which patients with PD are safe to drive, and predicting who is at risk for falling asleep while driving is difficult. Although sudden-onset sleep episodes are frequent enough to warrant serious concern, the true risk for such spells or related accidents in PD is not known. Furthermore, the impact of medications, particularly DA agonists and levodopa, remains controversial. Until these questions are answered, the clinician must remain vigilant to detect those who appear to be at high risk. In some cases, such as when there is a recent history of a sleep attack or when there is prominent EDS, driving restrictions are appropriate. For patients with a sufficiently long and mild warning, it may be reasonable to recommend extreme caution while driving and to discourage long drives and traveling alone. When an episode only occurs shortly after a dose of medicine, the timing of the dose may sometimes be changed to accommodate to the patient's schedule. Those receiving high-dose DA agonist therapy should also be extremely cautious, particularly during dose escalation. Finally, all driving patients should probably be educated about "sleep attacks," including the rare possibility of experiencing one without warning. Doing so may help the patient to identify the problem before it occurs while driving.

6. CONCLUSION

EDS is common, particularly in patients with PD, and screening for it helps to ensure patient safety and improve quality of life. The ESS provides a quantitative estimate of EDS and, when used in conjunction with a focused history, is the best screening instrument available. When EDS is present it is important to assess safety and minimize risks, which sometimes means driving restrictions. A good sleep history and examination often leads to an accurate diagnosis. In some cases, PSG may be required, particularly when an SRBD is suspected. Management of sleep hygiene and adjustment of medications may be sufficient for treatment in select patients. Otherwise, targeted therapies are usually available, depending on the underlying cause of EDS. When no cause can be identified, or treatment is unsuccessful, relief may be provided with wakefulness-promoting medications.

REFERENCES

1. Steadman's Medical Dictionary, 27th ed. Lippincott Williams and Wilkins, Philadelphia, PA, 2000.
2. Fabbrini G, Barbanti P, Aurilia C, et al. Excessive daytime sleepiness in de novo and treated Parkinson's disease. Mov Disord 2002;17:1026–1030.
3. Johns MW. Sensitivity and specificity of the multiple sleep latency test (MSLT), the maintenance of wakefulness test and the Epworth sleepiness scale: failure of the MSLT as a gold standard. J Sleep Res 2000;9:5–11.
4. National Sleep Foundation and WB&A Market Research. 2003 Sleep in America Poll – Executive Summary. 2004.
5. Tandberg E. Excessive daytime sleepiness and sleep benefit in Parkinson's disease; a community-based study. Mov Disord 1999;14:922–927.
6. Gjerstad MD, Aarsland D, Larsen JP. Development of daytime somnolence over time in Parkinson's disease. Neurology 2002;58:1544–1546.
7. Decker M, et al. Parkinsonian-like sleep-wake architecture in rats with bilateral striatal 6-OHDA lesions. Soc. Neurosci. Abstr. 2000;26:p1514.
8. Daley J, Turner RS, Bliwise DL, Rye DB. Nocturnal sleep and daytime alertness in the MPTP-treated primate. Sleep 1999;22:S218–S219.

9. Rye D, Jankovic J. Emerging views of dopamine in modulating sleep/wake state from an unlikely source: PD. Neurology 2002;58:341–346.
10. Wisor JP, Nishino S, Sora I, et al. Dopaminergic role in stimulant-induced wakefulness. J Neurosci 2001;21:1787–1794.
11. Frucht S, Rogers JD, Greene PE, et al. Falling asleep at the wheel: motor vehicle mishaps in persons taking pramipexole and ropinirole. Neurology 1999;52:1908–1910.
12. Ferreira JJ, Galitsky M, Montastruc JL, Rascol O. Sleep attacks and Parkinson's disease treatment. Lancet 2000;355:1333–1334.
13. Ferreira JJ, Galitzky M, Thalamas C, et al. Effect of ropinirole on sleep onset: a randomized, placebo-controlled study in healthy volunteers. Neurology 2002;58:460–462.
14. Rye D, Bliwise D, Dihenia B, Gurecki P. Daytime sleepiness in Parkinson's disease. J Sleep Res 2000;9:63–69.
15. Hauser RA, Gauger L, Anderson WM, Zesiewicz TA. Pramipexole-induced somnolence and episodes of daytime sleep. Mov Disord 2000;15:658–663.
16. Arnulf I, Konofal E, Merino-Andreu M, et al. Parkinson's disease and sleepiness: an integral part of PD. Neurology 2002;58:1019–1024.
17. Pal PK, Calne S, Samii A, Fleming JAE. A review of normal sleep and its disturbances in Parkinson's disease. Parkinsonism Relat Disord 1999;5:1–17.
18. Schapira AHV. Sleep attacks (sleep episodes) with pergolide. Lancet 2000;355:1331–1332.
19. Tan EK, Lum SY, Fook-Chong SM, et al. Evaluation of somnolence in Parkinson's disease: comparison with age- and sex-matched controls. Neurology 2002;58:465–468.
20. Johns MW. A new method for measuring daytime sleepiness: the Epworth sleepiness scale. Sleep 1991;14:540–545.
21. Johns M, Hocking B. Daytime sleepiness and sleep habits of Australian workers. Sleep 1997;20:844–849.
22. Sangal RB, Mitler MM, Sangal JM. Subjective sleepiness ratings (Epworth sleepiness scale) do not reflect the same parameter of sleepiness as objective sleepiness (maintenance of wakefulness test) in patients with narcolepsy. Clin Neurophysiol 1999;110:2131–2135.
23. Flemons WW. Clinical practice. Obstructive sleep apnea. N Engl J Med 2002;347:498–504.
24. Allen RP, Earley CJ. Restless legs syndrome: a review of clinical and pathophysiologic features. J Clin Neurophysiol 2001;18:128–147.
25. Earley CJ. Clinical practice. Restless legs syndrome. N Engl J Med 2003;348:2103–2109.
26. Tan EK, Lum SY,Wong MC. Restless legs syndrome in Parkinson's disease. J Neurol Sci 2002;196:33–36.
27. Chesson AL Jr, Wise M, Davila D, et al. Practice parameters for the treatment of restless legs syndrome and periodic limb movement disorder. An American Academy of Sleep Medicine report. Standards of Practice Committee of the American Academy of Sleep Medicine. Sleep 1999;22:961–968.
28. Overeem S, van Hilten JJ, Ripley B, et al. Normal hypocretin-1 levels in Parkinson's disease patients with excessive daytime sleepiness. Neurology 2002;58:498–499.
29. Overeem S, Mignot E, van Dijk JG, Lammers GJ. Narcolepsy: clinical features, new pathophysiologic insights, and future perspectives. J Clin Neurophysiol 2000;18:78–105.
30. Hogl B, Saletu M, Brandauer E, et al. Modafinil for the treatment of daytime sleepiness in Parkinson's disease: a double-blind, randomized, crossover, placebo-controlled polygraphic trial. Sleep 2002:25:905–909.
31. Mahowald MW, Schenck C. REM sleep disorder. In: Kryger M, Roth T, Dement W, eds. Principles and Practice in Sleep Medicine, 2nd ed. WB Saunders, Philadelphia, PA, 1994.
32. Olson EJ, Boeve BF, Silber MH. Rapid eye movement sleep behaviour disorder: demographic, clinical and laboratory findings in 93 cases. Brain 2000;123:331–339.
33. Hoehn MM. Falling asleep at the wheel: motor vehicle mishaps in people taking pramipexole and ropinirole. Neurology 2000;54:275.
34. Montastruc JL, Brefel-Courbon C, Senard JM, et al. Sudden sleep attacks and antiparkinsonian drugs: a pilot prospective pharmacoepidemiological study. Mov Disord 2000;15:130.
35. Montastruc JL, Brefel-Courbon C, Senard JM, et al. Sleep attacks and antiparkinsonian drugs: a pilot prospective pharmacoepidemiological study. Clin Neuropharmacol 2001;24:181–183.
36. Hobson DE, Lang AE, Martin WR, Razmy A, Rive J, Fleming J. Excessive daytime sleepiness and sudden onset sleep in Parkinson's disease: a survey by the Canadian Movement Disorders Group. JAMA 2002;287:455–463.
37. Merino-Andreu M, Arnulf I, Konofal E, et al. Unawareness of naps in Parkinson's disease and in disorders with excessive daytime sleepiness. Neurology 2003;60:1553–1554.
38. Lings S, Dupont E. Driving with Parkinson's disease. A controlled laboratory investigation. Acta Neurol Scand 1992;86:33–39.
39. Zesiewicz TA, Cimino CR, Malek AR, et al. Driving safety in Parkinson's disease. Neurology 2002;59:1787–1788.
40. Heikkila VM, Turkka J, Korpelainen J, et al. Decreased driving ability in people with Parkinson's disease. J Neurol Neurosurg Psychiatry 1998;64:325–330.

18
Sleep Apnea

Cheryl M. Carlucci and Robert A. Hauser

SUMMARY

Two types of sleep apnea have been identified: obstructive sleep apnea (OSA) and central sleep apnea (CSA). OSA occurs when the upper airway collapses; in OSA, there is no airflow, often despite great respiratory effort. In CSA, the transitory cessations of breathing are because of a drop in respiratory capacity—there is no airflow and no respiratory effort. Excessive daytime sleepiness is a consequence of both OSA and CSA. A comprehensive history, ideally obtained from both the patient and bed partner, is the essential first step in diagnosing sleep apnea, but the gold standard for assessing sleep apnea is the polysomnogram. Sleep apnea has not been extensively evaluated in the setting of Parkinson's disease (PD), but recent studies have suggested that OSA may be more common in PD than in age- and sex-matched controls, and obesity may not be as important a risk factor for OSA in PD as it is in the general population.

Key Words: Obstructive sleep apnea; central sleep apnea; polysomnography; snoring, excessive daytime sleepiness.

1. OVERVIEW

The word "apnea" comes from the Greek terms "a" for no and "pnea" for breath. Hence, apnea means "no breath" and sleep apnea, by definition, is apnea that occurs during sleep. Individuals with sleep apnea literally stop breathing for brief periods of time when asleep and must at least partially awake in order to resume breathing. Sleep is therefore fragmented.

Because there can be very brief episodes of decreased respiratory activity during normal sleep, criteria have been established for the diagnosis of sleep apnea. An apneic event is defined as cessation of airflow for 10 or more seconds *(1)*. Episodes of decreased, but not complete, cessation of flow are hypopneas. Hypopneas are defined as a decrease in airflow of at least 50% from the patient's baseline accompanied by either a drop in O_2 saturation of at least 3% or an arousal *(2)*.

Obstructive sleep apnea (OSA) and central sleep apnea (CSA) are two forms of sleep apnea. There is no airflow in OSA, often regardless of significant respiratory attempt. OSA arises with upper airway failure, either during inspiration or at the end of expiration, depending on the patient's upper airway anatomy. The patient is attempting to breathe against a closed airway (*see* Fig. 1). The transitory arrest of breathing in CSA are caused by reduced respiratory activity, where no airflow or respiratory effort exists (*see* Fig. 2).

Some apneic events are comprised of elements of both central apnea (i.e., the absence of effort) followed by obstructive apnea (increased effort in the absence of airflow). These events are mixed apneas and may be the predominant type for some patients (*see* Fig. 3). Notably, almost every obstructive apneic event appears to be preceded by a very brief decrease in effort.

From: *Current Clinical Neurology*
Parkinson's Disease and Nonmotor Dysfunction
Edited by: R. F. Pfeiffer and I. Bodis-Wollner © Humana Press Inc., Totowa, NJ

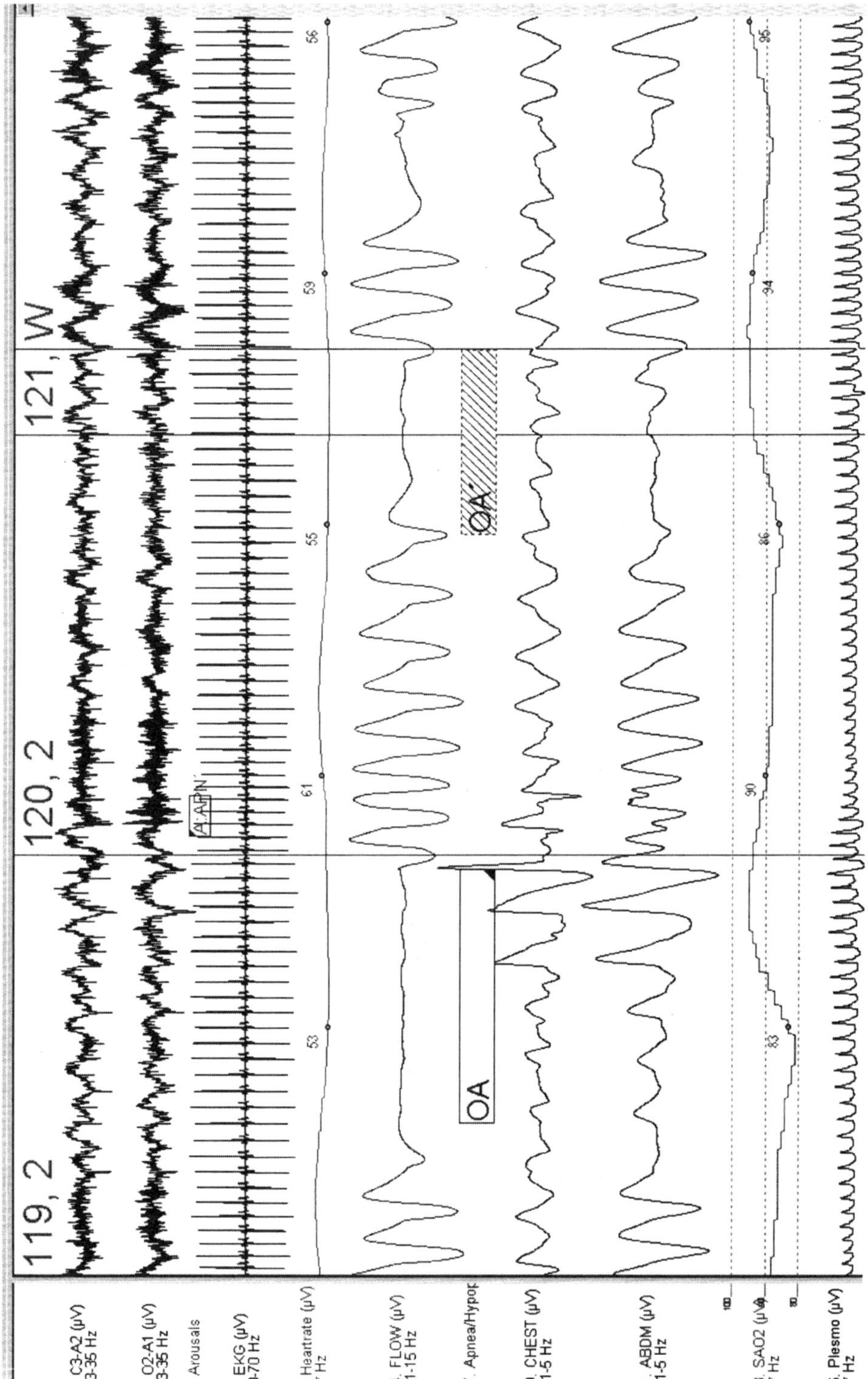

Fig. 1. Obstructive sleep apneas (OA and OA'). Figure courtesy of The Sleep Disorders Center at Tampa General Hospital.

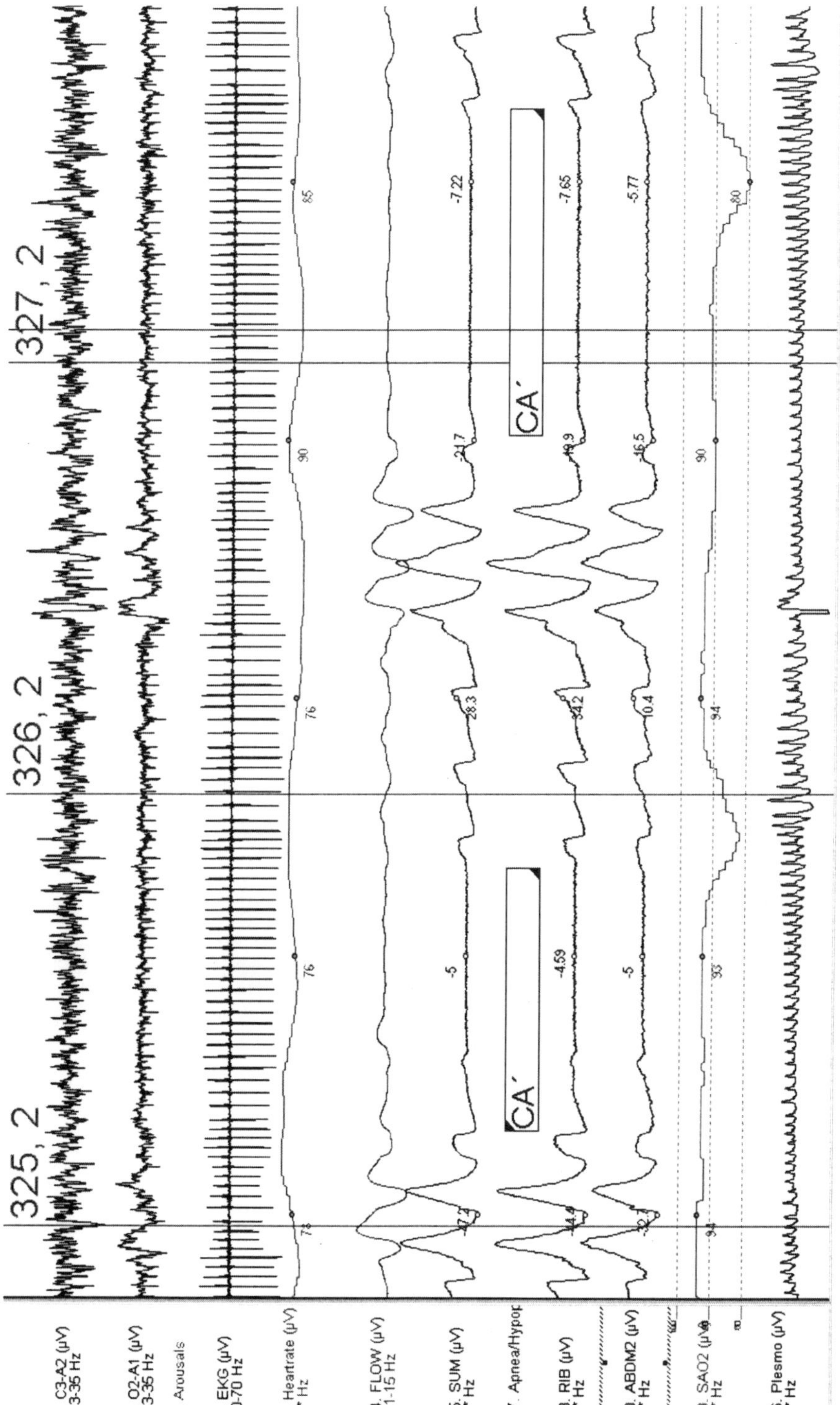

Fig. 2. Central sleep apnea (CA′). Figure courtesy of The Sleep Disorders Center at Tampa General Hospital.

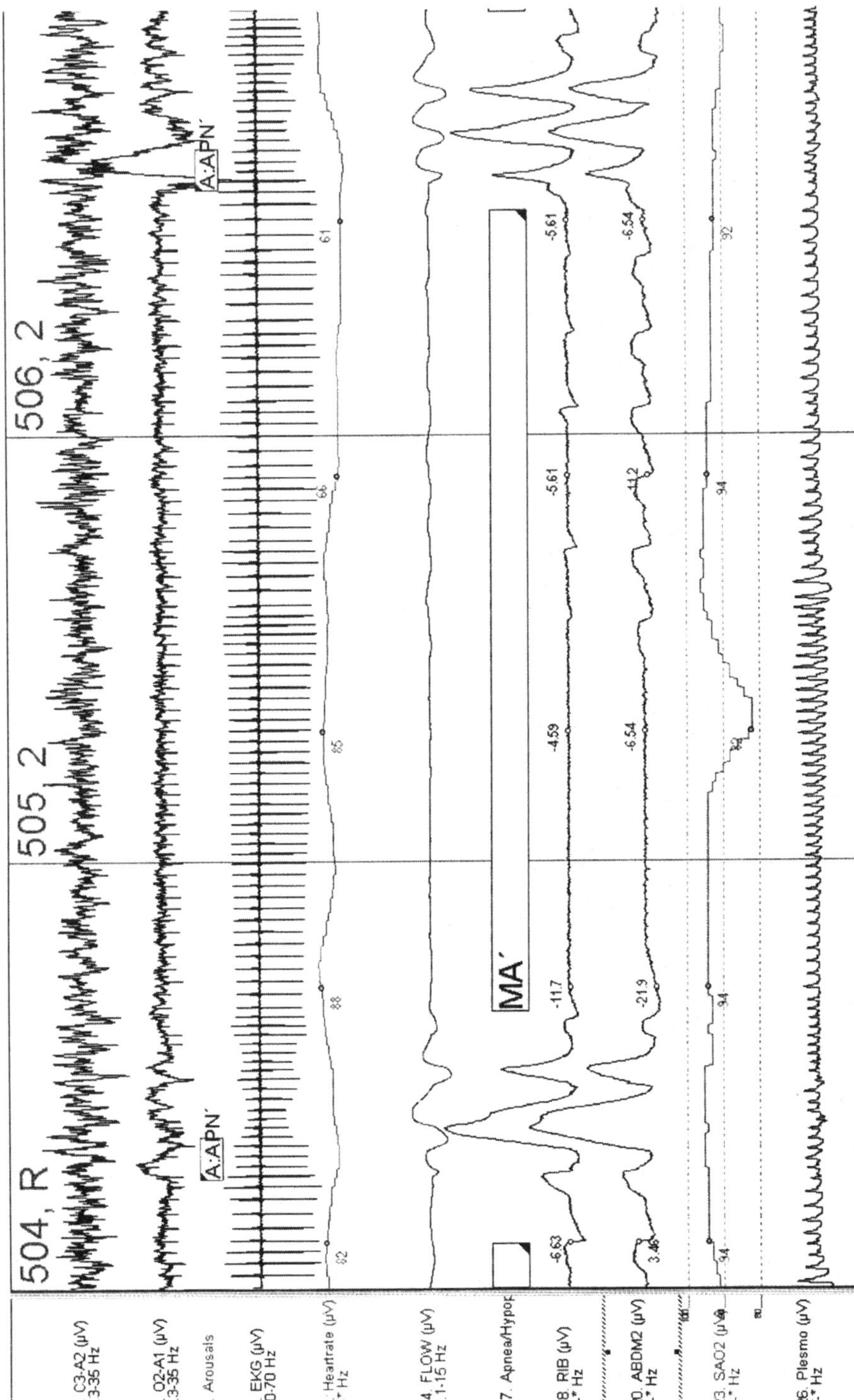

Fig. 3. Mixed apnea (MA´). Figure courtesy of The Sleep Disorders Center at Tampa General Hospital.

OSA is estimated to occur in approximately 4% of adult males and 2% of adult females *(3)*. OSA prevalence increases with age, and it is estimated that by age 60, 60% of men and 45% of women have symptoms (most commonly, snoring) suggestive of OSA *(4)*. Pure, or even primarily, CSA is considered rare and is generally reported to account for 4 to 10% of patients seen in sleep centers *(5)*. There are no general population statistics for CSA at this time.

2. OBSTRUCTIVE SLEEP APNEA

Although the nasal cavity accounts for half of the total resistance in the upper airway, its contribution is relatively constant *(6)*. In OSA in the general population, the main focus of concern is the pharynx, which can be divided into four segments: nasopharynx, velopharynx, oropharynx, and hypopharynx. Although most patients with OSA have several areas of pharyngeal collapse, the velopharynx (region immediately behind the uvula) and the oropharynx (region behind the oral cavity and tongue) are the primary sites involved.

Dilation of the upper airway is produced by over 20 skeletal muscles that surround the pharyngeal airway and stiffen the pharyngeal walls *(7)*. Control of these muscles is a complex process because any muscle action depends on the actions of other muscles and the state of the surrounding anatomical structures. For example, whether the mouth is open or shut affects the position of the tongue, and opening the mouth can destabilize the upper airway. The size of the tongue and position of the mandible can also have significant effects on the size of the pharyngeal airway. The functions of the various pharynx muscles are also affected by the status of the airway itself. If the pharyngeal constrictors are activated when there is a relatively high airway volume, the airway will be constricted. If they are activated at a low airway volume, the airway is dilated. Thus, the upper airway anatomy and functional state of the musculature determine the size of the pharyngeal airway.

Any factor that decreases muscle tone will also contribute to OSA. During rapid eye movement (REM) sleep, skeletal muscles other than the diaphragm show a marked decline in tone. This stage of sleep is normally characterized by virtual paralysis with very brief episodes of intermittent phasic activity. Hence, OSA is generally at its worst when the patient is in REM sleep.

In addition to the tone of the intrinsic upper airway muscles, positional factors have been found to be influential. Many patients experience upper airway restriction only when they are supine. Neck flexion predisposes to airway closure, whereas extension of the neck promotes a more open airway *(8)*. Kyphoscoliosis can also contribute to OSA.

Finally, no OSA discussion is complete without including obesity as a cause for OSA. Obesity is one of the cardinal risk factors for OSA and is believed to affect the process primarily by narrowing the upper airway.

3. CENTRAL SLEEP APNEA

Although many normal individuals exhibit irregular respiration at sleep onset with brief respiratory pauses, some individuals experience repeated episodes of CSA at sleep onset. In some cases, these events lead to arousals that awaken the patient, and it is not unusual for such patients to present with complaints of insomnia.

During sleep, metabolic mechanisms control ventilation and pCO_2 is the single most important factor *(9)*. A low pCO_2 reduces the drive for respiration. Hypocapnia can be the result of intrinsic disorders of chemosensitivity or hyperventilation. The latter is often associated with arousals and poor ventilatory control *(10)*. Severely diminished or absent sensitivity to pCO_2 results in sleep-disordered breathing, typically CSA *(11)*.

Nasal congestion is certainly associated with OSA, but it can also have a significant role in CSA. Possible impact may be owing to occlusion of nasal receptors that are instrumental in respiratory control and to pharyngeal collapse that can occur secondary to nasal obstruction *(12)*.

Various neurological disorders are related to CSA (*see* Table 1). The Shy-Drager syndrome (multiple system atrophy) has been associated with severe OSA with reports of death *(13)*. Brainstem infarc-

Table 1
Disorders Associated With Central Sleep Apnea

Autonomic dysfunction
Multiple system atrophy
Familial dysautonomia
Diabetes mellitus
Brainstem infarction
Cervical cordotomy
Muscular dystrophy
Myasthenia gravis
Postpolio syndrome

tion and medullary lesions from polio can lead to hypoventilation and abnormal ventilatory control, which predisposes to CSA. Even if the brainstem is intact, disruption of the neuronal control of the respiratory muscles ultimately affects the metabolic control of respiration. Neuromuscular disorders can cause decreased respiratory effort and waking hypoventilation, which can lead to loss of normal chemosensitvity and CSA *(14)*.

4. CLINICAL FEATURES OF SLEEP APNEA

Patients with OSA are typically unaware of their sleep problem. In contrast, the bed partner usually recognizes a sleeping problem because OSA is significantly associated with snoring. The snoring may be so loud that no one wants to share a bed or bedroom with an OSA patient. The bed partner may provide a highly suggestive description: the individual falls asleep, snores (typically very loudly), and then is silent. The silence lasts long enough for the observer to become aware of it, and the silence usually ends with a loud snorting sound. Bed partners frequently report having to hit or push the patient to get them to breathe again.

The most common complaint of patients with OSA is excessive daytime sleepiness (EDS). Indeed, the daytime sleep manifestations of severe OSA patients can be mistaken for narcolepsy to the extent that sleep is severely fragmented by frequent awakenings. Headache is another common complaint; morning headaches are especially frequent. However, many patients also report nocturnal headaches. Generally, the headache of OSA is dull, nonfocal, and lasts a few hours *(15; see* Table 2).

As noted previously, OSA is more common during REM sleep. Depression, personality changes, and psychomotor dysfunction may occur secondary to disruption of REM sleep, but hypoxemia may also be a factor. Night sweats, nocturia, and sexual dysfunction result from hemodynamic and autonomic changes that develop caused by apneic events.

The presentation of CSA can vary depending on whether or not there is hypercapnia. Hypercapnic CSA is characterized by respiratory failure, cor pulmonale, polycythemia, and daytime sleepiness. When hypercapnia is not present, daytime sleepiness and insomnia owing to restless sleep may also be accompanied by mild and intermittent snoring, awakenings that may be associated with choking, and a normal body habitus *(16)*.

5. DIAGNOSIS OF SLEEP APNEA

Similar to other medical disorders, a comprehensive history is the crucial first step in diagnosing sleep apnea. If possible, the history should be obtained with the bed partner or housemate present. Denial of daytime sleepiness is common, and patients hardly ever report hearing themselves snore. If they are aware of nocturnal arousals or awakenings, they can only rarely identify the triggering factor.

The gold standard for assessing sleep apnea is the polysomnogram (PSG), involving overnight monitoring of the patient, including electroencephalography, which is necessary for determining sleep

Table 2
Common Symptoms of Obstructive Sleep Apnea

Excessive daytime sleepiness
Psychomotor dysfunction
Decreased motor skills
Memory impairment
Depression
Headache
Night sweats
Nocturia
Personality changes
Sexual dysfunction

onset and sleep staging. Extraoccular eye movements are recorded (via electro-oculography), as is mentalis muscle tone (via electromyography), to help determine when the patient is in REM sleep. In addition to these specific sleep parameters, the study includes transducers to record airflow, respiratory effort, and cardiac rhythm. Pulse oximetry is obtained to assess the severity extent of oxygen desaturations associated with apneic events. Also, the motor activity of the legs is recorded with electrodes on the anterior tibialis muscles. The patient is usually videotaped during the PSG. Although somewhat involved and time-consuming, a full PSG allows identification of sleep-related breathing disorders, sleep-related cardiac arrythmias, and various movement disorders known to occur during sleep, including periodic limb movements of sleep, and REM behavior disorder.

More recently, portable equipment to assess sleep and respiration has been developed *(17)*. Although these studies have not replaced laboratory-based PSG, they offer the potential to reduce cost, inconvenience, and delays in obtaining sleep studies.

6. TREATMENT OF OSA

As with any other medical disorder, an understanding of the underlying pathophysiology provides the key to treatment. OSA can be successfully treated by alleviating the obstruction. There are two major ways to accomplish this goal; one is to remove the obstruction. Several surgical procedures have been developed that address the different areas of obstruction (*18; see* Table 3). Sufficiently aggressive surgery can effectively treat even the most severe OSA, but the patient must be willing to undergo the procedure indicated by the site of collapse.

The mainstay of OSA treatment is the use of nasally administered positive airway pressure. This is achieved by establishing a seal via a mask over the nose and administering room air under pressure sufficient to keep the airway patent during sleep. The earlier versions of these devices did so at a constant pressure and were therefore referred to as continuous positive airway pressure (CPAP) devices. Subsequently, bilevel positive airway pressure (BiPAP) devices, capable of varying the pressure to account for the decreased pressure needed to maintain the airway on expiration were developed. The latest advance is the use of autotitrating devices that adjust the pressure at the mask to account for changes in the resistance of the patient's upper airway.

Pressures required to maintain an open airway can range from as little as 3 to 5 mmHg up to 16 to 20 mmHg. As would be expected, compliance is generally better at lower pressures. At the highest pressures, serious consideration must be given to surgical interventions that may not cure the OSA, but can result in significantly lower pressure requirements for positive airway pressure treatment. Reducing pressures improves compliance and decreases the incidence of CPAP complications, such as nasal irritation, conjunctivitis from air leaks under the mask, aerophagy, and very rarely, pneumothorax or pneumoencephaly.

The use of positive airway pressure has been well-documented as an effective means of eliminating apnea during sleep. The major problem is that the device has to be used on a regular basis and for

Table 3
Surgical Procedures for the Treatment of Obstructive Sleep Apnea

Site of obstruction	Procedure
Nose	Deviated septal repair Turbonate resection Adenoidectomy (rare)
Velopharynx	Uvulopalatalpharyngoplasty Somnoplasty Tonsillectomy
Oropharynx	Mandibular osteotomy with genioglossis advancement
Hypopharynx	Hyoid myotomy with suspension Maxillomandibular advancement osteotomy Base of tongue resection
Bypass all upper airway obstruction	Tracheotomy

extended periods during sleep. Unfortunately, compliance is a major problem with reports of actual use typically varying from 65% to 80% *(19).*

Other techniques and devices are aimed at addressing specific problems. Nasal dilators, both intrinsic and extrinsic, have been used effectively to reduce snoring but cannot be regarded as sufficient treatment for OSA. Devices to train the patient not to sleep in a supine position have some benefit for positionally related OSA. Weight loss, if it can be achieved, is also very efficient in reducing the degree of OSA in obese patients.

7. TREATMENT OF CSA

Although it seems counter-intuitive, the use of positive airway pressure has been demonstrated to be a beneficial treatment for CSA. As noted previously, activation of nasal and pharyngeal receptors have a positive effect on respiration control. Typically, very low pressures are required, and BiPAP may be more effective for these patients as it reduces the work of breathing on expiration when compared to CPAP.

Prior to the advent of CPAP and BiPAP, several different medications were attempted to treat CSA. Acetazolamide, a carbonic anhydrase inhibitor, had been shown to reduce central apneas in a small number of patients, but long-term studies did not show continued efficacy, and exacerbation of mixed apneas was reported. In essence, none of the drug therapies that have been tried, including the progestational agent, medroxyprogesterone, or stimulants (e.g., theophylline) have proved effective *(20).*

8. SLEEP APNEA IN PARKINSON'S DISEASE

EDS in Parkinson's disease (PD) received very limited attention prior to the report by Frucht et al., which described eight patients taking pramipexole and one taking ropinirole who fell asleep while driving *(21).* This report sparked a series of investigations into the prevalence of EDS in PD and its causes. One recent survey of 303 patients who had PD found that 50.2% had EDS as defined by an abnormally high (>10) Epworth Sleepiness Scale score *(22).* Stepwise regression analysis revealed that sleepiness correlated with longer duration of PD ($p < .0001$), more advanced PD ($p < .0004$), male sex ($p < .0001$), and the use of any dopamine agonist ($p < .0004$).

Although many recent investigations have focused on anti-Parkinsonian medications as a cause of EDS, other potential causes must not be overlooked. Several early sleep surveys in patients who had PD indicated that overnight sleep disturbances, especially frequent awakenings (sleep fragmentation), were common in PD. Factor et al. noted that 88.5% of patients with PD reported difficulty maintaining sleep, and most awakened two to five times per night, whereas 74.4% of control subjects reported difficulty maintaining sleep and awakened one to three times nightly ($p < .005$; *23*). Similarly, Tandberg et al. found a significantly higher prevalence of frequent awakenings in patients who had PD (38.9%) than diabetes patients (21%) or healthy elderly controls (12%) ($p < .001$; *24*). It was speculated that frequent awakenings in PD might be owing to motor disability, depression, or pain. However, it is also possible that sleep disorders, including sleep apnea, may have a role in causing frequent awakenings in PD, because PSG evaluations were not included in these studies.

An early PSG study confirmed frequent and prolonged awakenings throughout the night in patients who had PD *(25)*. In this study, hypoventilation and sleep apnea were not observed in 12 patients with PD or 12 normal controls.

However, another early PSG study found more apneic episodes and desaturations in patients with PD than age- and sex-matched controls *(26)*. In this study, Efthimiou et al. studied 4 untreated patients who had PD, 6 treated patients who had PD, and 20 controls. The mean number of apneic episodes and mean number of desaturations during sleep were: treated PD, 48.5/26; untreated PD, 24/3; and normal controls, 10.8/0.7. The percentage of apneic episodes that were obstructive or mixed were: treated PD, 83.5%; untreated PD 93%; and normal controls, 9%. One patient with untreated PD fulfilled criteria for sleep apnea syndrome—interestingly, this patient was not obese.

In a more recent study employing contemporary electrophysiologic techniques, Arnulf et al. evaluated 54 consecutive levodopa-treated patients who had PD with a complaint of EDS *(27)*. Of these patients, 20% had moderate or severe sleep apnea, as defined by an apnea-hypopnea index more than 15 per hour. This prevalence is substantially greater than that in an elderly American population (2.5–4.4%; *28*). Obstructive apneas and hypopneas were typical, whereas central and mixed apneas were extremely rare. Patients with moderate or severe sleep apnea had body mass indices (25.3 ± 5.2 kg/m^2) and MSLs (5.3 ± 0.8 minutes) similar to patients with no or mild sleep apnea. These investigators also described a narcolepsy-like phenotype (≥ 2 sleep-onset REM periods) in 39% of subjects. These patients were sleepier than those without such a phenotype, as evidenced by shorter Multiple Sleep Latency Tests (MSLTs).

Therefore, preliminary information suggests that OSA may be more common in PD than age- and sex-matched controls, but this remains to be proven. There is also the suggestion that obesity may not be as important a risk factor for OSA in PD as it is in the general population, which may reflect a different physiologic basis for OSA, such as upper airway muscle dysfunction *(29)*.

The significance of OSA as a cause of sleepiness in PD remains to be determined. In the study by Arnulf at al., patients who had PD with a complaint of EDS with and without OSA were equally sleepy, as reflected by similar MSLTs. However, it is possible that the non-OSA group was preferentially affected by other causes of sleepiness. A beneficial response to CPAP would indicate that OSA is, in fact, causing or contributing to sleepiness. Clinical experience indicates that some patients who have PD with OSA do experience a substantial reduction in sleepiness with CPAP treatment. However, a definitive evaluation of response to CPAP in a large group of patients who have PD with EDS and OSA is necessary. Unfortunately, such a study may be complicated by issues like compliance, adequate pressure titration, and lack of benefit in CPAP response in some patients with OSA in the general population.

Currently, it seems likely that EDS in PD can be caused by the disease itself, dopaminergic medications, and sleep disorders (e.g., sleep apnea). In patients with PD who experience EDS, reversible or treatable conditions that might be the cause should be sought. Typically, dopaminergic medications are first considered. Dopamine agonists may be lowered or discontinued, and if necessary and feasible, the levodopa dose may be reduced. However, if there is no improvement in sleepiness when dopaminergic medications are lowered or if such manipulations are not possible, consideration should be given to obtaining an overnight PSG to exclude potentially treatable sleep disorders like OSA.

We and others have suggested that it may be possible to treat EDS in PD with modafinil, a novel wake-promoting agent *(30,31)*. However, we are concerned about the possibility that modafinil administration in patients with untreated OSA could lead to subjective improvement while still exposing the patient to potentially harmful physiologic consequences of OSA. Therefore, we usually attempt to obtain an overnight PSG to eliminate OSA prior to introducing modafinil or other wake-promoting agents.

Fatigue is a common complaint in PD, but its cause and treatment are uncertain. We recently conducted an open-label pilot evaluation of fatigue in PD *(32)*. Of 18 patients who completed baseline evaluations, 10 (56%) were found to have an apnea-hypopnea index more than 20 per hour. Of 13 subjects who completed the treatment phase of the study, 9 were judged to have clinically relevant OSA; 7 were treated with CPAP, and 2 refused. Four subjects treated with CPAP were also treated with modafinil, and four patients were treated with modafinil alone. The mean modafinil dose at endpoint was 271 ± 95 mg. Fatigue severity scores improved from 48.4 ± 8.8 at baseline to 40.2 ± 13.4 at endpoint ($p = .004$). One subject discontinued modafinil because of a headache, and one terminated early owing to worsening PD.

Although very preliminary, this study raises the question as to whether OSA might be a cause of fatigue in PD. To definitively answer that question, a comparison should be made of OSA prevalence in patients who have PD with and without fatigue. Further evaluations would be required to determine if CPAP could improve fatigue in such patients. Whether modafinil can improve fatigue in PD also awaits definitive study in an appropriately designed double-blind study.

9. SLEEP APNEA IN MSA

Numerous of studies have demonstrated a high prevalence of sleep-related respiratory disturbances and nocturnal stridor in multiple system atrophy (MSA; *33–34*). There is a high prevalence of vocal cord abductor dysfunction, and stridor may be caused by dystonia of the vocal cords rather than paralysis *(35)*.

Chokroverty et al. evaluated 10 men with olivopontocerebellar degeneration and found that 5 (50%) had sleep apnea *(34)*. Three had pure central sleep apnea, and two showed obstructive, central, and mixed apneas. The apneas occurred during non-REM sleep and lasted up to 45 seconds.

Munschauer et al. studied respiration during sleep in seven patients with MSA and autonomic failure (MSA-AF) and seven control subjects *(36)*. Although mean values for respiratory rate, tidal volume, and inspiratory flow rate were similar in both groups, the coefficients of variability were significantly greater in patients with MSA-AF. One patient had central apnea, five had loud snoring, and five had respiratory stridor during sleep. Four of the five patients with MSA examined had vocal cord paralysis, and four of five nontracheostomized patients had upper airway obstruction without significant oxygen desaturation. Three of these five patients subsequently died suddenly during sleep. The investigators concluded that MSA-AF is associated with upper airway dysfunction and disordered central respirations that can be life-threatening. They suggested that even mild obstruction during sleep may warrant tracheostomy.

Silber et al. compared 17 patients who had MSA with nocturnal stridor, including 7 with daytime stridor to 25 patients who had MSA without stridor *(33)*. Analysis of 30 patients with follow-up information showed a significantly shorter survival from the sleep evaluation (but not from disease onset) for patients with stridor when compared to those without. Of patients with stridor, 9 of 11 died a median of 2 years from presentation, and the only two survivors had undergone tracheostomy. Patients with daytime stridor and immobile vocal cords had especially poor prognoses. Based on these findings, the authors recommended tracheostomy for MSA patients with stridor. However, 2 of 4 patients with tracheostomies also died, as did 6 of 19 without stridor. The investigators postulated that central hypoventilation may have been responsible for many of these other deaths and therefore also recommended assessment for central hypoventilation and appropriate management if present.

Iranzo et al. studied sleep patterns and laryngeal function of 20 patients with MSA and found sleep disturbances in all and vocal cord abduction dysfunction in 14 (70%; *36*). In three patients with nocturnal stridor and complete vocal cord abductor dysfunction, CPAP eliminated laryngeal stridor, obstructive apnea, and oxygen desaturation.

Thus, OSA is common in MSA and appears to be closely related to vocal cord abductor dysfunction. Although CPAP can eliminate OSA in MSA, compliance may still be an issue. It is not clear if

CPAP can prolong survival, and some investigators have recommended tracheostomy if even mild obstruction is present. Patients with MSA may also experience central hypoventilation.

10. SUMMARY

OSA should not be overlooked as a potential cause of EDS in PD. Recent studies have demonstrated that approximately 20% of PD patients with complaints of EDS have OSA. Likely, OSA is more typical in PD than in matched controls, but this remains to be proven. Also, obesity may not be as serious a risk factor for OSA in PD as it is in the general population. Therefore, one should not discount the possibility of OSA in patients with PD who are not obese. In patients who have PD with EDS, we first consider manipulation of anti-Parkinsonian medications. If EDS cannot be adequately alleviated by reduction of anti-Parkinsonian medications, we generally then proceed with an overnight PSG to evaluate possible sleep disorders, including OSA. At this time, we believe it is prudent to obtain a PSG before the initiation of a wake-promoting medication.

REFERENCES

1. Standards of Practice Committee of the American Sleep Disorders Association. Practice Parameters for the Indications for Polysomnography and Related Procedures. American Sleep Disorders Association Report, 1997.
2. Sleep-Related Breathing Disorders in Adults: Recommendations for Syndrome Definition and Measurement Techniques in Clinical Research, The Report of an American Academy of Sleep Medicine Task Force. Sleep 1999;22:667–689.
3. Bassiri A, Guilleminault C. Clinical features and evaluation of obstructive sleep apnea-hypopnea syndrome. In: Kryger MH, Roth T, Dement WC, eds. Principles and Practice of Sleep Medicine, 3rd ed. W.B. Saunders, Philadelphia, PA, 2000, p. 869.
4. Dement WC, Miles LE, Carskaden MA. "White paper" on sleep and aging. J Am Geriatric Soc 1982;30:25–50.
5. White DP. Central sleep apnea. In: Kryger MH, Roth T, Dement WC, eds. Principles and Practice of Sleep Medicine, 3rd ed. W.B. Saunders, Philadelphia, PA, 2000, p. 827
6. Hudgel DW, Martin RJ, Johnson B, Hill P. Mechanics of the respiratory system and breathing pattern during sleep in normal humans. J Appl Physiol 1984;56:133–137.
7. Fouke JM, Teeter JP, Strohl KP. Pressure-volume behaviour of the upper airway. J Appl Physiol 1986;61:912–918.
8. Morikawa S, Safar P, DeCarlo J. Influence of the head-jaw position upon upper airway patency. Anesthesiology 1981;22:265–270.
9. Skatrud J, Dempsey J. Interaction of sleep state and chemical stimuli in sustaining rhythmic ventilation. J Appl Physiol 1983;55:813–822.
10. Xie A, Wong B, Phillipson EA, et al. Interaction of hyperventilation and arousal in the pathogenesis of idiopathic central sleep apnea. Am J Respir Crit Care Med 1994;150:489–495.
11. White DP. Central sleep apnea. In: Kryger MH, Roth T, Dement WC, eds. Principles and Practice of Sleep Medicine, 3rd ed. W.B. Saunders, Philadelphia, PA, 2000, pp. 830–831.
12. White DP. Ventilation and the control of respiration during sleep: normal mechanisms, pathologic nocturnal hypoventilation, and central sleep apnea. In: Martin R, ed. Cardiorespiratory Disorders During Sleep, 2nd ed. Futura, New York, 1990, p. 97.
13. Lockwood AH. Shy-Drager syndrome with abnormal respirations and antidiuretic hormone release. Arch Neurol 1976;33:292–295.
14. White DP. Central sleep apnea. In: Kryger MH, Roth T, Dement WC, eds. Principles and Practice of Sleep Medicine, 3rd ed. W.B. Saunders, Philadelphia, PA, 2000, p. 833.
15. American Sleep Disorders Association. The International Classification of Sleep Disorders, Revised Diagnostic and Coding Manual. American Sleep Disorders Association, Rochester, MN, 1997, pp. 52–58.
16. White DP. Central sleep apnea. In: Kryger MH, Roth T, Dement WC, eds. Principles and Practice of Sleep Medicine, 3rd ed. W.B. Saunders, Philadelphia, PA, 2000, p. 834.
17. ASDA practice parameters for the use of portable recordings in the assessment of obstructive sleep apnea. Sleep 1997;20:406–422.
18. Riley RW, Powell NB, Li KK, Guilleminault C. Obstructive sleep apnea syndrome: a surgical protocol for dynamic upper airway reconstruction. J Oral Maxillofacial Surg 1993;51:742–747.
19. Sin DD, Mayers I, Man G, Pawluk L. Long-term compliance rates to continuous positive airway pressure in obstructive sleep apnea: a population-based study. Chest 2002;121:430–435.
20. Sanders MH. The management of sleep-disordered breathing. In: Martin R, ed. Cardiorespiratory Disorders During Sleep, 2nd ed. Futura, New York, 1990, pp. 172–173.
21. Frucht S, Rogers JD, Greene PE, et al. Falling asleep at the wheel: motor vehicle mishaps in persons taking pramipexole and ropinirole. Neurology 1999;52:1908–1910.

22. Ondo WG, Dat Vuong K, Khan H, et al. Daytime sleepiness and other sleep disorders in Parkinson's disease. Neurology 2001;57:1392–1396.
23. Factor SA, McAlarney T, Sanchez-Ramos JR, Weiner WJ. Sleep disorders and sleep effect in Parkinson's disease. Mov Disord 1990;5:280–285.
24. Tandberg E, Larsen JP, Karlsen. A community-based study of sleep disorders in patients with Parkinson's disease. Mov Disord 1998;13:895–899.
25. Apps MCP, Sheaff PC, Ingram DA, et al. Respiration and sleep in Parkinson's disease. J Neurol Neurosurg Psych 1985;48:1240–1245.
26. Efthimiou J, Ellis SJ, Hardie RJ, Stern GM. Sleep apnea in idiopathic and postencephalitic Parkinsonism. Adv Neurol 1986;45:275–276.
27. Arnulf I, Konofal E, Merino-Andreu M, et al. Parkinson's disease and sleepiness: an integral part of PD. Neurology 2002;58:1019–1024.
28. Bixler EO, Vgontzas A, Ten Have T, Tyson, Kales A. Effects of age on sleep apnea in men. Am J Respir Crit Care Med 1998;157:144–148.
29. Vincken WG, Gauthier SG, Dollfuss RE, et al. Involvement of upper-airway muscles in extrapyramidal disorders. A cause of airflow limitation. N Engl J Med 1984;311:438–442.
30. Hauser RA, Wahba MN, Zesiewicz TA, Anderson WM. Modafinil treatment of pramipexole-associated somnolence. Mov Disord 2000;15:1269–1271.
31. Adler CH, Caviness JN, Hentz JG, et al. Randomized trial of modafinil for treating subjective daytime sleepiness in patients with Parkinson's disease. Mov Disord 2003;18:287–293.
32. Hauser RA, Zesiewicz TA, Delgado HM, et al. Evaluation and treatment of fatigue in Parkinson's disease. Neurology 2002;58(Suppl 3):A433.
33. Silber MH, Levine S. Stridor and death in multiple system atrophy. Mov Disord 2000;15:699–704.
34. Chokroverty S, Sachdeo R, Masdeu J. Autonomic dysfunction and sleep apnea in olivopontocerebellar degeneration. Arch Neurol 1984;41:926–931.
35. McNicholas WT, Rutherford R, Grossman R, et al. Abnormal respiratory pattern generation during sleep in patients with autonomic dysfunction. Am Rev Respir Dis 1983;128:429–433.
36. Munschauer FE, Loh L, Bannister R, Newsome-Davis J. Abnormal respiration and sudden death during sleep in multiple system atrophy with autonomic failure. Neurology 1990;40:677–679.
37. Kneisley LW, Rederich GJ. Nocturnal stridor in olivopontocerebellar atrophy. Sleep 1990;13:362–368.
38. Isozaki E, Hayashi M, Hayashida T, et al. Vocal cord abductor paralysis in multiple system atrophy—paradoxical movement of vocal cords during sleep. Rinsho Shinkeigaku 1996;36:529–533.
39. Blumin JH, Vberke GS. Bilateral vocal cord paresis and multiple system atrophy. Arch Otolaryngol Head Neck Surg 2002;128:1404–1407.
40. Merlo IM, Occhini, Paccheti C. Not paralysis, but dystonia causes stridor in multiple system atrophy. Neurology 2002;58:649.
41. Iranzo A, Santamaria J, Tolosa E. Continuous positive air pressure eliminates nocturnal stridor in multiple system atrophy. Lancet 2000;356:1329–1330.

IV Sensory Dysfunction in Parkinson's Disease

19
Visual Dysfunction

Robert L. Rodnitzky

SUMMARY

Various abnormalities of visual function have been documented in Parkinson's disease (PD). Levodopa-responsive abnormalities of visual-evoked potentials (VEP) and electroretinographic patterns have been demonstrated in PD patients as well as in primates with experimental Parkinsonism. Dopamine is found within several structures subserving vision, including the visual cortex, lateral geniculate, and retina, but retinal dopaminergic dysfunction is likely the greatest contributor to visual syndromes associated with PD. Abnormalities of color perception, especially in the blue–green axis, and visual-contrast sensitivity (VCS) are two of the most important and well-documented visual aberrations related to PD. Although VCS impairment seems largely related to retinal dopaminergic dysfunction, the observation that this form of visual impairment is orientation-specific raises the possibility of visual cortex involvement as well. Visual abnormalities in PD are seldom clinically apparent and not likely to be discovered during the routine neurological examination using ordinary high-contrast visual acuity testing. However, it is important to recognize that several types of disability, ranging from gait freezing to visual hallucinations or impaired driving, may be related to an underlying impairment of visual function in PD.

Key Words: Parkinson's disease (PD); visual dysfunction; dopamine; color vision; contrast sensitivity; visual acuity; hallucinations.

1. INTRODUCTION

A wide range of visual dysfunction is common in patients with Parkinson's disease (PD; *1,2*). Most of these abnormalities are relatively subtle from a clinical point of view, but all can have practical consequences under certain circumstances. Despite the potential functional implications of visual symptoms in PD, they are seldom of sufficient severity to replace motoric dysfunction as a patient's primary clinical complaint. Most of the visual abnormalities linked to PD are demonstrable in the very early clinical phase of the illness and are presumably present in the preclinical phase of PD as well. As PD is predominantly a disorder of the elderly, it is not surprising that patients in this age group are often aware of declining visual function. When symptoms (e.g., visual blurring, difficulty reading, impaired near vision, or abnormal light sensitivity) appear in a patient with PD, it prompts both the patient and the clinician to wonder what, if any, relationship these symptoms have to the underlying neurological disorder. When complaints referred to the visual system are specifically solicited from patients who have PD, the most common are tired eyes or blurred vision when reading and diplopia *(3)*. Can complaints like this be logically associated to the known pathophysiology of PD? In this chapter, the known aberrations of visual function that occur in PD are discussed as well as their pathogenesis. In the course of the discussion, it becomes apparent that several forms of visual dysfunction in PD are very subtle and more easily demonstrated through electrophysiologic or psychophysical testing than by clinical means.

From: *Current Clinical Neurology*
Parkinson's Disease and Nonmotor Dysfunction
Edited by: R. F. Pfeiffer and I. Bodis-Wollner © Humana Press Inc., Totowa, NJ

Prior to discussing clinical dysfunction of the visual system in PD, it is useful to first review the role of dopamine in the visual system and abnormalities of this neurotransmitter that have been shown within this context.

2. DOPAMINE AND THE VISUAL SYSTEM

Dopamine is found in several anatomical structures that subserve vision; its localization within the amacrine and interplexiform cells of the retina is perhaps the most important *(4)*. In an autopsy study of patients with PD, retinal dopamine concentration was shown to be decreased *(5)* but was normal in those who had received levodopa therapy shortly before death, suggesting that this therapy might be instrumental in reversing visual dysfunction related to retinal dopamine deficiency. Several observations support the concept that dopamine has a specific function in the retina of primates. The chemical protoxin 1-methyl-4-phenyl-1-2-5-6-tetrahydropyridine (MPTP) produces a clinical parkinsonian syndrome when injected into primates and significantly lowers retinal dopamine. These changes are associated with abnormalities in the latency and amplitude of both the pattern visual-evoked potential (VEP) and the electroretinogram, both of which can be reversed by levodopa administration *(6)*. Similarly, intravitreal injection of the neurotoxin 6-hydroxydopamine into aphakic monkeys results in abnormalities in both the phase and amplitude of the pattern electroretinogram (PERG) and VEP pattern, particularly for stimuli with higher spatial frequencies *(7)*. This finding suggests dopamine as a factor in retinal spatial tuning. The visual-evoked response *(8)* and PERG *(9)* are abnormal in idiopathic PD as well, and both can be improved with levodopa, especially the latter *(10)*.

Other structures within the visual system also have dopaminergic innervation, including the lateral geniculate *(11)* and visual cortex *(12)*. Recordings from single units in the lateral geniculate body of cats during simultaneous iontophoretic application of dopamine have implied that dopamine controls visual activity in this structure in several ways, e.g., direct inhibition of relay cells through D1 receptors, and both direct facilitation of relay cell function and excitation of inhibitory neurons through D2 receptors *(13)*. Asymmetric primary visual cortex glucose hypometabolism has been demonstrated in PD, where the most severe abnormality appears ipsilateral to the most severe motoric dysfunction *(14)*. The laterality of this abnormality indicates that it is more likely related to dysfunction in the nigrostriatal system than the retina because the former structure is asymmetrically involved in PD, whereas the latter, even if asymmetrically affected, has bilateral input to the visual cortices and is expected to result in symmetrical hypometabolism.

Notwithstanding dopamine's potential widespread influence within the visual system, its role in the retina seems to be the most significant. Dopamine content in the retina exhibits distinct circadian rhythms that can be driven by light–dark cycles or, in total chronic darkness, by the cyclic presence of melatonin *(15,16)*. Dopaminergic neurons are thought to subserve a modulatory influence in the retina and may mediate center-surround functions important to receptive field organization *(17)*. An investigation in which the PERG spatial-contrast response was recorded after taking dopamine D1 or D2 antagonists or a D1 agonist suggested that D1 receptors may be the most important for surround organization of retinal ganglion cells, and D2 receptors may contribute to the center response amplification of other ganglion cells *(18)*. The neurobiology of retinal dopamine has recently been thoroughly reviewed *(19)*.

3. VISUAL ACUITY

Although common clinical experience suggests that there is not a severe and clinically impressive decline of visual acuity in PD, group comparisons between PD patients and controls do reveal a difference. Repka et al. *(3)* tested high-contrast visual acuity in 39 patients who had PD and an equal number of age-matched controls. A small, but statistically significant, difference in visual acuity was found between the groups, the mean value in PD being 20/39 and in controls 20/28. Visual acuity decline in patients with PD correlated with increasing disease severity, further supporting the notion that this abnormality is linked to the evolving pathology of the underlying PD. Whether loss of visual acuity in PD is related to retinal or cortical dysfunction is uncertain, but the authors speculated that the known reduction of retinal dopamine in PD might result in an increase of the receptive field size, leading to a decrease in visual function. Despite that severity of visual acuity loss in PD appears to be associated to advancing disease, it does not appear to be reversible with treatment because high-contrast visual acuity has been demonstrated to be similarly impaired whether patients are "on" or "off" dopaminergic drugs *(20)*. One other link between dopamine and visual acuity is the clinical observation that levodopa administration improves human amblyopia in both children and adults *(21)*.

Although not directly related to visual acuity, one common efferent visual problem in PD that can significantly reduce visual efficiency (especially for reading) is convergence insufficiency *(3)*. This extremely common condition in PD is associated with an abnormally distant near point of convergence, greater than 10 cm, and slow convergence amplitude. It is typically linked with the subjective complaint of asthenopia, or eyestrain, and is especially bothersome for patients using bifocal eyeglasses for reading because their proper use requires intact convergence. Near vision may be functionally impaired in such patients but amenable to correction with the use of prisms to compensate for impaired convergence or by instruction in the practice of monocular occlusion when reading. A recent report suggests that convergence insufficiency in PD can be improved by therapy with levodopa *(22)*, strengthening the connection between this form of dysfunction and dopamine deficiency.

4. COLOR VISION

Abnormal color discrimination has frequently been reported in patients with PD *(23,24)*. The impairment is typically most prominent in the tritan (blue–yellow) axis *(25,26)*. Abnormalities of color perception have been demonstrated using both bedside clinical testing techniques, such as the Farnsworth-Munsell (FM) 100-hue test *(26)*, or more elaborate psychophysical means, e.g., computer-generated assessment of color-contrast sensitivity *(25)*. Haug et al. offered an explanation as to why the tritan-contrast threshold is most affected in PD. Generally, the blue cone system is preferentially affected in retinal disease because its response range is limited and has the greatest vulnerability. The relatively selective involvement in PD can be explained by the fact that these short-wavelength–sensitive cones are relatively scarce in the retina and spaced widely apart, such that maintenance of their large-receptive fields is dependent on interaction across considerable distances, a function mediated by the dopaminergic interplexiform and amacrine cells of the retina, the precise retinal elements most affected in PD.

The abnormality of color vision seen in PD can be demonstrated very early in patients prior to receiving pharmacological therapy for their condition. It can be reversed by treatment with levodopa and other dopaminergic drugs *(27,28)*. When color vision was tested in untreated patients with PD a significant correlation was noted between the error score of the FM test and the severity of clinical parkinsonian signs measured by the motor and activities of daily living subscales of the Unified Parkinson's Disease Rating Scale *(29)*. Furthermore, when patients who have PD are followed longitudinally over time, color discrimination scores decline progressively as the underlying disease progresses *(30)*. Despite the apparent correlation with disease severity, one investigation found that color vision abnormalities in PD do not correlate with dopaminergic nigral degeneration as measured by I^{123} β-CIT single-photon emission tomography of the dopamine transporter, suggesting that this visual abnormality is extranigral in origin *(31)*. A unifying reason why color discrimination does not correlate with nigral degeneration, yet parallels the clinical severity of PD, is that retinal dopamine depletion (the probable cause of the abnormality in color vision), albeit independent of nigral dopamine depletion, occurs contemporaneously at a relatively constant pace over time. Regan et al. *(32)* questioned whether abnormalities of color discrimination tests in PD are real or just an epiphenomenon related to the motor disability of PD. Used to demonstrate impaired color vision in many studies of PD, the FM test requires the patient to execute a motor response to correctly identify varying color hues. They questioned whether it is the motor disability of patients who have PD rather than a primary visual disorder, that causes these patients to fail this test, and at the same time explains why levodopa (which corrects the motoric abnormality) improves the color vision score. These investigators utilized a computer-controlled test of color vision that did not require a motor response and found no difference between patients who had PD and a control group. However, their hypothesis fails to explain why other investigators *(25)* uncovered abnormalities of color vision in PD, when utilizing computerized-testing techniques, or why most studies have revealed a preferential loss in the tritan-color axis with little or no abnormality in the protan (red–green) axis, both of which should have been similarly affected if the abnormal test scores were simply a reflection of parkinsonian motor impairment. Additional evidence that supports the validity of color vision dysfunction in PD is the fact that abnormalities of the visual-evoked response produced by color pattern stimuli are more responsive to levodopa therapy than are those evoked by black-and-white stimuli *(33)*. Similarly, color-contrast sensitivity in patients with PD is most impaired along the tritan axis *(25)*. Lastly, other medical conditions characterized by impairment of dopaminergic transmission have been associated with color vision abnormalities. In patients undergoing cocaine withdrawal, a hypodopaminergic state, a similar tritan-axis deficit in color discrimination has been noted that is not seen during the hyperdopaminergic intoxication phase *(34)*. In contrast, color discrimination abnormalities in schizophrenia have been found to be general and not hue-specific, leading to the hypothesis that axis-specific color discrimination abnormalities are a reflection of depletion of dopamine, not its general deregulation *(35)*.

5. VISUAL-CONTRAST SENSITIVITY

Visual-contrast sensitivity (VCS) is a function not traditionally considered or tested in the clinical realm, yet it is an important sensory function that pervades many activities of daily living. VCS is a visual function consistently found to be abnormal in PD and is measured by determining the minimal contrast allowed to distinguish objects from one another presented at a given spatial frequency. Visual targets spaced very closely together are said to have a high-spatial frequency, and those spaced farther apart represent a low-spatial frequency. Another way to depict VCS is to ask how close in contrast adjacent images displayed at a given spatial frequency must be before they are indistinguishable from a visually homogeneous field. Typically, sinusoidal gratings of various spatial frequencies are used to test this function in humans. In this context, the term "sinusoidal" refers to the gradual diminution of contrast between adjacent targets, not a precipitous contrast change, such as would be seen between adjacent black-and-white squares on a checkerboard. In PD, VCS is most severely reduced at intermediate-spatial frequencies *(36,38)*, and the abnormality is most exaggerated when the gratings are temporally modulated at medium frequencies of 4–8 Hz *(36)*. Additionally, VCS is sometimes less attenuated at lower spatial frequencies in PD than it is in normal individuals *(39)*. These abnormalities are different from those of the VCS changes that are associated with normal aging *(40)*. In some studies, VCS loss has correlated with the overall severity of PD *(41)* but not in others *(38)*. However, on an hourly basis over the course of an individual day, there appears to be a more consistent correlation with the severity of parkinsonian symptoms. VCS exhibits a circadian variability that conforms to the common pattern of improved morning and worsened afternoon motoric disability seen in PD *(38)*. Recent evidence describing the circadian cycles of retinal dopamine content are consistent with this observation *(15,16)*. Similarly, VCS function can change in parallel to motor symptoms during transient "on" and "off" phases in fluctuating patients who have PD *(42)* and can be improved with levodopa *(43)*. VCS loss that is spatial frequency-selective and orientation-dependent is also seen in patients with drug-induced Parkinsonism, suggesting that dopamine deficiency of other causes can result in visual dysfunction similarly to that seen in idiopathic PD *(44)*.

Whether the basic abnormality underlying abnormal VCS in PD resides in the retina, visual cortex, or both is still unclear. The presence of interocular differences in VCS *(38,45)* indicates a link to retinal pathology. Moreover, the PERG, which largely reflects retinal ganglion cell activity, has been found to be abnormal in PD *(46,47)* with a characteristic amplitude loss at intermediate-spatial frequencies like those associated with the greatest VCS abnormality in PD *(46)*. As is the case with VCS, levodopa therapy improves the PERG abnormality in PD *(46,47)*. In a recent study, the demonstration that contrast-discrimination threshold in patients who had PD correlated with frequency-specific PERG abnormalities (a retinal phenomenon), but not VEPs (a cortical phenomenon), was viewed as further evidence that the VCS abnormality in these patients is predominantly a result of retinal dopamine deficiency *(48)*. However, some evidence also supports a cortical abnormality as a cause of VCS dysfunction in PD. VCS impairment in patients with PD is orientation-specific, in that the VCS deficit is more severe for horizontally oriented patterns than those arrayed vertically *(36,37)*. Orientation specificity may be partially subserved by the lateral geniculate, *(49)*, but mostly this perceptual function is believed to reside in the orientation-tuned receptive fields of the visual cortex *(50)*. This observation clearly raises the possibility of a central contribution to the VCS abnormality in PD as well. On the other hand, preservation of the cortically mediated function of contrast adaptation in PD has been considered evidence that cortical pathology is not significant in this condition and is not likely to have a major role regarding the reduced-contrast sensitivity seen in these patients *(51)*.

Like color vision abnormalities in PD, VCS impairment progressively increases over time as the underlying neurologic condition worsens *(30)*. This worsening appears at the intermediate-spatial frequencies known to be most affected in PD, rather than at higher spatial frequencies, which would be expected to show the greatest decline if the progressive worsening were solely a result of aging *(52)*. Consonant with this decline in VCS over time is a progressive reduction in latency amplitude and lengthening of the ERG in PD, once again linking abnormal VCS in this patient population to retinal dysfunction *(53)*.

VCS in patients with PD is not commonly tested for, and abnormalities that might be present often go unnoticed. Such abnormalities are typically present despite the normal visual acuity measured by standard Snellen chart testing *(54,55)*, which is confined to extremely high-contrast visual stimuli. The use of lower contrast letter charts in patients with PD and other medical conditions has been found to detect visual loss that was not appreciated through the use of standard visual acuity charts *(54)*. Although patients with PD and their physicians may not be aware of a contrast-sensitivity abnormality unless specifically tested for it, functional correlates of this deficit might exist. Intact spatiotemporal vision is functionally important on a daily basis because much of the visual world is periodic in array *(56)*. For example, intact-contrast sensitivity is important for the normal perception of depth and depth discrimination *(57)*. In patients who have PD, abnormal-contrast sensitivity might predispose to gait freezing. Mestre et al. *(58)* described a patient with gait freezing who exhibited increased contrast sensitivity to low- and intermediate-spatiotemporal frequencies, in the presence of environmental stripes arrayed at this frequency, but not at higher spatial frequencies or with his eyes closed. They postulated that a hypersensitivity to these low-frequency visual stimuli resulted in an adaptive "braking" reflex, leading to gait freezing. Other investigators have demonstrated that the gait of patients with PD improves in the presence of well-illuminated periodic stimuli (lines) in the visual environment *(59)*, and parameters of gait, such as stride length, are related to visual cues *(60)*. It is not unreasonable to hypothesize that abnormal VCS in patients who have PD might lead to impaired function in certain other circumstances, such as driving a motor vehicle in a low-contrast environment that can exist at dusk or dawn.

6. VISUAL HALLUCINATIONS

Visual hallucinations occur frequently in PD. They were reported by over 25% of individuals in a recent evaluation of 214 consecutive patients with this condition *(61)*. In addition to known risk factors, such as age, dementia, and therapy with anticholinergic or dopaminergic drugs, visual loss may also contribute to complex visual hallucinations *(62–64)*. The occurrence of visual hallucinations in visually impaired, but psychologically normal, individuals is considered a form of the Charles Bonnet syndrome *(65,66)*.

Because patients afflicted with this syndrome are cognitively intact and have retained insight, this form of hallucinosis, which is usually devoid of personal meaning, tends to be somewhat less emotionally upsetting. Functional magnetic resonance imaging of patients with the Charles Bonnet syndrome has revealed increased activity in the ventral extrastriate region *(67),* but whether this abnormal signal and the associated clinical syndrome reflect abnormal cortical excitation, a release phenomenon, or disrupted re-entry signals is not yet known. Although visual hallucinosis is most typically associated with significant visual loss *(63,65,68),* in PD it has been associated with several relatively mild visual abnormalities, including abnormal color discrimination, reduced visual-contrast sensitivity *(64),* and impaired color-contour perception *(62).* In these studies, patients with the Charles Bonnet syndrome had otherwise normal visual acuity, indicating that relatively minimal visual abnormalities only need to be present to predispose a patient who has PD to hallucinosis. The appearance of Charles Bonnet syndrome in patients who have PD with somewhat subtle visual loss, and its predominance in elderly individuals, has led to speculation that some degree of underlying cerebral degeneration is critical to development of the syndrome *(68).* Treatment of the Charles Bonnet syndrome can be difficult, and therapy with neuroleptics that improve other forms of PD-related hallucinosis has been generally unpromising *(69).* Alternatively, improvement in the syndrome has been reported after institution of optical aids that result in improved functional vision *(70).*

7. CONCLUSION AND PRACTICAL CLINICAL SIGNIFICANCE

Abnormalities of electrophysiologic tests, such as the VEP and PERG, as well as psychophysical tests of VCS and color discrimination leave little doubt that the visual system is involved in PD. Reversal of these deficits with levodopa and the correlation of abnormal electrophysiologic tests with reduced retinal dopamine in experimental Parkinsonism establish a compelling link between deficiencies in this neurotransmitter and the visual abnormalities of PD. The role of retinal dysfunction seems certain, but the contribution of cortical- and lateral-geniculate impairment to these visual symptoms is yet unclear.

The potential clinical relevance of these visual abnormalities in PD is not widely appreciated. Abnormalities (e.g., impaired VCS and abnormal color discrimination) are unlikely to be clearly apparent to the patient, but it is important for the clinician to realize that a variety of more subtle and indirect forms of dysfunction as diverse as gait freezing, impaired depth perception, and visual hallucinations might be related to these categories of visual impairment. Another issue of clinical importance that emerges from these findings is the extent to which documenting abnormalities of vision might be diagnostically significant in identifying early or presymptomatic PD or distinguishing PD from various other parkinsonian syndromes. The differentiation between idiopathic PD and multiple system atrophy has been investigated in this regard, and distinct group differences between the two conditions have been identified in mean VEP latency and visual-contrast thresholds *(45,51).* As these are group differences, they are not very useful in making a clinical distinction between the two conditions in individual patients. In progressive supranuclear palsy, mean VCS performance has been noted to be more severely impaired than in PD but not so consistently abnormal in individual patients to be useful in distinguishing this syndrome from other parkinsonian conditions *(48).* Regarding color testing as a diagnostic aid, Birch et al. *(26)* found that 23% of PD patients had tritan color vision deficits, whereas none of 40 age-matched controls were abnormal. These results suggest that impaired blue–yellow vision supports a PD diagnosis, but a normal result does not rule it out.

Using visual tests to identify PD in its earliest stage or even prior to the onset of motoric symptoms is slightly more promising. Indications suggest that abnormalities of color vision and VCS may be present prior to the typical PD clinical presentation. Color vision has been found to be abnormal in mild and untreated patients with PD, very early in the course of illness, implying that the abnormality may have antedated clinical diagnosis of PD *(24).* Perhaps the most useful application of VCS testing in the identification and diagnosis of PD is its use in association with other assessments as part of a battery. Camicioli et al. *(71)* found that a battery consisting of tapping rate combined with either olfactory assessment or measurement of visual-contrast sensitivity discriminated between patients who had mild PD and control subjects with greater than 90% accuracy.

The continuous unraveling of the anatomic, neurochemical, and neurophysiologic substrates of the visual impairment typical of PD will not only advance our understanding of the mechanisms that underly this dysfunction but likely will enhance our ability to derive useful diagnostic, therapeutic, and prognostic information from its clinical investigation. Clearly visual dysfunction in the various forms seen in PD constitutes a less serious form of disability than the motoric impairment that is typical of this disorder, but there can be little doubt that it contributes in the aggregate to overall functional impairment. This fact alone should provide significant impetus for continued investigation of visual dysfunction mechanisms in PD and renewed interest in analyzing its mechanisms and clinical significance.

REFERENCES

1. Rodnitzky RL. Visual dysfunction in Parkinson's disease. Clin Neurosci 1998;5:102–106.
2. Bodis-Wollner I. Visualizing the next steps in Parkinson disease. Arch Neurol 2002;59:1233–1234.
3. Repka MX, Claro MC, Loupe DN, Reich SG. Ocular motility in Parkinson's disease. J Pediatr Ophthalmol Strabismus 1996;33:144–147.
4. Frederick JM, Rayborn ME, Laties AM, et al. Dopaminergic neurons in the human retina. J Comp Neurol 1982;210:65–79.
5. Harnois C, Di Paolo T. Decreased dopamine in the retinas of patients with Parkinson's disease. Invest Ophthalmol Vis Sci 1990;31:2473–2475.
6. Ghilardi MF, Chung E, Bodis-Wollner I, et al. Systemic 1-methyl,4-phenyl,1-2-3-6-tetrahydropyridine (MPTP) administration decreases retinal dopamine content in primates. Life Sci 1988;43:255–262.
7. Ghilardi MF, Marx MS, Bodis-Wollner I, et al. The effect of intraocular 6-hydroxydopamine on retinal processing of primates. Ann Neurol 1989;25:357–364.
8. Bodis-Wollner I, Yahr MD. Measurements of visual evoked potentials in Parkinson's disease. Brain 1978;101:661–671.
9. Peppe A, Stanzione P, Pierelli F, et al. Low contrast stimuli enhance PERG sensitivity to the visual dysfunction in Parkinson's disease. Electroencephalography Clinical Neurophysiology 1992;82:453–457.
10. Peppe A, Stanzione P, Pierelli F, et al. Visual alterations in de novo Parkinson's disease: pattern electroretinogram latencies are more delayed and more reversible by levodopa than are visual evoked potentials. Neurology 1995;45:1144–1148.
11. Papadopoulos GC, Parnavelas JG. Distribution and synaptic organization of dopaminergic axons in the lateral geniculate nucleus of the rat. J Comp Neurol 1990;294:356–361.
12. Parkinson D. Evidence for a dopaminergic innervation of cat primary visual cortex. Neuroscience 1989;30:171–179.
13. Zhao Y, Kerscher N, Eysel U, Funke K. D1 and D2 receptor-mediated dopaminergic modulation of visual responses in cat dorsal lateral geniculate nucleus. J Physiol 2002;539:223–238.
14. Bohnen NI, Minoshima S, Giordani B, et al. Motor correlates of occipital glucose hypometabolism in Parkinson's disease without dementia. Neurology 1999;52:541–546.
15. Doyle SE, McIvor WE, Menaker M. Circadian rhythmicity in dopamine content of mammalian retina: role of the photoreceptors. J Neurochem 2002;83:211–219.
16. Doyle SE, Grace MS, McIvor W, Menaker M. Circadian rhythms of dopamine in mouse retina: the role or melatonin. Vis Neurosci 2002;19:593–601.
17. Bodis-Wollner I, Tagliati M. The visual system in Parkinson's disease. Adv Neurol 1993;60:390–394.
18. Bodis-Wollner I, Tzelepi A. The push-pull action of dopamine on spatial tuning of the monkey retina: the effects of dopaminergic deficiency and selective D1 and D2 receptor ligands on the pattern electroretinogram. Vision Res 1998;38:1479–1487.
19. Djamgoz MB, Hankins MW, Hirano J, Archer SN. Neurobiology of retinal dopamine in relation to degenerative states of the tissue. Vision Res 1997;37:3509–3529.
20. Jones RD, Donaldson IM, Timmings PL. Impairment of high-contrast visual acuity in Parkinson's disease. Mov Disord 1992;7:232–238.
21. Pandey PK, Chaudhuri Z, Kumar M, et al. Effect of levodopa and carbidopa in human amblyopia. J Pediatr Ophthalmol Strabismus 2002;39:81–89.
22. Racette BA, Gokden MS, Tychsen LS, Perlmutter JS. Convergence insufficiency in idiopathic Parkinson's disease responsive to levodopa. Strabismus 1999;7:169–174.
23. Buttner T, Kuhn W, Klotz P, et al. Disturbance of colour perception in Parkinson's disease. J Neural Transm 1993;6:11–15.
24. Buttner T, Kuhn W, Muller T, et al. Distorted color discrimination in 'de novo' parkinsonian patients. Neurology 1995;45:386–387.
25. Haug BA, Kolle RU, Trenkwalder C, et al. Predominant affection of the blue cone pathway in Parkinson's disease. Brain 1995;118:771–778.
26. Birch J, Kolle RU, Kunkel M, et al. Acquired colour deficiency in patients with Parkinson's disease. Vision Res 1998;38:3421–3426.

27. Buttner T, Kuhn W, Patzold T, Przuntek H. L-Dopa improves colour vision in Parkinson's disease. J Neural Transm Park Dis Dement Sect 1994;7:13–19.
28. Buttner T, Kuhn W, Muller T, et al. Color vision in Parkinson's disease: missing influence of amantadine sulphate. Clin Neuropharmacol 1995;18:458–463.
29. Muller T, Kuhn W, Buttner T, Przuntek H. Distorted colour discrimination in Parkinson's disease is related to severity of the disease. Acta Neurol Scand 1997;96:293–296.
30. Diederich NJ, Raman R, Leurgans S, Goetz CG. Progressive worsening of spatial and chromatic processing deficits in Parkinson disease. Arch Neurol 2002;59:1249–1252.
31. Muller T, Kuhn W, Buttner T, et al. Colour vision abnormalities do not correlate with dopaminergic nigrostriatal degeneration in Parkinson's disease. J Neurol 1998;245:659–664.
32. Regan BC, Freudenthaler N, Kolle R, et al. Colour discrimination thresholds in Parkinson's disease: results obtained with a rapid computer-controlled colour vision test. Vision Res 1998;38:3427–3431.
33. Barbato L, Rinalduzzi S, Laurenti M, et al. Color VEPs in Parkinson's disease. Electroencephalogr Clin Neurophysiol 1994;92:169–172.
34. Desai P, Roy M, Brown S, Smelson D. Impaired color vision in cocaine-withdrawn patients. Arch Gen Psychiatry 1997;54:696–699.
35. Shuwairi SM, Cronin-Golomb A, McCarley RW, O'Donnell BF. Color discrimination in schizophrenia. Schizophr Res 2002;55:197–204.
36. Regan D, Maxner C. Orientation-selective visual loss in patients with Parkinson's disease. Brain 1987;110:415–432.
37. Bulens C, Meerwaldt JD, van der Wildt GJ. Effect of stimulus orientation on contrast sensitivity in Parkinson's disease. Neurology 1988;38:76–81.
38. Struck LK, Rodnitzky RL, Dobson JK. Circadian fluctuations of contrast sensitivity in Parkinson's disease. Neurology 1990;40:467–470.
39. Bodis-Wollner I. The visual system in Parkinson's disease. In: Cohen B, Bodis-Wollner I, eds. Vision and the Brain. Raven Press, New York, 1990, pp. 297–316.
40. Mestre D, Blin O, Serratrice G, Pailhous J Spatiotemporal contrast sensitivity differs in normal aging and Parkinson's disease. Neurology 1990;40:1710–1714.
41. Hutton JT, Morris JL, Elias JW, et al. Spatial contrast sensitivity is reduced in bilateral Parkinson's disease. Neurology 1991;41:1200–1202.
42. Bodis-Wollner I, Marx MS, Mitra S, et al. Visual dysfunction in Parkinson's disease. Loss in spatiotemporal contrast sensitivity. Brain 1987;110:1675–1698.
43. Hutton JT, Morris JL, Elias JW. Levodopa improves spatial contrast sensitivity in Parkinson's disease. Arch Neurol 1993;50:721–724.
44. Bulens C, Meerwaldt JD, van der Wildt GJ, Keemink CJ. Visual contrast sensitivity in drug-induced Parkinsonism. J Neurol Neurosurg Psychiatry 1989;52:341–345.
45. Delalande I, Hache JC, Forzy G, et al. Do visual-evoked potentials and spatiotemporal contrast sensitivity help to distinguish idiopathic Parkinson's disease and multiple system atrophy? Mov Disord 1998;13:446–452.
46. Tagliati M, Bodis-Wollner I, Yahr MD. The pattern electroretinogram in Parkinson's disease reveals lack of retinal spatial tuning. Electroencephalogr Clin Neurophysiol 1996;100:1–11.
47. Peppe A, Stanzione P, Pierantozzi M, et al. Does pattern electroretinogram spatial tuning alteration in Parkinson's disease depend on motor disturbances or retinal dopaminergic loss? Electroencephalogr Clin Neurophysiol 1998;106:374–382.
48. Langheinrich T, Tebartz van Elst L, Lagreze WA, et al. Visual contrast response functions in Parkinson's disease: evidence from electroretinograms, visually evoked potentials and psychophysics. Clin Neurophysiol 2000;111:66–74.
49. Xu X, Ichida J, Shostak Y, et al. Are primate lateral geniculate nucleus (LGN) cells really sensitive to orientation or direction? Vis Neurosci 2002;19:97–108.
50. Hubel DH, Wiesel TN, Stryker MP. Orientation columns in macaque monkey visual cortex demonstrated by the 2-deoxyglucose autoradiographic technique. Nature 1977;269:328–330.
51. Tebartz van Elst L, Greenlee MW, Foley JM, Lucking CH. Contrast detection, discrimination and adaptation in patients with Parkinson's disease and multiple system atrophy. Brain 1997;120:2219–2228.
52. Kline DW. Ageing and the spatiotemporal discrimination performance of the visual system. Eye 1987;1:323–329.
53. Ikeda H, Head GM, Ellis CJ. Electrophysiological signs of retinal dopamine deficiency in recently diagnosed Parkinson's disease and a follow up study. Vision Res 1994;34:2629–2638.
54. Regan D, Neima D. Low-contrast letter charts in early diabetic retinopathy, ocular hypertension, glaucoma, and Parkinson's disease. Br J Ophthalmol 1984;68:885–889.
55. Kupersmith MJ, Shakin E, Siegel IM, Lieberman A. Visual system abnormalities in patients with Parkinson's disease. Arch Neurol 1982;39:284–286.
56. DeValois R, DeValois K. Spatial Vision. Oxford University Press, Inc., New York, 1988.
57. Rohaly AM, Wilson HR. The effects of contrast on perceived depth and depth discrimination. Vision Res 1999;39:9–18.
58. Mestre D, Blin O, Serratrice G. Contrast sensitivity is increased in a case of nonparkinsonian freezing gait. Neurology 1992;42:189–194.

59. Azulay JP, Mesure S, Amblard B, et al. Visual control of locomotion in Parkinson's disease. Brain 1999;122:111–120.
60. Lewis GN, Byblow WD, Walt SE. Stride length regulation in Parkinson's disease: the use of extrinsic, visual cues. Brain 2000;123:2077–2090.
61. Sanchez-Ramos JR, Ortoll R, Paulson GW. Visual hallucinations associated with Parkinson disease. Arch Neurol 1996;53:1265–1268.
62. Buttner T, Kuhn W, Muller T, et al. Visual hallucinosis: the major clinical determinant of distorted chromatic contour perception in Parkinson's disease. J Neural Transm Gen Sect 1996;103:1195–1204.
63. Lepore FE. Visual loss as a causative factor in visual hallucinations associated with Parkinson disease. Arch Neurol 1997;54:799.
64. Diederich NJ, Goetz CG, Raman R, et al. Poor visual discrimination and visual hallucinations in Parkinson's disease. Clin Neuropharmacol 1998;21:289–295.
65. Pfeiffer RF, Bodis-Wollner I. Charles Bonnet syndrome. J Am Geriatr Soc 1996;44:1128–1129.
66. Teunisse RJ, Cruysberg JR, Hoefnagels WH, et al. Visual hallucinations in psychologically normal people: Charles Bonnet's syndrome. Lancet 1996;347:794–797.
67. Ffytche DH, Howard RJ, Brammer M, et al. The anatomy of conscious vision: an fMRI study of visual hallucinations. Nat Neurosci 1998;1:738–742.
68. Manford M, Andermann F. Complex visual hallucinations. Clinical and neurobiological insights. Brain 1998;121:1819–1840.
69. Batra A, Bartels M, Wormstall H. Therapeutic options in Charles Bonnet syndrome. Acta Psychiatr Scand 1997;96:129–133.
70. Pankow L, Luchins DJ. An optical intervention for visual hallucinations associated with visual impairment in an elderly patient. Optom Vis Sci 1997;74:138–143.
71. Camicioli R, Grossmann SJ, Spencer PS, et al. Discriminating mild Parkinsonism: methods for epidemiological research. Mov Disord 2001;16:33–40.

20
Primary Visual and Visuocognitive Deficits

Ivan Bodis-Wollner and Andrea Antal

SUMMARY

Visual abnormalities in individuals with Parkinson's disease (PD) are unlikely to be uncovered during routine neurological examination. However, more sophisticated electrophysiological testing using techniques, such as the visual-evoked potential and pattern electroretinogram, confirms the presence of visual system involvement in PD. Progressive select pathology of dopaminergic neuronal processing in the retina, leading to loss of spatiotemporal tuning and distorted retinal input to higher visual centers, is present.

With its dopaminergic deficiency, the retina may not be the only site of visual pathology in PD. More complex visuocognitive difficulties, e.g., impairment of consciously controlled visual information processing, have also been identified in PD. Visual event-related potential testing in patients with PD demonstrates a delay in the P300 component, suggesting slowness of visual information processing. Whereas some investigators have noted this abnormality only in demented patients with PD, others have indicated its presence in both demented and nondemented individuals. The visuospatial sketchpad, a component of the working memory system, shows a specific selective impairment in PD, and visual categorization deficits (suggesting involvement of posterior parietal cortex) have also been found. Concurrent electrophysiological recordings of primary and visuocognitive responses reveal that the impairment of higher order visual processing in PD is not simply a consequence of retinal dopaminergic deficiency. Electrophysiological, neuropsychological, and functional neuroimaging data imply that both frontal and posterior cortico–subcortical circuits may be involved.

Key Words: Vision; Parkinson's disease (PD); pattern electroretinogram; visual-evoked potential; visuocognitive; event-related potential; working memory.

1. INTRODUCTION

Parkinson's disease (PD) is generally known as a movement disorder resulting from dopaminergic deficiency that affects the basal ganglia. Therapy with dopaminergic agents reliably improves motor symptoms. Although dopaminergic deficit is the pathogenomic feature of the disease, dopaminergic deficits and the clinical manifestations of the disease extend beyond the motor system. In the last two decades, it has become apparent that beyond or parallel with progressive motor impairments, nonmotor symptoms are also present. One well-explored area of nonmotor dysfunction in PD is vision. Visual perceptual, visuospatial, visuomotor, and visuocognitive dysfunctions have been studied by various techniques in PD. This chapter discusses the relationship of visual and visuocognitive abnormalities to motor symptoms and visual response to dopaminergic therapy. Visual electrodiagnostic, psychophysical, and whenever possible, imaging data on visual and visuocognitive processing in PD is described.

Because PD is predominantly a disease of the elderly, it is not surprising that many patients have visual complaints. They may represent various etiologies, and clinicians do not relate these nonspecific symptoms to a primarily motor disease. Indeed, visual abnormalities in PD are probably not uncovered during a routine neurological examination. Vision assessment relying on ordinary high-contrast visual

From: *Current Clinical Neurology*
Parkinson's Disease and Nonmotor Dysfunction
Edited by: R. F. Pfeiffer and I. Bodis-Wollner © Humana Press Inc., Totowa, NJ

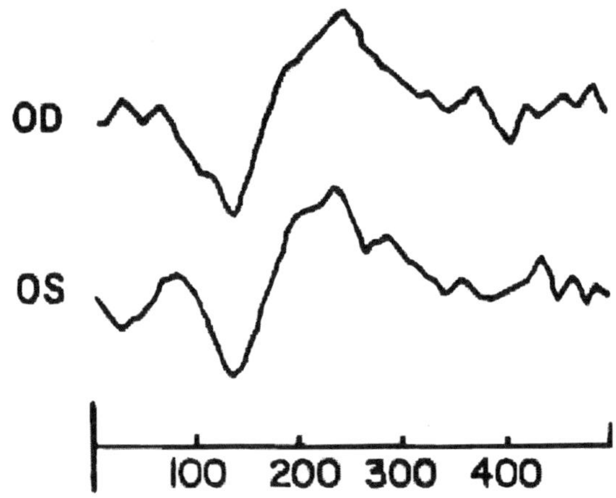

Fig. 1. Increased P100 latency in the right eye (140 ms) and in the left eye (142 ms) of a 75-year-old PD patient. Positivity is downward. From ref. *1* with permission of Brain.

acuity (VA) and visual field testing are unlikely to capture the visual deficit in PD. In this disorder, evidence exists for intrinsic retinal dopaminergic deficiency, affecting intraretinal processing of spatial and temporal contrast. To strengthen the case for considering certain visual deficits in PD germane to the disease, the evidence for retinal dopamine (DA) deficiency as a cause of visual impairment in PD is summarized. However, aside from primary visual impairments, visuocognitive difficulties, such as impairment of consciously controlled visual information processing (including sustained and selective attention) and visual categorization are also among the common cognitive symptoms observed in PD. Dopaminergic dysregulation of the prefrontostriatal circuits and related posterior cortical areas in patients who have PD also has to be considered in the higher levels of cognitive dysfunction. Experiments that show high levels of visual processes possibly linked to dopaminergic deficiency independently of retinal dysfunction are discussed.

2. BACKGROUND: PRIMARY VISUAL DYSFUNCTION AND THE ROLE OF DOPAMINERGIC VISUAL PROCESSES

2.1. *Retina*

Originally, it was reported by Bodis-Wollner and Yahr *(1)* that over 50% of treated patients with PD had delayed visual-evoked potential (VEP) (Fig. 1). Not only the prevalence, but the finding itself remained controversial until a number of electrophysiological and psychophysical studies addressed the importance of the specificity of the visual stimulus used for testing (for reviews, *see* refs. *2–4*). The VEP and pattern electroretinogram (PERG) abnormality in PD is most evident for foveal stimuli of medium and high spatial frequencies. (>2 cycles/degree [cpd]). This stimulus type is optimal for healthy observers, i.e., they require the least contrast to see them among any other stimulus patterns *(5–7;* Fig. 2). The psychophysically determined contrast sensitivity (CS) reveals the same stimulus-specific abnormality: it is the most reduced above 2 cpd *(2,6,8–14)*. However, visual impairment remains clinically undocumented in the majority of patients, as many vision care specialists are unaware of testing for a potentially profound CS deficit in any patient with near normal VA.

CS loss in PD becomes more profound when the stimulus grating is temporally modulated at 4 to 8 Hz *(10,15,16)*, suggesting that a dopaminergic deficiency state also affects distal temporal processing *(17)*. In summary, the spatial and temporal selectivity of visual losses detected with CS in PD is consistent with the results of electrophysiological tests (PERG and VEP). The interpretation of visual

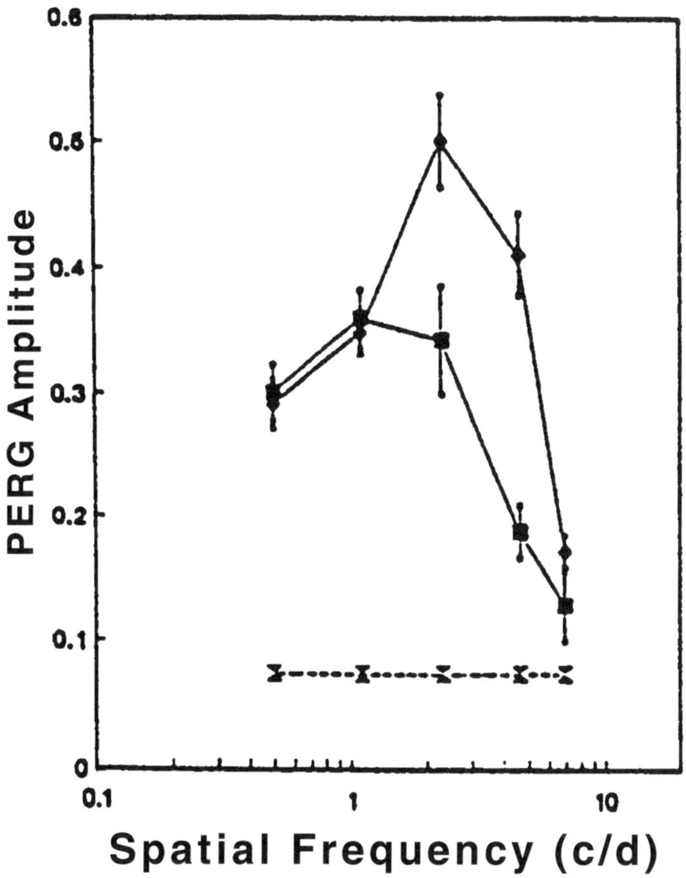

Fig. 2. The PERG tuning function in PD: PERG spatial-transfer function obtained in patients (squares) and age-matched subjects (diamonds). The functions are parallel at lower SF and very close at the higher SF tested (6.9 cpd). Note lack of tuning of the PERG transfer function in PD. From ref. *7* with permission of Clinical Neurophysiology.

deficits in PD suggests that the disease process causes progressive, select pathology of dopaminergic neuronal processing in the human retina, leading to loss of spatiotemporal tuning and distorted retinal input to higher visual centers.

VEP delay (P100 component) is observed in *de novo* and also in treated patients who have PD using stimuli at middle (2–6 cpd) spatial frequencies *(18–20)*. However, one study *(20)*, reported that treated patients have more delayed VEPs than untreated patients have. This result could possibly suggest that levodopa therapy has a deleterious effect on vision. Yet, this apparently paradoxical result may indicate that treated patients have more advanced disease, which results in worse retinal visual responses *per se (7,14)*. Generally, although both pattern electroretinogram (PERG) and VEP improve with therapy, there is an apparent difference: levodopa therapy improves PERG abnormalities to a higher degree than it does VEP deficits *(19,21,22)*. One possible interpretation is that VEP changes in PD represent secondary nondopaminergic, and therefore more chronic, alterations in visual processing.

Essential proof of visual system involvement in PD was recently provided by a longitudinal study of visual dysfunction: CS impairs in parallel with the worsening of motor score *(14)*. These results therefore suggest that the visual system shares progressive degeneration of dopaminergic neurons and/or progressive failure of the effect of L-dopa therapy with the motor system.

The foregoing discussion makes a case for the conclusion that visual dysfunction is an *integral* part of PD: the deficit fluctuates with motor symptoms in "on-off" patients and worsens with the progression of motor symptoms. The role of DA deficiency is strongly implied by all these studies, but DA deficiency may not be *exclusively* responsible for visual changes in PD.

2.2. Cortex

PERG changes in PD are caused by retinal dopaminergic deficiency. However, the retina may not be the only site of visual pathology in PD; there are other dopaminergic loci. The lateral geniculate nucleus (LGN) *(23)* and visual cortex have dopaminergic innervation *(24)*. Asymmetrically lateralized primary visual cortex glucose hypometabolism has been demonstrated in PD. The most severe abnormalities are contralateral to the most severe motoric dysfunction *(25)*. It is therefore possible that occipital hypometabolism indirectly reflects basal ganglia dysfunction, rather than being consequent to disordered retinal input. Another possibility is that occipital hypometabolism represents intrinsic cortical pathology.

Consistent with the notion of intrinsic cortical pathology are the reported pattern orientation-dependent CS losses in PD *(10,12)*. Orientation selectivity of visual neurons is first established in the primary visual cortex of primates and most mammalians *(26,27)*. The PD deficit is more severe for horizontal patterns than for vertical patterns *(12)*. This finding is not explained by retinal dopaminergic deficiency. One possible explanation may be visual cortical pathology in PD. The presence of intraocular differences in CS and VEP in PD is consistent with either retinal pathology *(13)* or with pathology affecting monocular columns in V1. Alternatively, orientation-dependent CS abnormality in PD suggests cortical pathology. However, contrast adaptation, which has a cortical origin, is spared in PD *(28)*. Studying the effect of dopaminergic therapy on orientation-selective losses in PD may be valuable.

3. VISUOCOGNITIVE PROCESSING

Besides the distal regulatory and modulatory role of DA in the visual process, a correlation possibly exists between cortical DA innervation and expression of cognitive capacities *(29)*. This is not surprising because of the known widespread cortical ascending systems and loops connecting the basal ganglia and various sensory cortical areas *(30)*. However, DA is apparently involved in much more than just "gating" bottom-up visual information flow. Several aspects of consciously controlled information processing, such as planning, problems solving, decision making, and response selection are associated with the function of frontostriatal circuits *(31–36)*. A dopaminergic dysregulation of this subcortico-cortical system in PD leads to apparent higher level cognitive dysfunctions *(32,35,37–39)*. Recent electrophysiological, neurophysiological, and functional imaging studies attempt to link cognitive symptoms and specific neuronal circuits of the basal ganglia and its connections.

3.1. Electrophysiology: P300 Deflection of Event-Related Potentials and the Clinical Neuropharmacology of P300 Abnormalities

Identifiable positive and negative deflections of event-related potentials (ERPs) have been implicated to provide indices for the timing of stages in information processing, which include stimulus evaluation, response selection and context updating *(40)*. ERPs are recorded in response to an external stimulus or event to which the subject is consciously paying attention. They are often elicited when the subject distinguishes one stimulus (target) from other stimuli (nontargets). The most extensively studied ERP component is the P300, appearing 300 to 400 ms after the onset of the target stimulus *(41)*. P300 amplitude is maximal at the midline electroencephalographic electrodes (Cz and Pz) and is inversely related to the probability of the eliciting event.

Many visual ERP studies yielded a delayed P300 only in demented patients suffering from PD *(42–46)*, but other studies reported a delayed P300 in nondemented patients *(47–51)*. This suggests the slowness of visual information processing may be independent or precedes global dementia. Although it is uncertain why visual P300 latency is reported to be affected in some but not in all studies of non-

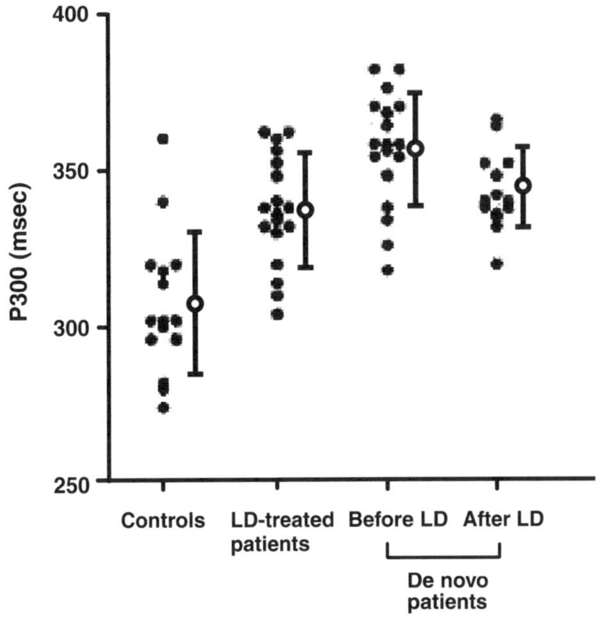

Fig. 3. Comparisons of the P300 latencies in controls and patient groups. Open circles with bars show mean and SDs. LD indicates levodopa. From ref. *58* with permission of Journal of Neurological Science.

demented patients with PD, there may be some rational explanations. First, differences in visual stimuli and experimental paradigms should be taken into account. Wang et al. *(52)* have observed that different interstimulus intervals (ISI) could distinguish patients with PD from controls: cognitive processes reflected by P300 latency to rare target stimuli were influenced by longer ISI in patients who had PD but not in control subjects. Second, P300 latency during the oddball paradigm in PD was also influenced by age at test, age at onset, and duration of illness *(47,49,52)*.

Differences in the type of medication that patients receive should also be considered. Studies in 1-methyl-1,4 phenyl-1,2,3,6-tetra-hydropyridine (MPTP)-treated monkeys suggest that levodopa therapy alone does not affect the visual P300 *(53);* however D2 receptor blockade can be an influence *(54)*. D1 receptor is involved in visual working memory (WM) in the prefrontal area (for review, *see* ref. *55*), which was also identified as one of the generators of P300 *(56)*. It has been shown that to improve motor symptoms of PD, the activation of both D1 and D2 receptor subtypes is needed *(57)*. Therefore, it is conceivable that the synergistic action of D1 and D2 receptors is needed to improve the visual P300. Levodopa treatment has been found to shorten the latency of P300 in patients (*42,58;* Fig. 3). However, some investigators have described a prolonged P300 latency in medicated patients *(59,60)*. One possibility is that medicated patients are more severely affected to start with, and P300 correlates with disease severity. (Such correlation has not been studied in detail.)

Another possibility is that cognitive slowing in PD is caused by abnormalities of nondopaminergic systems *(61)*, but there is little direct evidence of correlation of the P300 in PD with cholinergic or other types of neurotransmitter alterations. Pretreatment-delayed P300 improved in patients who had PD following treatment with amantadine, a low-affinity uncompetitive *N*-methyl-D-aspartate receptor antagonist *(62)*. Amantadine is closely related to memantine, advocated for the treatment of cognitive impairment in Alzheimer's disease. Amantadine's effect was noticeable not only as a monotherapy, but also in patients treated with levodopa. It is unknown how amantadine exercised this beneficial effect. A frequent assertion is that amantadine has DA-mimetic properties; therefore; it cannot be excluded that amantadine improves cognitive ERPs in PD as a DA-mimetic agent.

3.1.1. *Does P300 Abnormality Reflect Working Memory Impairment?*

WM refers to the short-term, attention-demanding maintenance and manipulation of information for purposeful actions *(63)*. WM is closely related to the notions of stimulus-representation matching and decision making. In the previously mentioned experiments, in which classic oddball paradigm is used to elicit the P300 component, a target stimulus has to be stored in the active memory to compare that with subsequently presented stimuli for a same-different decision making. Additionally, cortical areas identified as generators of P300 (dorsolateral prefrontal and parietal cortices) have also rules in WM processes *(56)*. One part of the WM system, the visuospatial sketchpad that relates to the maintaining of visual information *(63)*, shows a specific selective impairment in PD. The visual subsystem responsible for the object-related visual analysis seems to be spared until the later stages of the disease, whereas the visual processing of spatial location, motion, and three-dimensional properties is impaired early *(35,64–66)*. For example, in delayed-response tests, patients who had PD with mild symptoms were unable to briefly maintain the memory trace of spatial locations of irregular polygons, whereas they successfully kept online the shapes of the same stimuli *(66)*. Patients with PD also make significantly more errors in mental rotation of three-dimensional wireframe figures *(65)*.

Wang et al. *(52)* has combined the oddball paradigm with a delayed-response test (S1-S2 paradigm). In this procedure, a simple geometric design is first presented (S1), followed by another (S2) stimulus that can be the same as S1. P300 is recorded only for S2 stimuli. It was shown that when the time interval between S1 and S2 increases, nondemented patients with PD show particular deficits, suggesting impaired working memory for visual shapes.

3.1.2. *The Relationship of Primary Visual-Evoked Potentials and the Concurrently Obtained P300*

3.1.2.1. Latency

Comparing the P100 and P300 of the concurrently obtained visual ERP resulted in a somewhat surprising finding in two independent and ethnically different groups of patients with PD. A prolongation of the normalized P300 latency (P300–P100 latency difference, called central processing time) differentiated younger patients who had PD from controls *(47)*. These data suggest that younger patients with PD could be differentiated from other types of PD patients using a concurrent VEP and visual P300 recording, but were confirmed in non-Caucasian patients with PD *(49)*. Amantadine also shortened the latency of the visual P300 with little or no effect on the primary VEP component *(62)*.

3.1.2.2. Amplitude

Although numerous studies have analyzed P300 latency, only a few have examined P300 amplitude in PD. P300 amplitude increases when more attention is allocated, as when performing unexpected or complex tasks. However, it is conceivable that the interpretation of raw amplitude can be misleading, because a nonspecific, age-related low-voltage EEG recording could cause low P300 amplitude *(47)*. Measuring the P300:P100 amplitude ratio could give a more reliable measure on amplitude alterations. Indeed, it was found that this individually normalized P300 amplitude provided a significant distinction of younger nondemented patients with PD than from older patients and age-matched control subjects *(47,49)*.

3.1.3. *The Passive P300*

Most of the studies have used an active condition to evoke the P300 component (silent count or button press to the target stimuli). However, there is another positive wave termed "P3a" or "passive P300," which is elicited by unexpected neutral stimuli under conditions of passive attention. Although this component did not distinguish between demented patients who had PD and age-matched controls, it separated the group of demented patients with PD from Alzheimer's patients *(43)*. This result suggests that an abnormality of the passive P300 may depend on the specific underlying neuropathology of dementia.

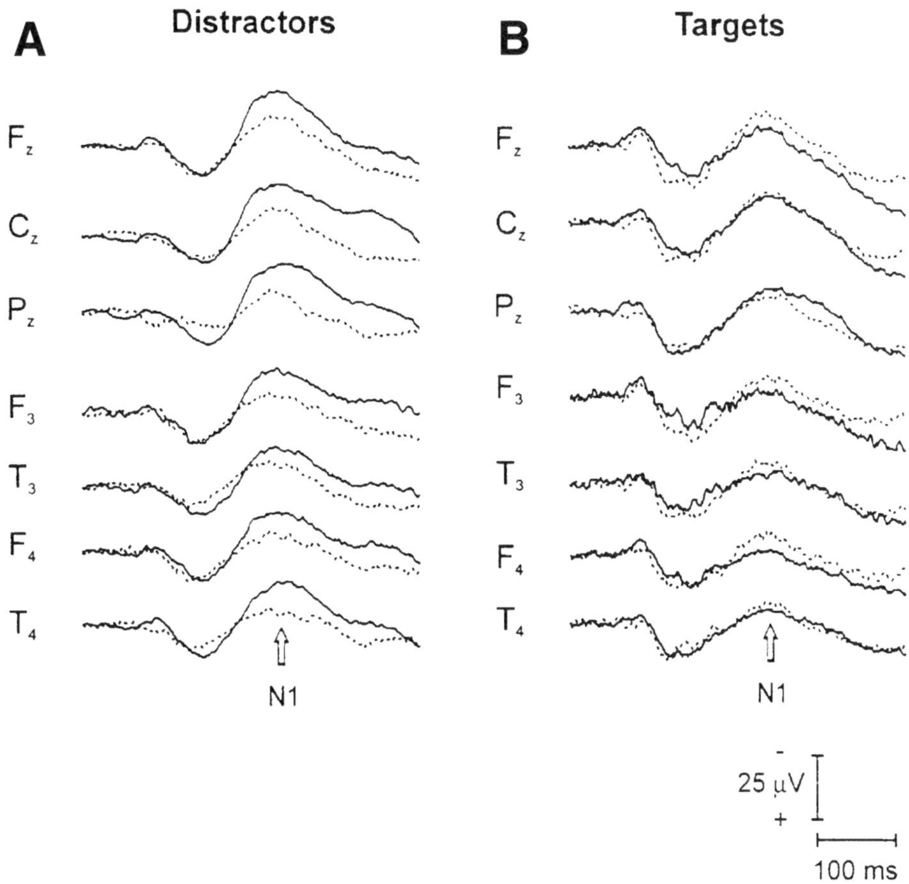

Fig. 4. Grand averaged ERPs for **(A)** nonanimal/distractor and for **(B)** animal/target stimuli in the control group (continuous line) and PD group (dotted line). Note that there is an amplitude difference of N1 component for distractors, but there is no N1 difference for targets. From ref. *75* with permission of Cognitive Brain Research.

3.2. N200 of the Visual ERP

Apparently P100 and P300 are independently affected in PD. Thus, it would be relevant to know the stage of visual processing where their independence becomes established. The analysis of earlier cognitive ERP components, such as N200, showed that this component is also independently changing from P300 *(47)*. The visual N200 that follows P100 and precedes P300 is probably a visual form of the auditory mismatch negativity *(67)*. This component is more negative for the infrequent deviant stimuli and distributed over the extrastriate visual areas and posterior-temporal cortex. N200 latency was delayed in nondemented patients with PD, even when P300 was not prolonged with a simple visual paradigm *(47)*. In a semantic discrimination task, the same result was found *(48)*. This further suggests that visual deficits and processes indexed by the P300 may reflect processing that is either parallel or well beyond the interface of bottom-up and top-down visual inputs *(68,69)*.

3.3. Electrophysiological Evidence of Visual Categorization Impairment

Although previous studies have suggested that the visual subsystem responsible for object-related visual analysis is spared until the later stages of PD *(35,64–66)*, recent electrophysiological studies have found it is otherwise.

The vast majority of human mental activities are based on categorical processes that serve adaptive and purposeful behavior *(70)*. Basic visual feature encoding and initial stages of perceptual categorization occur in the first 200-ms poststimulus, whereas conceptual and semantic properties are represented in later stages of information processing *(71,72)*. Thorpe and his associates found that nonanimal scenes elicited more negative responses than images with animals, even at 150 ms following stimulus onset (N1; *73,74*). Despite relatively preserved P100, this difference was not observable in patients with PD (*75,76;* Fig. 4). However, the exact psychological and physiological mechanisms of this difference are not well-established. It is hypothesized that the neostriatum may mediate feature weighting and extraction processes, and the differential N1 may refer to this function. This hypothesis is consistent with multiunit recording data from the basal ganglia of human volunteers. Electrophysiological responses revealed different neuronal responses when the subjects paid attention to select stimulus features (e.g., shape, orientation, and brightness; for review, *see* ref. *77*). This top-down attentional bias, probably mediated by frontostriatal circuits, can facilitate object categorization by feature weighting. In PD, a possible dysfunctional weighting and selecting process is reflected by the diminished differential N1.

In addition to frontostriatal circuits, one should consider other possible circuits of visual categorization should be considered. It has been suggested *(78)* that analysis of form and color of category exemplars takes places in the occipitotemporal extrastriate visual cortex. Support for the role of the occipitaltemporal areas in visual categorical perception is underlined by electrophysiological studies showing that response properties of monkey anterior inferior temporal (IT) neurons cannot account for all aspects of the categorical representation *(79)*. The prefrontal cortex contains category-specific units and receives input from the neostriatum, which receives inputs from large populations of IT neurons *(80)*.

Similarly to the previously described N1 effects, the amplitude of the N400 component is reduced in patients who have PD *(81,82)*. The ERP N400 component has been extensively investigated as an indicator of semantic relatedness: pictures and words appearing in an incongruent semantic context elicit more negative N400 *(83–85)*. Thus, an attenuated N400 may refer to impaired working memory functions responsible for the maintenance of context *(35,86)*.

3.4. Electrophysiological Deficits in Distributed Mechanisms of Visual Perception

There is growing evidence that cognitive processes require the interaction between distributed neuronal groups. The "binding hypothesis" essentially assumes that it is not feasible to provide specialized brain areas for each of the multitude of different tasks. Rather, different areas have to be "bound" together within very short time intervals to solve perceptual tasks likely by synchronized or desynchronized activities of neuronal assemblies. The frequency range around 20 to 60 Hz is known as "gamma-band" activity. This rhythm exists spontaneously and/or can be evoked, induced, or emitted in different structures of the central nervous system in response to olfactory, auditory, somatosensory and visual stimuli or in concomitance with attentional/perceptual-cognitive processes. In normal observers, γ-band activity has been shown to accompany primary visual-evoked responses and be suppressed during the P300 period of the VEP *(51,87)*. However, this suppression in PD does not exist *(51)*. Generally, this cortical suppression is thought to reflect competitive hippocampal gamma activation associated with P300 target processing *(88);* therefore, hippocampal gamma activation may be caused by short-term memory updating. In patients who have PD the lack of "cognitive" γ suppression may reflect on visuocognitive processing deficits during performance of the task *(51)*. Additionally, it was observed that cortico–cortical frequency coherence can be modified by levodopa therapy in patients with PD *(89)*. Using a simple visual-tracking task, coherence increase was found after levodopa therapy, whereas without levodopa, the coherence was much reduced. It appears that ascending dopaminergic projections from the mesencephalon may modulate the pattern and extent of cortico–cortical coupling in visuomotor tasks. Additionally, it seems that time-frequency analysis of visual ERPs might contribute to differentiate patients with and without hippocampal dysfunction or, more generally, it could help bring better understanding of the binding of different cortical areas in dysfunctional cognitive processing in PD.

4. CONCLUSION

In the last two decades, an increasing body of evidence has revealed specific and nonspecific visual abnormalities in patients with PD. Most prominently, the abnormal and levodopa-sensitive PERG tuning *(7,42,90),* levodopa-sensitive delayed VEPs *(1),* and reduced CS that fluctuates with the dopaminergic state *(2,9,16,17)* provide evidence of a specific parkinsonian retinopathy. Improvements of these abnormalities by levodopa therapy in humans and in the PD monkey model have established a link between the visual symptoms observed in PD and retinal pathology. However, beyond the retina, electrophysiological, neuropsychological, and functional neuroimaging data suggest dopaminergic dysregulation of a higher level of visuocognitive functions in the cortico–subcortical system in PD. Recent studies of visual categorization deficits imply that the posterior parietal cortex is involved in this disease. A wealth of cognitive studies in PD are consistent with the hypothesis of Brown and Marsden *(91),* who proposed that patients who have PD are particularly impaired in self-initiated, effort-demanding tasks. At this point, it is clear that visuocognitive impairment is not a passive or predictable consequence of retinal dopaminergic deficiency. However, the anatomical site(s), particularly the exclusive role of the frontal cortex, has to be modified in view of recent studies implying a posterior stream of visual-working memory.

Some overwhelming, human and electrophysiological evidence indicates that dopaminergic therapy improves visuocognitive impairment, at least in the initial phase of PD. As the disease progresses, this treatment type seems to be less effective, possibly because of the nondopaminergic disturbances of PD (noradrenergic, serotonergic, and cholinergic deficits and cortical Lewy bodies; *35,87*). In the future, novel pharmacological methods targeting the neurodegenerative process itself (e.g., compounds acting on the glutaminergic *N*-methyl-D-aspartate and growth-factor receptors) may become warranted.

REFERENCES

1. Bodis-Wollner I, Yahr MD. Measurements of visual evoked potentials in Parkinson's disease. Brain 1978;101:661–671.
2. Bodis-Wollner I. Visual deficits related to dopamine deficiency in experimental animals and Parkinson's disease patients. Trends Neurosci 1990;13:296–302.
3. Bodis-Wollner I, Tzelepi A. The push-pull action of dopamine on spatial tuning of the monkey retina: the effects of dopaminergic deficiency and selective Dl and D2 receptor ligands on the pattern electroretinogram. Vision Res 1998;38:1479–1487.
4. Bodis-Wollner I, Tzelepi A. Push-pull model of dopamine's action in the retina. In: Hung GK, Ciuffreda KC, eds. Models of the Visual System. Kluwer Academic Publishers, New York, 2000, pp. 191–214.
5. Bodis-Wollner I. Pattern evoked potential changes in Parkinson's disease are stimulus-dependent. Neurology 1985;35:1675–1676.
6. Stanzione P, Piereli F, Peppe A, et al. (1989) And Bernardi G. Pattern visual evoked potential abnormalities in Parkinson's disease: effects of L-Dopa therapy. Clin Vis Sci 1989;4:115–127.
7. Tagliati M, Bodis-Wollner I, Yahr M. The pattern electroretinogram in Parkinson's disease reveals lack of retinal spatial tuning. Electroencephalogr Clin Neurophysiol 1996;100:1–11.
8. Tartaglione A, Pizio N, Bino G, et al. VEP changes in Parkinson's disease are stimulus dependent. J Neurol Neurosurg Psychiatry 1984;47:305–307.
9. Bodis-Wollner I, Marx MS, Mitra S, et al. Visual dysfunction in Parkinson's disease. Loss in spatiotemporal contrast sensitivity. Brain 1987;110:1675–1698.
10. Regan D, Maxner C. Orientation-selective visual loss in patients with Parkinson's disease. Brain 1987;110:415–432.
11. Mestre D, Blin O, Serratrice G, Pailhous J. Spatiotemporal contrast sensitivity differs in normal aging and Parkinson's disease. Neurology 1990;40:1710–1714.
12. Bulens C, Meerwaldt JD, van der Wildt GJ. Effect of stimulus orientation on contrast sensitivity in Parkinson's disease. Neurology 1988;38:76–81.
13. Delalande I, Hache JC, Forzy G, et al. Do visual-evoked potentials and spatiotemporal contrast sensitivity help to distinguish idiopathic Parkinson's disease and multiple system atrophy? Mov Disord 1998;13:446–452.
14. Diederich NJ, Raman R, Leurgans S, Goetz CG. Progressive worsening of spatial and chromatic processing deficits in Parkinson disease. Arch Neurol 2002;59:1249–1252.
15. Bodis-Wollner I. Visual contrast sensitivity. Neurology 1988;38:336–337.
16. Masson G, Mestre D, Blin O. Dopaminergic modulation of visual sensitivity in man. Fundam Clin Pharmacol 1993;7:449–463.

17. Marx M, Bodis-Wollner I, Bobak P, et al. Temporal frequency-dependent VEP changes in Parkinson's disease. Vision Res 1986;26:185–193.
18. Gottlob I, Schneider E, Heider W, Skrandies W. Alteration of visual evoked potentials and electroretinograms in Parkinson's disease. Electroencephalogr. Clin Neurophysiol 1987;66:349–357.
19. Peppe A, Stanzione P, Pierelli F, et al. Visual alterations in de novo Parkinson's disease, pattern electroretinogram latencies are more delayed and more reversible by levodopa than are visual evoked potentials. Neurology 1995;45:1144–1148.
20. Okuda B, Tachibana H, Kawabata K, et al. Visual evoked potentials (VEPs) in Parkinson's disease: correlation of pattern VEPs abnormality with dementia. Alzheimer. Dis Assoc Disord 1995;9:68–72.
21. Bhaskar PA, Vanchilingam S, Bhaskar EA, et al. Effect of L-dopa on visual evoked potential in patients with Parkinson's disease. Neurology 1986;36:1119–1121.
22. Peppe A, Stanzione P, Pierantozzi M, et al. Does pattern electroretinogram spatial tuning alteration in Parkinson's disease depend on motor disturbances or retinal dopaminergic loss? Electroencephalogr Clin Neurophysiol 1998;106:374–382.
23. Albrecht D, Quaschling U, Zippel U, Davidowa H. Effects of dopamine on neurons of the lateral geniculate nucleus: an iontophoretic study. Synapse 1996;23:70–78.
24. Reader TA, Quesney LF. Dopamine in the visual cortex of the cat. Experientia 1986;42:1242–1244.
25. Bohnen NI, Minoshima S, Giordani B, et al. Motor correlates of occipital glucose hypometabolism in Parkinson's disease without dementia. Neurology 1999;52:541–546.
26. Blakemore C, Campbell FW. On the existence of neurones in the human visual system selectively sensitive to the orientation and size of retinal images. J Physiol 1969;203:237–260.
27. Zeki S. The distribution of wavelength and orientation selective cells in different areas of monkey visual cortex. Proc R Soc Lond B Biol Sci 1983;217:449–470.
28. Tebartz van Elst L, Greenlee MW, Foley JM, Lucking CH. Contrast detection, discrimination and adaptation in patients with Parkinson's disease and multiple system atrophy. Brain 1997;120:2219–2228.
29. Nieoullon A. Dopamine and the regulation of cognition and attention. Prog Neurobiol 2002;67:53–83.
30. Wichmann T, DeLong MR. Functional neuroanatomy of the basal ganglia in Parkinson's disease. Adv Neurol 2003;91:9–18.
31. Goldman-Rakic PS, Lidow MS, Smiley JF, Williams MS. The anatomy of dopamine in monkey and human prefrontal cortex. J Neural Transm Suppl 1992;36:163–177.
32. Gabrieli JD. Memory systems analyses of mnemonic disorders in aging and age-related diseases. Proc Natl Acad Sci USA 1996;93:13534–13540.
33. LeBras C, Pillon B, Damier P, Dubois B. At which steps of spatial working memory processing do striatofrontal circuits intervene in humans? Neuropsychologia 1999;37:83–90.
34. Owen AM, Downes JJ, Sahakian BJ, et al. Planning and spatial working memory following frontal lobe lesions in man. Neuropsychologia 1990;28:1021–1034.
35. Owen AM, Iddon JL, Hodges JR, et al. Spatial and non-spatial working memory at different stages of Parkinson's disease. Neuropsychologia 1997;35:519–532.
36. Grossman M, Zurif E, Lee C, et al. Information processing speed and sentence comprehension in Parkinson's disease. Neuropsychology 2002;16:174–181.
37. Mattay VS, Tessitore A, Callicott JH, et al. Dopaminergic modulation of cortical function in patients with Parkinson's disease. Ann Neurol 2002;51:156–164.
38. Cools R, Stefanova E, Barker RA, et al. Dopaminergic modulation of high-level cognition in Parkinson's disease: the role of the prefrontal cortex revealed by PET. Brain 2002;125:584–594.
39. Owen AM, James M, Leigh PN, et al. Fronto-striatal cognitive deficits at different stages of Parkinson's disease. Brain 1992;115:1727–1751.
40. Kutas M, McCarthy G, Donchin E. Augmenting mental chronometry: the P300 as a measure of stimulus evaluation time. Science 1977;197:792–795.
41. Sutton S, Braren M, Zubin J, John ER. Evoked-potential correlates of stimulus uncertainty. Science 1965;150:1187–1188.
42. Stanzione P, Fattapposta F, Giunti P, et al. P300 variations in parkinsonian patients before and during dopaminergic monotherapy: a suggested dopamine component in P300. Electroencephalogr Clin Neurophysiol 1991;80:446–453.
43. Tachibana H, Toda L, Sugita M. Actively and passively evoked P3 latency of event-related potentials in Parkinson's disease. J Neurol Sci 1992;111:134–142.
44. Goodin DS, Aminoff LM. Electrophysiological differences between demented and nondemented patients with Parkinson's disease. Ann Neurol 1987;21:90–94.
45. Toda K, Tachibana H, Sugita M, Konishi K. P300 and reaction time in Parkinson's disease. J Geriatr Psychiatry Neurol 1993;6:131–136.
46. Wang L, Kuroiwa Y, Li M, et al. The correlation between P300 alterations and regional cerebral blood flow in non-demented Parkinson's disease. Neurosci Lett 2000;282:133–136.
47. Antal A, Pfeiffer R, Bodis-Wollner I. Simultaneously evoked primary and cognitive visual evoked potentials distinguish younger and older patients with Parkinson's disease. J Neural Transm 1996;103:1053–1067.
48. Tachibana H, Aragane K, Miyata Y, Sugita M. Electrophysiological analysis of cognitive slowing in Parkinson's disease. J Neurol Sci 1997;149:47–56.

49. Sagliocco L, Bandini F, Pierantozzi M, et al. Electrophysiological evidence for visuocognitive dysfunction in younger non Caucasian patients with Parkinson's disease. J Neural Transm 1997;104:427–439.
50. Bodis-Wollner I, Borod JC, Cicero B, et al. Modality dependent changes in event-related potentials correlate with specific cognitive functions in nondemented patients with Parkinson's disease. J Neural Transm Park Dis Dement Sect 1995;9:197–209.
51. Bodis-Wollner I, Tzelepi A, Sagliocco L, et al. Visual processing deficit in Parkinson disease. In: Koga Y, Nagata K, Hirata K, eds. Brain Topography Today. Elsevier, Amsterdam, 1998, pp. 606–611.
52. Wang L, Kuroiwa Y, Kamitani T, et al. Effect of interstimulus interval on visual P300 in Parkinson's disease. J Neurol Neurosurg Psychiatry 1999;67:497–503.
53. Glover A, Ghilardi MF, Bodis-Wollner I, Onofrj M. Alterations in event-related potentials (ERPs) of MPTP-treated monkeys. Electroencephalogr Clin Neurophysiol 1988;71:461–468.
54. Antal A, Keri S, Bodis-Wollner I. Dopamine D2 receptor blockade alters the primary and cognitive components of visual evoked potentials in the monkey, Macaca fascicularis. Neurosci Lett 1997;232:179–181.
55. Goldman-Rakic PS. The cortical dopamine system: role in memory and cognition. Adv Pharmacol 1998;42:707–711.
56. Halgren E, Marinkovic K, Chauvel P. Generators of the late cognitive potentials in auditory and visual oddball tasks. Electroencephalogr Clin Neurophysiol 1998;106:156–164.
57. Chase TN, Mouradian MM, Fabbrini G, Juncos JL. Pathogenetic studies of motor fluctuations in Parkinson's disease. J Neural Transm Suppl 1988;27:3–10.
58. Sohn YH, Kim GW, Huh K, Kim JS. Dopaminergic influences on the P300 abnormality in Parkinson's disease. J Neurol Sci 1998;158:83–87.
59. Hansch EC, Syndulko K, Cohen SN, et al. Tourtellotte WW. Cognition in Parkinson disease: an event-related potential perspective. Ann Neurol 1982;11:599–607.
60. Prasher D, Findley L. Dopaminergic induced changes in cognitive and motor processing in Parkinson's disease: an electrophysiological investigation. J Neurol Neurosurg Psychiatry 1991;54:603–609.
61. Pillon B, Deweer B, Vidailhet M, et al. Is impaired memory for spatial location in Parkinson's disease domain specific or dependent on "strategic" processes? Neuropsychologia 1998;36:1–9.
62. Bandini F, Pierantozzi M, Bodis-Wollner I. The visuo-cognitive and motor effect of amantadine in non-Caucasian patients with Parkinson's disease. A clinical and electrophysiological study. J Neural Transm 2002;109:41–51.
63. Baddeley A. Recent developments in working memory. Curr Opin Neurobiol 1998;8:234–238.
64. Lee AC, Harris JP, Calvert JE. Impairments of mental rotation in Parkinson's disease. Neuropsychologia 1998;36:109–114.
65. Moreaud O, Fournet N, Roulin JL, et al. The phonological loop in medicated patients with Parkinson's disease: presence of phonological similarity and word length effects. J Neurol Neurosurg Psychiatry 1997;62:609–611.
66. Postle BR, Jonides J, Smith EE, et al. Spatial but not object, delayed response is impaired in early Parkinson's disease. Neuropsychology 1997;11:171–179.
67. Tales A, Newton P, Troscianko T, Butler S. Mismatch negativity in the visual modality. Neuroreport 1999;10:3363–3367.
68. Coull JT. Neural correlates of attention and arousal: insights from electrophysiology, functional neuroimaging and psychopharmacology. Prog Neurobiol 1998;55:343–361.
69. Kotchoubey B, Lang S. Parallel processing of physical and lexical auditory information in humans. Neurosci Res 2003;45:369–374.
70. Harnad S. Categorical Perception: The Groundwork of Cognition. Cambridge University Press, New York, 1987.
71. Hillyard SA, Teder-Salejarvi WA, Münte TF. Temporal dynamics of early perceptual processing. Curr Opin Neurobiol 1998;8:202–210.
72. Schendan HE, Ganis G, Kutas M. Neurophysiological evidence for visual perceptual categorization of words and faces within 150 ms. Psychophysiology 1998;35:240–251.
73. Thorpe S, Fize D, Marlot C. Speed of processing in the human visual system. Nature 1996;381:520–522.
74. VanRullen R, Thorpe SJ. The time course of visual processing: from early perception to decision-making. J Cogn Neurosci 2001;13:454–461.
75. Antal A, Keri S, Dibo G, et al. Electrophysiological correlates of visual categorization: evidence for cognitive dysfunctions in early Parkinson's disease. Brain Res Cogn Brain Res 2002;13:153–158.
76. Antal A, Keri S, Kincses T, et al. Corticostriatal circuitry mediates fast-track visual categorization. Brain Res Cogn Brain Res 2002;13:53–59.
77. Kropotov JD, Etlinger SC. Selection of actions in the basal ganglia-thalamocortical circuits: review and model. Int J Psychophysiol 1999;31:197–217.
78. Farah M, Humphreys GW, Rodman HR. Object and face recognition. In: Zigmond MJ, Bloom FE, Landis SC, et al., eds. Fundamental Neuroscience. Academic Press, New York, 1999, pp. 1339–1361.
79. Vogels R. Categorization of complex visual images by rhesus monkeys. Part 2: single-cell study. Eur J Neurosci 1999;11:1239–1255.
80. Cheng K, Saleem KS, Tanaka K. Organization of corticostriatal and corticoamygdalar projections arising from the anterior inferotemporal area TE of the macaque monkey: a Phaseolus vulgaris leucoagglutinin study. J Neurosci 1997;17:7902–7925.
81. Miyata Y, Tachibana H, Sugita M. Memory function in aging and Parkinson's disease—an event-related potential study. Nippon Ronen Igakkai Zasshi 1998;35:464–471.

82. Tachibana H, Miyata Y, Takeda M, et al. Event-related potentials reveal memory deficits in Parkinson's disease. Brain Res Cogn Brain Res 1999;8:165–172.
83. Barrett SE, Rugg MD. Event-related potentials and the semantic matching of pictures. Brain Cogn 1990;14:201–212.
84. Friedman D. Cognitive event-related potential components during continuous recognition memory for pictures. Psychophysiology 1990;27:136–148.
85. Kutas M, Hillyard SA. Brain potentials during reading reflect word expectancy and semantic association. Nature 1984;307:161–163.
86. Cohen JD, Servan-Schreiber D. Context, cortex and dopamine: a connectionist approach to behavior and biology in schizophrenia. Psychol Rev 1992;99:45–77.
87. Bodis-Wollner I. Visualizing the next steps in Parkinson Disease. Arch Neurol 2002;59:1233–1234.
88. Basar-Eroglu C, Basar E. A compound P300–40 Hz response of the cat hippocampus. Int J Neurosci 1991;60:227–237.
89. Cassidy M, Brown P. Task-related EEG-EEG coherence depends on dopaminergic activity in Parkinson's disease. Neuroreport 2001;12:703–707.
90. Peppe A, Stanzione P, Pierelli F, et al. Low contrast stimuli enhance PERG sensitivity to the visual dysfunction in Parkinson's disease. Electroencephalogr Clin Neurophysiol 1992;82:453–457.
91. Brown RG, Marsden CD. Cognitive function in Parkinson's disease: from description to theory. Trends Neurosci 1990;13:21–29.

21
Olfactory Dysfunction

Sarah Furtado and Zbigniew K. Wszolek

SUMMARY

Numerous studies have established the presence of olfactory dysfunction in Parkinson's disease (PD), which includes deficits in odor identification, threshold detection, and odor recognition memory. Sniff vigor may also have an important role in PD, but this is not typically assessed. Regardless, the olfactory deficit in PD typically ranges from moderate hyposmia to anosmia and is therefore more severe than the milder hyposmia (or even normosmia) found in patients with other Parkinsonian syndromes, such as multiple system atrophy, progressive supranuclear palsy, and corticobasal ganglionic degeneration. Patients with inherited Parkinsonism also have significant deficits in olfactory function. Lastly, this chapter reviews the neuropathology of olfactory dysfunction in PD.

Olfactory dysfunction in PD may precede the onset of motor dysfunction by many years. This information may become important in (1) making a clinical diagnosis of PD, (2) distinguishing PD from other Parkinsonian syndromes, and (3) making decisions regarding the utilization of potential neuroprotective therapies when they become available.

This chapter reviews the nature of olfactory dysfunction in PD. Neuroanatomical aspects of olfaction are first considered.

Key Words: Parkinson's disease (PD); olfaction; olfactory nerve; hyposmia; sniff vigor.

1. INTRODUCTION

Olfactory dysfunction has long been recognized as one of the nonmotor complications of Parkinson's disease (PD) and may precede the onset of the motor disorder. Recent advances in neuroimaging and anatomy have further elucidated the nature of the impairment. The purpose of this chapter is to review this literature and discuss the utility of this information for advancing research and developing therapies for PD.

2. OLFACTION IN HUMANS: ANATOMICAL AND CLINICAL CONSIDERATIONS

The olfactory epithelium in the posterior nasal cavity is a specialized sensory epithelium responsible for carrying information regarding the plethora of odorants encountered by humans. This specialized epithelium contains bipolar receptor cells: the short process extends to the mucosal surface, and the long process forms the olfactory nerve (cranial nerve I), which projects to the olfactory bulb beneath each hemisphere. These bipolar cells undergo regeneration approximately every 60 days from precursor basal cells (also in the epithelium), necessitating the continuous formation of connections between the epithelia and olfactory bulb *(1)*.

Odorants are absorbed into the mucous layer overlying the receptor cell through the aid of olfactory-binding protein, which facilitates interaction of the odorant with receptor cell cilia. This interac-

From: *Current Clinical Neurology*
Parkinson's Disease and Nonmotor Dysfunction
Edited by: R. F. Pfeiffer and I. Bodis-Wollner © Humana Press Inc., Totowa, NJ

tion results in increased frequency of action potentials, usually increasing the level of cyclic adenosine monophosphate through adenyl cyclase; this stimulation is odorant potency-dependent. Single neurons may respond to multiple odorants, enabling humans to detect hundreds of different odorants. However, individual neurons express distinct receptor molecules, and up to 1000 odorant receptors are thought to exist. Research suggests that nasal mucosae are organized topographically; e.g., certain odorants preferentially activate the anterior mucosae, whereas others activate posterior regions *(1,2)*.

The unmyelinated axons of the roughly 6 million bipolar receptor cells form the olfactory nerve, traversing the cribriform plate of the ethmoid bone to terminate in the olfactory bulb on the dendritic arbor of mitral cells and tufted cells. The specialized clusters in the area of termination are collectively referred to as glomeruli; dopamine and γ-aminobutyric acid are known transmitters in this area *(2,3)*. Neurons are also generated from the subventricular zone in the brain and migrate rostrally to the olfactory bulb, where differentiation occurs into local interneurons. The olfactory tract (axons of mitral and tufted cells) then continues to the primary olfactory cortex (without relay in the thalamus). Synapses are located in the anterior olfactory nucleus (caudal to the olfactory bulb with some neurons in the olfactory tract), olfactory tubercle, pyriform cortex (receptor of dopaminergic projections from the midbrain *[3]*), cortical nucleus of the amygdala, and entorhinal area. The entorhinal area projects to the hippocampus; the olfactory tubercle projects to the medial dorsal nucleus of the hippocampus, then projects to the orbitofrontal cortex and is thought to be involved in the conscious perception of smell. The amygdala projects to the hypothalamus and midbrain and is believed to be related to the emotional perception of smell *(1,2)*. The connections of the olfactory system are shown in Fig. 1.

The study of olfaction in humans involves the use of tests that assess odor threshold detection, odor discrimination, odor identification, and odor memory. An example of a commonly used test (for assessing odor identification) is the University of Pennsylvania Smell Identification Test (UPSIT; Sensonics, Haddon Heights, NJ), which asks subjects to identify 40 odors in a multiple-choice paradigm. This test is widely available, easy to use, has standardized normative data with reproducible results, and is available in multiple languages. The Cross-Cultural Smell Identification Test combines a simplified version of the UPSIT with odor threshold detection *(4)*. Other less commonly used techniques involve recording olfactory event-related potentials in response to different odorants, morphological evaluation of the olfactory epithelium performed during local or generalized anesthesia, and postmortem pathological analysis of olfactory structures *(4)*.

Through the use of these tests and others, certain discoveries have been made regarding human olfaction: (1) generally, women have a better sense of smell than men; (2) odor identification is mediated partly by a heritable component; (3) a significant loss in sense of smell occurs after 65 years of age; (4) this loss occurs earlier in men than in women; (5) olfaction is compromised by smoking and urban living conditions *(2)*.

Functional neuroimaging obtained during olfactory testing showed activation of primary olfactory forebrain structures with expected changes (less activation in men than in women and less activation with increasing age). Functional magnetic resonance imaging techniques showed that amygdala activation was associated with odor intensity, whereas orbitofrontal cortex activation was associated with odor valence *(5)*. Odorants may activate posterior lateral areas of the cerebellum, whereas the act of sniffing activates the anterior cerebellar areas *(6)*.

This chapter focuses on the main olfactory system (cranial nerve I and its connections). The vomeronasal/accessory olfactory system and trigeminal somatosensory systems *(2),* which have not been well-studied in humans, are not discussed here.

3. OLFACTION AND PD

The first study of olfaction in PD was that of Ansari and Johnson *(7),* who conducted a test of odor detection threshold in 22 men treated for PD. Study criteria excluded patients with head trauma, nasal

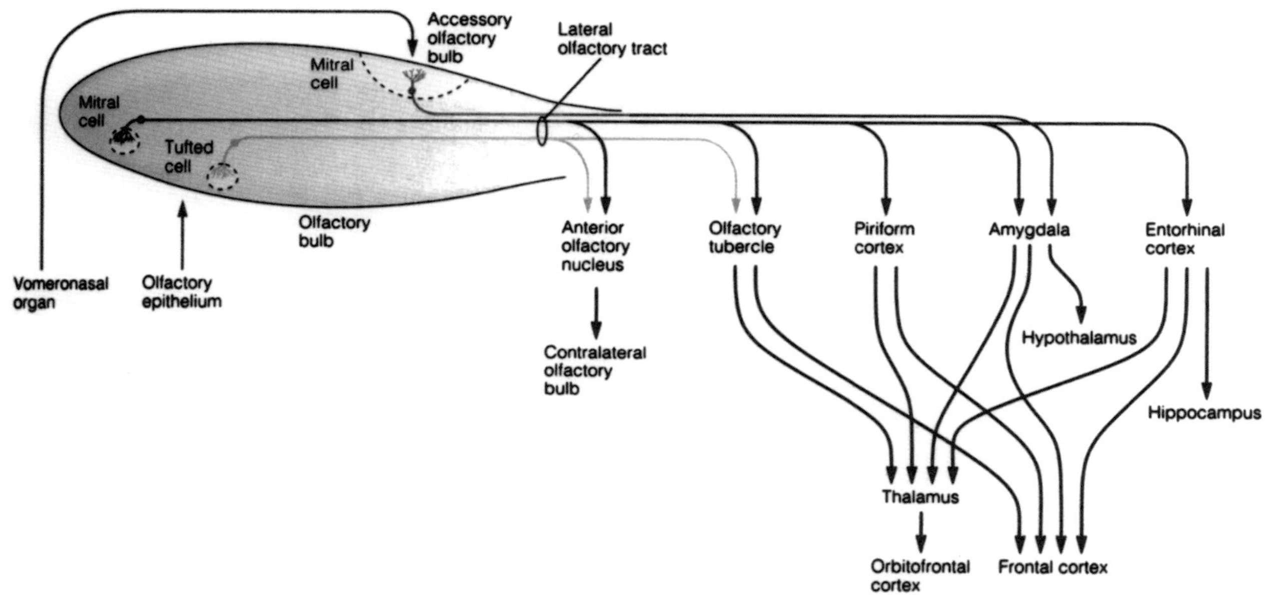

Fig. 1. Connections of the olfactory system. From Kandel ER, Schwartz JH, Jessell TM, eds. Principles of Neurol Science, 4th ed. New York: McGraw-Hill, 2000: 633, with permission of McGraw-Hill Companies.

injury, or other significant comorbidity. When compared to control subjects with other neurologic disorders (e.g., seizure, multiple sclerosis, stroke, or headache), patients with PD were impaired in their detection of amyl acetate. The odor detection threshold appeared to be related to the rate of disease progression but not to treatment *(7)*.

In another early description of olfactory dysfunction in PD, Ward et al. *(8)* tested patients with PD for odor detection threshold as well as the discrimination of common odorants. Patients who had PD were significantly impaired in both tests; some were anosmic. Treatment and PD duration had no influence on olfactory dysfunction.

Tissingh et al. *(9)* assessed odor detection, discrimination (without naming), and identification in patients with treated or early untreated PD in comparison to healthy controls. Both the treated and the untreated patients with PD showed significant impairment in all three tests. Because a deficit in odor detection may influence odor discrimination and identification, data from these tests were corrected for odor detection before analysis. With this correction, medicated patients did not perform as well as unmedicated patients on tests of odor discrimination or identification, possibly because of disease progression.

Similarly, Muller and colleagues *(10,11)* conducted tests of odor threshold detection, discrimination, and identification in 50 patients with treated or untreated PD. All PD patients demonstrated moderate-to-complete anosmia, but no relationship was found between anosmia and PD subtype or duration of disease. Deficits were maintained over time.

Olfactory dysfunction in patients with PD has been reported extensively *(12–14)*. The findings are generally robust with dysfunction demonstrated in the areas of odor identification, threshold detection, and odor recognition memory *(15)*. However, variable findings remain in the following areas: (1) stage of disease *(7,12)*, (2) treatment status *(8,9)*, (3) degree of olfactory impairment in each nostril *(9,16,17)*, and (4) possible disease subtype *(10,11,18)*. This variability may be related to methodological issues (whether some or all tests of olfaction are used; whether patients with head injury, active smoking, or dementia have been excluded; or whether the diagnosis of PD is accurate). Interestingly, olfactory dysfunction in PD does not respond to apomorphine *(19)*, which suggests that this dysfunction is not mediated by the dopaminergic system.

The importance of methodological considerations is reflected in investigations by Sobel and colleagues *(20)* into potential causes of olfactory dysfunction in PD. Patients who had PD indicated a significant deficit in sniffing ability as assessed by reduced sniff airflow rate and volume; this dysfunction influenced their ability to perform on olfactory function tests. Increasing sniff vigor improved olfactory performance in patients with the poorest olfaction. Because vigor of sniffing is not usually measured in tests of olfactory function, there may be an overestimation of the olfactory deficit in PD.

The olfactory deficit may precede the onset of motor deficit in PD by many years, which has implications for early diagnosis *(12,21)* and potential neuroprotective medications. Montgomery et al. *(21)* found a higher proportion of abnormal scores on a PD battery, including studies of olfaction in first-degree and clinically unaffected relatives of patients with PD than in controls with no family history of PD. Some of these first-degree relatives later developed PD.

In the aforementioned study by Ward et al. *(8)*, a considerable proportion of the control group was either a clinically unaffected monozygotic or same-sex dizygotic twin of the proband. In the case of one set of twins, the olfactory deficit was more marked in the unaffected cotwin than in the affected subject. Subsequent research indicates that longitudinal follow-up increases the likelihood of PD diagnosis in the cotwin *(22)*, along with the finding (described in Chapter 4) that olfactory dysfunction may precede the onset of motor abnormalities of PD by several years. In light of this research, one wonders whether the study by Ward et al. *(8)* may have underestimated the severity of the olfactory deficit in PD and whether the olfactory deficit described in the unaffected cotwin may have been an early marker of PD in this particular individual.

Berendse et al. *(23)* studied 25 hyposmic and 23 normosmic relatives of patients with PD through the use of single-photon emission-computed tomography (SPECT) with 2(β)-carboxymethoxy-3(β)(4-iodophenyl) tropane (β-CIT). They found reductions in striatal dopamine transporter binding in 4 of 25 hyposmic relatives but in none of the 23 normosmic relatives. Clinical Parkinsonism developed in 2 of the 4 hyposmic relatives with abnormal SPECT scans 6–12 months after the SPECT studies. A unilateral resting tremor developed in a third hyposmic relative, but no other features of Parkinsonism were observed *(23)*.

4. OLFACTION IN OTHER PARKINSONIAN SYNDROMES AND INHERITED PD

The demonstration of olfactory dysfunction in PD has raised questions regarding the specificity of this dysfunction for PD. Various studies have examined olfactory dysfunction in other Parkinsonian syndromes. Generally, a mild deficit has been shown (i.e., mild hyposmia in patients with multiple system atrophy and normosmia in patients with progressive supranuclear palsy [PSP] or corticobasal ganglionic degeneration [CBGD]), but the deficit in PD is more severe *(10,11,24)*. Normosmia has also been found in Parkinsonism induced by 1-methyl-4-phenyl-1,2,3,6-tetrahydropyridine *(25)*. These findings have raised the possibility that olfactory testing may provide another tool in the clinical armamentarium to distinguish idiopathic PD from other Parkinsonian syndromes.

In contrast, Ahlskog et al. *(26)* showed a marked impairment on the UPSIT in patients with various subtypes of the amyotrophic lateral sclerosis-Parkinsonian complex found in the native Chamorro population of Guam. Lesser deficits of olfactory function were also shown in the Chamorro control group, raising the potential of presymptomatic disease in these individuals.

Olfactory dysfunction in familial Parkinsonism has also been addressed. Markopoulou et al. *(27)* administered the UPSIT to affected members of various large Parkinsonian kindreds with either idiopathic PD (families B, D, and H) or Parkinsonism-plus phenotypes (family G, pallido-ponto-nigral degeneration [PPND] family). In the idiopathic PD kindreds, four of the six affected individuals were anosmic and two were microsmic; three of the four at-risk individuals were microsmic, and one was normosmic. In the Parkinsonism-plus families, five of the six affected individuals were anosmic, and one was microsmic; six of the eight at-risk individuals were normosmic, and two were microsmic. As expected, the clinically affected individuals demonstrated greater olfactory dysfunction than the at-risk individuals. Among anosmic or microsmic patients, those with the PD phenotype were similar to those with the Parkinsonism-plus phenotype in degree of olfactory impairment. However, affected or at-risk individuals from the families with the Parkinsonism-plus phenotype were less likely to be anosmic or microsmic and more likely to be normosmic than those with the PD phenotype. Olfactory dysfunction appeared to present at early stages of the illness. Notably, the genetic defects are known in two of these families (in the gene for α-synuclein in family H and tau in the PPND family), suggesting that olfactory dysfunction in these families is part of an inherited disorder.

We have shown significant deficits on the UPSIT in affected members of the Alberta family, a family with Parkinsonism-predominant spinocerebellar ataxia type 2 *(28)*. Two affected family members also had changes on positron emission tomography scanning (decreased fluorodopa striatal uptake, normal-to-increased raclopride binding) that were reminiscent of idiopathic PD. In the patients we examined, there is a possible relationship between the olfactory deficit and disease duration, but the number of patients available for examination was small.

A summary of the findings on Parkinsonism associated with olfactory dysfunction is given in Table 1.

5. PATHOLOGY OF OLFACTORY DYSFUNCTION IN PD

Crino et al. *(29)* used β-amyloid staining to examine olfactory epithelium from three patients with PD. In two of these patients, dystrophic neurites without Lewy bodies were found, occurring largely in the basal portions of the olfactory epithelium and suggesting localization to basal cells, the precursors of the olfactory neurons. This finding suggests that β-amyloid may participate in the production of olfactory neurons. It should be noted that similar staining was also found in patients with Alzheimer's disease and Down's syndrome *(29)*.

Table 1
Parkinsonism Associated With Olfactory Dysfunction

Disease	Olfactory function	References
Parkinson's disease	Impaired	Numerous
Progressive supranuclear palsy	Normal	Wenning et al. *(24)*
Corticobasal ganglionic degeneration	Normal	Wenning et al. *(24)*
Multiple system atrophy	Mild impairment	Wenning et al. *(24)* Muller et al. *(10,11)*
MPTP-induced Parkinsonism	Normal	Doty et al. *(25)*
Guamanian ALS-Parkinsonism complex	Impaired	Ahlskog et al. *(26)*
Familial Parkinson's disease		Markopoulou et al. *(27)*
Family H (α-synuclein)	Impaired	
Family B	Impaired	
Family D	Impaired	
Familial Parkinsonism		Markopoulou et al. *(27)*
Family G	Impaired	
PPND family (tau)	Impaired	
Alberta family (spinocerebellar ataxia type 2)	Impaired	Furtado et al. *(28)*

ALS, amyotrophic lateral sclerosis; MPTP, 1-methyl-4-phenyl-1,2,3,6-tetrahydropyridine; PPND, pallido-ponto-nigral degeneration.

Hawkes et al. *(13)* examined the olfactory bulbs in a postmortem study of patients who had PD. Lewy bodies were seen in every olfactory bulb examined, including the anterior olfactory nucleus, and were sufficiently distinctive to allow a presumptive diagnosis of PD. Pearce et al. *(30)* reviewed the anterior olfactory nucleus of the olfactory bulb in PD. On gross neuropathologic examination, the olfactory bulbs were flattened and shrunken, and the tracts were markedly thinned. Notable neuronal loss was observed in the anterior olfactory neurons of the olfactory bulbs and tracts; neuronal loss correlated strongly with disease duration but not with age of onset. Lewy bodies were found in all areas, as confirmed by staining for ubiquitin. The typical trilaminar structure was lacking, and the Lewy bodies found resembled cortical Lewy bodies (Fig. 2). Similar findings in the anterior olfactory nucleus of the olfactory bulb were found by Hawkes et al. *(13)*. Keeping with the normosmia demonstrated in PSP and CBGD, Tsuboi and colleagues *(31)* found minimal tau pathology in the olfactory bulbs in 28 cases of PSP and 3 cases of CBGD.

Harding et al. *(32)* examined the amygdala in postmortem analysis of brains from nondemented patients with PD at various disease stages. Amygdala volume was reduced in PD by about 20%. Lewy bodies were found throughout the various nuclei of the amygdala in PD, including the cortical nucleus, and present in approximately 4% of neurons with the concentration of Lewy bodies in the cortical and basolateral nuclei. A significant loss of neurons was also observed in the cortical nucleus of the amygdala, but importantly, these patients had not been examined for olfactory dysfunction.

6. OLFACTORY DYSFUNCTION AND ADVANCES IN RESEARCH AND THERAPY FOR PD

How can this information about the olfactory deficit in PD be used to help patients with the disorder? Olfactory dysfunction may provide clues to the pathogenesis of PD. Early olfactory dysfunction in PD may suggest a potential route for pathogenesis related to virus or neurotoxin inhalation and subsequent olfactory dysfunction; alternatively, olfactory dysfunction may be secondary to a primary degenerative process in PD *(9)*.

The diagnostic accuracy for PD, even with experienced neurologists specialized in movement disorders, is in the range of 65 to 75% when neuropathologic data from autopsy are available *(33,34)*.

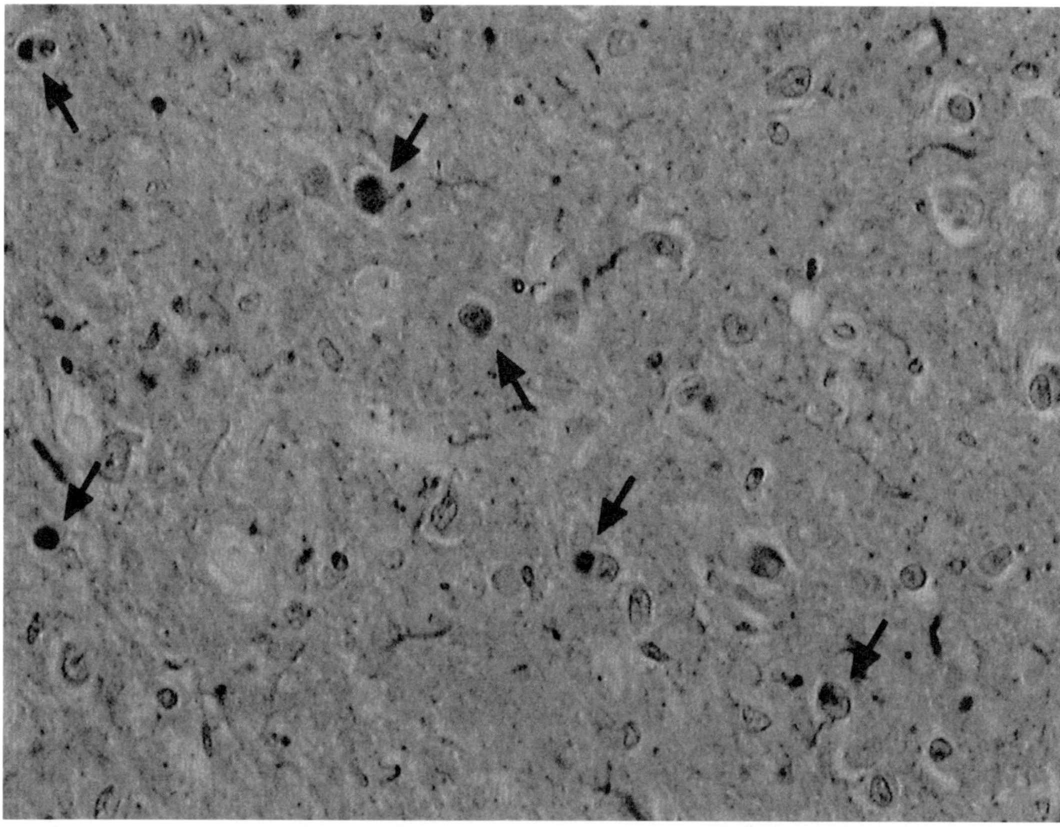

Fig. 2. Micrograph of anterior olfactory nucleus from a patient with a pathologic diagnosis of transitional Lewy body disease. Arrows indicate Lewy bodies of the cortical type. (Immunochemistry staining with α-synuclein antibody; ×200.) Figure courtesy of Drs. Y. Tsuboi and D. Dickson, Mayo Clinic, Jacksonville, FL.

However, routine incorporation of olfactory testing into the clinical battery, combined with functional neuroimaging, may increase diagnostic accuracy. Such an approach may also identify those at risk for idiopathic PD *(23,35)*.

What about patients who already have a diagnosis of PD? As described previously in Chapter 3, it is known that neurogenesis in the area of the olfactory epithelium and olfactory bulb (from the subventricular zone) is a lifelong process. Furthermore, experiential *(36,37)* and hormonal *(38)* influences modify neurogenesis in laboratory animals. Such manipulations may eventually become useful in the treatment of humans with PD.

7. CONCLUSION

Patients with PD have long been known to show olfactory dysfunction. This deficit appears to be present at an early stage of the illness and may precede the onset of the motor disorder. A portion of the deficit appears to be related to impairment in sniff vigor. Olfactory dysfunction has been found not only in inherited PD but also in some inherited Parkinsonism syndromes. However, when olfactory dysfunction occurs in Parkinsonism syndromes, the deficit is not as severe as that in idiopathic PD.

The olfactory dysfunction in PD has been characterized at a neuropathologic level regarding gross and microscopic atrophy of olfactory structures and the presence of Lewy bodies and dystrophic neurites in these structures. The potential for using this information to obtain clinical benefits for patients is discussed.

REFERENCES

1. Dodd J, Castellucci VF. Smell and taste: the chemical senses. In: Kandel ER, Schwartz JH, Jessell TM, eds. Principles of Neural Science, 3rd ed. Elsevier, New York, 1991, pp. 512–529.
2. Doty RL. Olfaction. Annu Rev Psychol 2001;52:423–452.
3. Liberini P, Parola S, Spano PF, Antonini L. Olfaction in Parkinson's disease: methods of assessment and clinical relevance. J Neurol 2000;247:88–96.
4. Wszolek ZK, Markopoulou K. Olfactory dysfunction in Parkinson's disease. Clin Neurosci 1998;5:94–101.
5. Anderson AK, Christoff K, Stappen I, et al. Dissociated neural representations of intensity and valence in human olfaction. Nat Neurosci 2003;6:196–202.
6. Sobel N, Prabhakaran V, Hartley CA, et al. Odorant-induced and sniff-induced activation in the cerebellum of the human. J Neurosci 1998;18:8990–9001.
7. Ansari KA, Johnson A. Olfactory function in patients with Parkinson's disease. J Chronic Dis 1975;28:493–497.
8. Ward CD, Hess WA, Calne DB. Olfactory impairment in Parkinson's disease. Neurology 1983;33:943–946.
9. Tissingh G, Berendse HW, Bergmans P, et al. Loss of olfaction in de novo and treated Parkinson's disease: possible implications for early diagnosis. Mov Disord 2001;16:41–46.
10. Muller A, Reichmann H, Livermore A, Hummel T. Olfactory function in idiopathic Parkinson's disease (IPD): results from cross-sectional studies in IPD patients and long-term follow-up of de-novo IPD patients. J Neural Transm 2002;109:805–811.
11. Muller A, Mungersdorf M, Reichmann H, et al. Olfactory function in Parkinsonian syndromes. J Clin Neurosci 2002;9:521–524.
12. Doty RL, Deems DA, Stellar S. Olfactory dysfunction in Parkinsonism: a general deficit unrelated to neurologic signs, disease stage, or disease duration. Neurology 1988;38:1237–1244.
13. Hawkes CH, Shephard BC, Daniel SE. Olfactory dysfunction in Parkinson's disease. J Neurol Neurosurg Psychiatry 1997;62:436–446.
14. Quinn NP, Rossor MN, Marsden CD. Olfactory threshold in Parkinson's disease. J Neurol Neurosurg Psychiatry 1987;50:88–89.
15. Mesholam RI, Moberg PJ, Mahr RN, Doty RL. Olfaction in neurodegenerative disease: a meta-analysis of olfactory functioning in Alzheimer's and Parkinson's diseases. Arch Neurol 1998;55:84–90.
16. Zucco G, Zeni MT, Perrone A, Piccolo I. Olfactory sensitivity in early-stage Parkinson patients affected by more marked unilateral disorder. Percept Mot Skills 2001;92:894–898.
17. Doty RL, Stern MB, Pfeiffer C, et al. Bilateral olfactory dysfunction in early stage treated and untreated idiopathic Parkinson's disease. J Neurol Neurosurg Psychiatry 1992;55:138–142.
18. Stern MB, Doty RL, Dotti M, et al. Olfactory function in Parkinson's disease subtypes. Neurology 1994;44:266–268.
19. Roth J, Radil T, Ruzicka E, et al. Apomorphine does not influence olfactory thresholds in Parkinson's disease. Funct Neurol 1998;13:99–103.
20. Sobel N, Thomason ME, Stappen I, et al. An impairment in sniffing contributes to the olfactory impairment in Parkinson's disease. Proc Natl Acad Sci USA 2001;98:4154–4159.
21. Montgomery EB. Jr, Baker KB, Lyons K, Koller WC. Abnormal performance on the PD test battery by asymptomatic first-degree relatives. Neurology 1999;52:757–762.
22. Dickson D, Farrer M, Lincoln S, et al. Pathology of PD in monozygotic twins with a 20-year discordance interval. Neurology 2001;56:981–982.
23. Berendse HW, Booij J, Francot CM, et al. Subclinical dopaminergic dysfunction in asymptomatic Parkinson's disease patients' relatives with a decreased sense of smell. Ann Neurol 2001;50:34–41.
24. Wenning GK, Shephard B, Hawkes C, et al. Olfactory function in atypical parkinsonian syndromes. Acta Neurol Scand 1995;91:247–250.
25. Doty RL, Singh A, Tetrud J, Langston JW. Lack of major olfactory dysfunction in MPTP-induced Parkinsonism. Ann Neurol 1992;32:97–100.
26. Ahlskog JE, Waring SC, Petersen RC, et al. Olfactory dysfunction in Guamanian ALS, Parkinsonism, and dementia. Neurology 1998;51:1672–1677.
27. Markopoulou K, Larsen KW, Wszolek EK, et al. Olfactory dysfunction in familial Parkinsonism. Neurology 1997;49:1262–1267.
28. Furtado S, Farrer M, Tsuboi Y, et al. SCA-2 presenting as Parkinsonism in an Alberta family: clinical, genetic and PET findings. Neurology 2002;59:1625–1627
29. Crino PB, Martin JA, Hill WD, et al. β-Amyloid peptide and amyloid precursor proteins in olfactory mucosa of patients with Alzheimer's disease, Parkinson's disease, and Down syndrome. Ann Otol Rhinol Laryngol 1995;104:655–661.
30. Pearce RK, Hawkes CH, Daniel SE. The anterior olfactory nucleus in Parkinson's disease. Mov Disord 1995;10:283–287.
31. Tsuboi Y, Wszolek ZK, Graff-Radford NR, et al. Tau pathology in the olfactory bulb correlates with Braak stage, Lewy body pathology and apolipoprotein epsilon4. Neuropathol Appl Neurobiol 2003;29:503–510.
32. Harding AJ, Stimson E, Henderson JM, Halliday GM. Clinical correlates of selective pathology in the amygdala of patients with Parkinson's disease. Brain 2002;125:2431–2445.
33. Rajput AH, Rozdilsky B, Rajput A. Accuracy of clinical diagnosis in Parkinsonism—a prospective study. Can J Neurol Sci 1991;18:275–278.

34. Hughes AJ, Daniel SE, Kilford L, Lees AJ. Accuracy of clinical diagnosis of idiopathic Parkinson's disease: a clinico-pathological study of 100 cases. J Neurol Neurosurg Psychiatry 1992;55:181–184.
35. Camicioli R, Grossmann SJ, Spencer PS, et al. Discriminating mild Parkinsonism: methods for epidemiological research. Mov Disord 2001;16:33–40.
36. Gheusi G, Cremer H, McLean H, et al. Importance of newly generated neurons in the adult olfactory bulb for odor discrimination. Proc Natl Acad Sci USA 2000;97:1823–1828.
37. Rochefort C, Gheusi G, Vincent JD, Lledo PM. Enriched odor exposure increases the number of newborn neurons in the adult olfactory bulb and improves odor memory. J Neurosci 2002;22:2679–2689.
38. Shingo T, Gregg C, Enwere E, et al. Pregnancy-stimulated neurogenesis in the adult female forebrain mediated by prolactin. Science 2003;299:117–120.

22

Pain Syndromes and Disorders of Sensation

Blair Ford and Ronald F. Pfeiffer

SUMMARY

Although routine clinical neurological examination generally does not reveal any abnormality of sensation in persons with Parkinson's disease (PD), subjective sensory symptoms are quite frequently present, and objective abnormalities of proprioceptive function and sensorimotor integration have been demonstrated with sophisticated testing. Primary sensory symptoms of PD may include paresthesias of varied descriptions (numbness, tingling, and burning).

Painful symptoms in PD can be classified into five categories: musculoskeletal pain, radicular or neuropathic pain, dystonia-related pain, primary (central) pain, and akathitic discomfort. Musculoskeletal pain in the form of shoulder stiffness frequently develops in persons with PD, often preceding the development of more classic motor features of the condition. Spinal deformities and painful contractures may also complicate the clinical picture in individuals with PD. The postural PD deformities may predispose to the development of compressive radiculopathy and sciatica. Dystonic spasms are among the most painful symptoms that a patient with PD may experience. Dystonia most often appears as an "off" phenomenon, but medication-induced dystonia may also occur. Primary or central pain is generated within the brain itself and is commonly characterized by bizarre, disagreeable painful sensations that are resistant to treatment. Parkinsonian akathisia is characterized by subjective inner restlessness that manifests as a constant need to move or change position, typically during "off" periods. The recognition and differentiation of parkinsonian pain from pain owing to other coincident medical conditions is vitally important for the effective diagnosis and treatment of pain in PD.

Key Words: Sensorimotor integration; pain; musculoskeletal; dystonia; central pain; akathisia.

1. INTRODUCTION

In his landmark description of what he labeled "the shaking palsy," James Parkinson provided an amazingly perceptive cataloging of the clinical characteristics of what is now known as Parkinson's disease (PD; *1*). His focus was on the motor features of the illness, yet, the information in this chapter demonstrates that abnormalities of sensation and sensory processing, evident with sophisticated measuring techniques unavailable in Parkinson's era, also occur in PD and that pain can be an important, and sometimes devastating, feature of the malady.

2. SENSORY IMPAIRMENT

2.1. *Historical Aspects*

If only the routine sensory testing performed during the usual clinical neurological examination is considered, James Parkinson's assertion that sensation is spared in PD is correct. On routine clinical testing, objective sensory loss is not apparent in patients with PD *(2)*. However, that is not the entire

From: *Current Clinical Neurology*
Parkinson's Disease and Nonmotor Dysfunction
Edited by: R. F. Pfeiffer and I. Bodis-Wollner © Humana Press Inc., Totowa, NJ

story. Subjective sensory symptoms are actually frequently present, and more sophisticated sensory testing does indeed demonstrate the presence of impairment of some aspects of sensation in PD.

In the years following Parkinson's original treatise, descriptions of subjective sensory phenomena in PD make their appearance. Hammond, in his 1871 textbook, maintains that "sensibility is rarely affected" in PD *(3),* whereas Charcot details the presence of "disagreeable sensations of a special order" that include not only "a nearly permanent sense of tension and traction in most of the muscles" and "an indefinable uneasiness, which shows itself in a perpetual desire for change of posture," but also "an habitual sensation of excessive heat," often associated with profuse perspiration *(4).* Gowers, while commenting that "cutaneous sensibility is never affected in paralysis agitans," goes on to add that "subjective sensations are frequent." Like Charcot, he describes "some abnormal sensation of temperature" in 75% of the 80 cases on which he had notes and a "sense of heat" in 22 of 47 individuals (47%) in whom the symptom was investigated *(5).*

2.2. Subjective Sensory Symptoms

In the modern era, attention was drawn to the presence of sensory symptoms in PD by Snider and colleagues *(6).* They noted the presence of sensory symptoms, not attributable to non-neurogenic causes, in 43 of 101 (43%) of the patients they studied and labeled them "primary sensory symptoms." Similar symptoms were present in only 8% of 64 controls. Although pain was the most frequently described sensory symptom, experienced by 29 (67%) of the 43 patients reporting sensory phenomena, tingling sensations were noted by 22 patients (51%), and 21 (49%) reported numbness. In their entire group of patients, 32% (32/101) admitted to the presence of paresthesia-like sensations not linked with sensory loss. In some individuals, sensory symptoms preceded development of the more classic motor features of PD. Koller subsequently reported that 38% (19/50) of patients with PD studied experienced sensory symptoms consisting of "true paresthesias" (numbness, tingling, and burning), compared with none of 15 individuals with essential tremor *(2).*

2.3. Objective Sensory Abnormalities

In recent years, more sophisticated sensory testing has demonstrated that objective sensory abnormalities may also be present in PD. Using sensitive techniques to study touch pressure and vibration perception on the plantar aspect of the foot, Pratorius et al. *(7)* demonstrated significantly higher thresholds (at least 2 times) in patients with PD in comparison to controls and suggested that this reduced sensitivity in the plantar foot might contribute to impaired balance control. Impaired joint position sense has also been demonstrated in PD, such that individuals with PD have more difficulty than controls in discriminating differences in the static angular position of their elbow joints *(8).* Tactile discrimination, studied by testing the ability to differentiate rectangular parallelepipeds (six-faced polyhedrons, all of whose faces are parallelograms) differing only in oblongness, is also diminished in persons with PD *(9).* Patients with PD also are impaired in their ability to discriminate differences in the location of simultaneously applied bilateral tactile stimuli *(10),* and elevated thresholds for two-point discrimination have been noted in the index fingers of patients who have PD *(11).*

Abnormalities in sensorimotor integration have also been clearly delineated in PD. When making slow, active pointing movements, individuals with PD tended to make hypometric movements and undershoot the target when deprived of the ability to watch their moving hand *(12).* This abnormality was present with both active and passive arm movement, suggesting the presence of a defect of kinesthesia to the investigators. Further support for the presence of a deficit in kinesthetic processing in PD has been provided by the demonstration that PD patients have impaired ability to accurately move the index finger from one target to another when vision is occluded (after the target location has been shown by passive movement of the finger; *13*). Using a testing paradigm in which vibration is applied to the antagonist muscle, investigators have demonstrated that patients with PD display less pronounced vibration-induced undershooting of both wrist and ankle movements than do normal controls

(14,15). In patients with asymmetric disease, this abnormality (reduced undershooting) was more evident on the more involved side, and tended to be less apparent when patients were in the "on" state in individuals with motor fluctuations *(14).* These findings were attributed to a disturbance in proprioceptive guidance, likely owing to impaired central processing of proprioceptive input by the basal ganglia. The investigators also suggested that this impairment of processing proprioceptive information might contribute to the motor abnormalities evident in PD *(14,15).* Depressed frontal responsiveness to sensory stimuli, as tested by somatosensory-evoked potentials, has also been demonstrated in PD, further implicating a disturbance in sensorimotor integration *(16).*

Thus, a considerable body of evidence has accumulated that documents the presence of subtle, but potentially significant, abnormalities of sensory function and sensorimotor integration in PD.

3. PAIN

3.1. Background

Pain is an important, but under-recognized, symptom in PD. This lack of recognition is often shared by both patients and physicians. For most individuals with PD, the clinical features of bradykinesia, rigidity, tremor, postural instability, dementia, and other impairments dominate the clinical perspective. However, many patients, when questioned directly, report painful symptoms or discomfort that they regard as connected to their PD.

The causes of chronic pain in PD are protean, which renders accurate diagnosis difficult. Virtually every type of pain sensation has been described in PD. For many, painful symptoms fluctuate in parallel with motor symptoms of the disorder and are designated as nonmotor sensory fluctuations *(17).* Although pain is often an inconsequential component of the overall clinical view, in a minority of patients with PD, pain is so severe and intractable that it overshadows the motor symptoms of the disease.

3.2. Historical Aspects

Despite not being considered as a major feature of the disorder, pain is listed prominently in many of the early descriptions of PD *(1,4,5,18–20).* James Parkinson wrote in his famous monograph that painful symptoms may be the first sign of the disorder *(1),* and Gowers noted "aching pains in the limbs" to be an occasional early clinical feature *(5).*

3.3. Prevalence of Pain

The true prevalence of pain in PD remains unknown, but it might be suspected to be higher than in the general population because of the rigidity, dystonia, physical restraints, and motor complications that the disease imposes. Painful or unpleasant sensations in patients with PD are, in fact, more common than expected. In five recent surveys of painful sensations in patients with PD, the percentage of patients who acknowledged the presence of pain ranged from 38% to 54% *(2,6,17,21,22).*

The challenge for the clinician is to recognize when a patient's complaint of pain requires further evaluation and to categorize the painful symptoms of PD into a framework for diagnosis and treatment. One study classified painful sensations by etiology *(22).* In this survey, 43 of 95 patients with PD experienced pain. Muscle cramps occurred in 32 (74%), dystonia-associated pain occurred in 12 (28%), radicular or neuritic pain developed in 6 (14%), and joint pains were present in 6 (14%). Other investigators have reported a higher incidence of central or primary parkinsonian pain *(2)* or akathisia *(17).*

3.4. Classification of Pain

The presence of pain in a patient with PD poses a considerable diagnostic and therapeutic dilemma to the clinician. The protean presentations and variable characteristics of pain in the PD setting can easily lead to diagnostic confusion and inappropriate treatment. Thus, a useful and practical system of pain classification in PD would be of great value. (Some attempts at this have been undertaken.)

Sigwald and Solignac *(21)* studied 203 randomly selected patients with PD and documented the presence of painful symptoms in 108. Symptoms were subdivided into paresthesias and pain symptoms. Painful sensations were classified by body region; the legs were the most frequently involved region, followed by arms, neck, lumbar region, epigastrium, and abdomen. No attempt was made to systematically classify painful symptoms by etiology.

As noted earlier, in the survey of Snider and colleagues *(6)*, 67% of individuals (29/43) who experienced primary sensory symptoms as part of their PD classified the symptom as pain. The pain was typically described as an intermittent poorly localized aching or cramp-like sensation more likely to affect the proximal portion of a limb and involve the limb with the greatest motor deficit. There were 11 patients that described burning paresthesias sometimes aggravated by levodopa. Painful muscle cramps or spasms were not counted as primary sensory symptoms in this study.

Koller considered all abnormal sensations to be primary sensory symptoms and, as noted previously, documented the presence of sensory symptoms in 38% (19/50) of the patients with PD studied *(2)*. Patients were further classified as having numbness (12), tingling (8), pain and achiness (6), coldness (6), and burning (1).

Goetz and colleagues *(22)* documented pain directly attributable to PD in 43 (45%) of the 95 subjects in their study. They divided patients' description of pain into five categories: 32 patients (74%) had pain of muscular origin; 12 (28%) experienced pain owing to dystonia; 6 (14%) were felt to have joint pain; 6 (14%) had radicular or neuritic pain; and diffuse "akathitic" pain occurred in 1 patient (2%). Symptoms suggestive of central or thalamic pain were not described in this series.

More recently, in a series of 50 patients with PD who were experiencing motor fluctuations, only 5 patients had no sensory symptoms *(17)*. Sensory symptoms were divided into seven categories: akathisia, tightening sensation, tingling sensation, diffuse pain, restlessness, neuralgic pain, and burning sensation. Diffuse pain was experienced by 54% of the 50 patients, neuralgic pain by 18%, and burning sensations by 8%. The vast majority of sensory symptoms, including those that might be considered painful, appeared during "off" states, but sometimes both diffuse pain and neuralgic pain were experienced during periods of dyskinesia.

Considering this background, painful symptoms can be classified into one or more of the following five categories: musculoskeletal pain, radicular or neuropathic pain, dystonia-related pain, primary (central) parkinsonian pain, and akathitic discomfort. Pain from mechanisms and sources outside of PD also may certainly occur in patients with PD. However, a discussion of this aspect of pain in PD is beyond the scope of this chapter.

4. SPECIFIC PAIN SYNDROMES

As a general approach, painful symptoms should be considered in relation to the cardinal symptoms of tremor, rigidity, akinesia, dystonia, and akathisia. It is important to note whether anti-Parkinsonian medications induce, exacerbate, or relieve PD-associated pain. Most painful symptoms in PD are more prominent during "off" motor fluctuations and therefore represent nonmotor fluctuations. However, not all pain experienced in the "off" state is a direct result of dopamine deficiency. For many patients, "off" pain represents a secondary consequence of increased rigidity and immobility. Pain caused by dystonia can be diagnosed when there is visible twisting, cramping, or posturing of the painful extremity or body part. Dystonia that develops during the "off" state may be painful, but medication-induced dystonia, occurring while the patient is "on" or during transitions between states, may be equally uncomfortable. Deep-brain stimulation may also induce painful dystonic muscle spasms, possibly from the spread of discharge to the corticospinal tract. A careful appraisal of possible musculoskeletal or rheumatologic pain mechanisms is important in patients with PD. Akathisia, although not painful, is intensely unpleasant and is a rare, but distinctive, symptom that occurs in PD. Primary parkinsonian pain, unrelated to a disturbance in motor function, is presumed to be of central origin and may be inferred partly by the nature of its clinical features and partly through exclusion of other causes. In the sections that follow, categories of painful symptoms in PD are described in further detail.

4.1. Musculoskeletal Pain

4.1.1. Mechanisms of Musculoskeletal Pain

In individuals with PD, pain of musculoskeletal origin mostly appears to be related to rigidity and bradykinesia. Deformities of posture, stiffness of limb movements and gait, and awkward mechanics for body motion and tasks may also place unusual stresses on the musculoskeletal system, and muscle cramps and joint-based pain may further fuel the discomfort. Aching, cramping, and joint pains in patients with PD presumably result from diminished mobility of affected limbs and joints. Muscle cramps and tightness typically involve the neck, arms, paraspinal, or calf muscles; joint pain most frequently originates in shoulders, hips, knees, and ankles *(22)*. Musculoskeletal discomfort in PD tends to be most evident during periods of increased Parkinsonism *(22)*.

4.1.2. Shoulder Stiffness

One of the most common musculoskeletal afflictions in PD is shoulder stiffness; a stiff shoulder may be the first sign of PD. The prevalence of the "frozen shoulder," also called periarthritis or adhesive capsulitis, is higher in patients with PD than in age-matched subjects without PD *(23)*. Among 150 consecutive patients with PD followed in a movement disorders clinic, 65 (43%) related a history of some type of shoulder disturbance, including shoulder trauma, which had preceded the development of their Parkinsonism. Six patients provided a history of spontaneous pain and restricted mobility regarding the shoulder joint. The peak incidence of frozen shoulder occurred in the 2 years *preceding* the first symptoms of PD, and in almost all cases, the initial PD symptoms developed in the upper limb ipsilateral to the frozen shoulder. Moreover, among patients with frozen shoulder, akinesia was the first PD symptom, occurring twice as frequently as tremor *(23)*.

4.1.3. Spinal Deformities

Spinal deformities are well-described in PD and may be responsible for pain. The typical posture of the individual with PD is stooped forward with the neck held in flexion. Some patients develop a fixed postural deformity, whereas others have an apparent truncal or neck dystonia that varies with posture and activity. In extreme cases, the spinal deformity in PD patients may become sufficiently severe to merit the label "camptocormia" or "bent spine" *(24)*. Individuals with camptocormia may have thoracolumbar spinal curvature so significant that the upper body is bent forward into a horizontal position. In such a position, upward gaze may be severely limited or even impossible. One of the hallmarks of camptocormia is that the deformity is not fixed; it completely disappears when the individual assumes the recumbent position. The pathogenesis of camptocormia in PD is uncertain. Camptocormia has been suggested to be a dystonic phenomenon, and levodopa has been reported both to accentuate and ameliorate the condition *(24)*. In contrast, a recent report described camptocormic posture in a patient as a result of focal myositis of the paraspinal muscles *(25)*.

There does not appear to be a specific or effective treatment for camptocormia. With advancing disease, the flexion deformity only worsens, despite treatment with anti-Parkinsonian agents. It is tempting to speculate that insertion of spinal rods might straighten the curvature, but anecdotal evidence suggests that this often fails owing to hardware disruption or migration or the development of infection. Deep-brain stimulation does not seem to ameliorate severe truncal flexion.

Scoliosis occurs more often in PD than in the elderly general population *(26,27)*. In one study, scoliosis was present in 62 of 103 (60%) patients with PD; the side of the convexity was unrelated to that of maximal deficit *(28)*.

4.1.4. Rheumatological and Orthopedic Abnormalities

An astounding array of rheumatological and orthopedic symptoms may be encountered in patients with PD, including temporomandibular joint disease, bursitis, arthritis, Baker's cyst, plantar fasciitis, stress fractures, cervical spondylosis, spinal stenosis, sciatica, ankylosing spondylitis, contractures, and others. The incidence of these conditions in PD has not been studied, and it is not possible to conclude a statistical or causal association with PD because rheumatologic conditions are common in the PD age range. In women, the combination of osteoporosis and PD, especially when postural instability is present, is particularly dangerous.

4.1.5. Painful Contractures

Painful contractures, the consequence of immobility, are yet another important source of pain in PD. Contractures result from a pathological shortening of muscle fibers, tendons, or ligaments and may involve the ankles, knees, hips, fingers, hands, wrists, elbows, or neck. Contractures can result from the characteristic flexed attitude of the disease and represent a complication of immobility. They may form surprisingly rapidly, sometimes within a matter of weeks.

Hand and foot deformities have typically been described in persons with PD, both by the neurological masters of the 19th century *(4,5)* and more recently *(29–32)*. The clenched fist in Parkinsonism may begin as a dystonic posture, but it leads to contractures, usually within several months of sustained hand and finger flexion. The clenched fist is often extremely painful and leads to loss of hand function, poor hand hygiene, and palmar infections *(32)*. Pain may result from the initial sustained dystonic contractions of the fingers in flexion or eventual consequent contractures, from joint disease, or from the nails piercing the skin of the palm.

In PD, the risk of developing contractures appears proportional to the amount of rigidity and bradykinesia. Limb contractures may represent a side effect of bromocriptine *(33)*, an agent that may cause fibrosis, but there are too few cases to substantiate this.

4.1.6. Diagnosis of Musculoskeletal Pain

When patients with PD develop what appears to be musculoskeletal pain, careful assessment of the muscles and tendons, bones, and joints is necessary. Painful symptoms must be considered in relation to Parkinsonian signs, range of motion, posture, activity, and anti-Parkinsonian medication. It should be possible to arrive at an accurate diagnosis on the basis of the history and exam, but ancillary testing, including serological tests, X-rays, bone scans, ultrasound, or rheumatological or orthopedic consultation, are occasionally needed. The presence of joint deformities or a concurrent rheumatological condition should be obvious. Differentiating between Parkinsonian rigidity, painful cramping, contracture, dystonia, and a fixed skeletal deformity can all be done on clinical examination.

4.1.7. Treatment of Musculoskeletal Pain

Treatment of musculoskeletal pain in PD depends on its cause. If Parkinsonian rigidity is the primary cause, dopaminergic therapy, physical therapy, and an exercise program are indicated. The goal of treatment is to restore mobility. Once this is achieved, an exercise program can be invaluable in maintaining mobility and preventing further musculoskeletal problems.

Nonsteroidal anti-inflammatory drugs (NSAIDs) and analgesics are helpful for rheumatological and orthopedic conditions in tandem with physical therapy. Passive range of motion exercises are important to prevent contractures in patients with limited mobility, but once formed, a contracture generally requires surgical intervention.

4.2. Radicular and Neuritic Pain

4.2.1. Mechanisms of Radicular and Neuritic Pain

Pain and discomfort that is well-localized to the territory of a nerve or nerve root is described as radicular or neuritic pain and accounted for 14% of the pain syndromes experienced by patients with PD in one survey *(22)*. However, most case reports and surveys do not permit detailed evaluation of this type of pain because the descriptions do not provide adequate clinical information or neuroimaging data to confirm the pathological process. Thus, the true incidence of radicular and neuritic pain in PD is uncertain.

It is also unclear whether PD itself actually fosters the development of neuritic or radicular pain. Postural deformities of PD might conceivably predispose to the development of compressive radiculopathy, sciatica, or myelopathy. Immobility is certainly a risk factor for the evolution of compressive focal neuropathy. A traumatic radial nerve palsy was described in one report *(34)*. Peak-effect dyskinesias may exacerbate radicular and neuritic pain *(22,35)*. Both tremor and dyskinesia involving the wrist may possibly promote development of carpal tunnel syndrome. Trigeminal neuralgia has been described in PD *(36)*.

4.2.2. Diagnosis and Treatment of Radicular and Neuritic Pain

Evaluation and treatment of pain in this category begins with careful clinical examination supplemented (if needed) by electrodiagnostic studies and neuroimaging. Radicular pain can often be treated with a judicious mobility program, NSAIDs, and pain medication. In one interesting case report describing two individuals whose sciatica was exacerbated by dyskinesia, morphine treatment not only reduced the sciatica pain but also suppressed the dyskinesias *(35)*. In the presence of refractory pain, or a severe or worsening neurological deficit that coincides with an abnormality on the radiological studies, decompressive surgery may be indicated. For a compressive peripheral neuropathy, avoidance of aggravating postures is important, sometimes with the aid of splints or braces. Decompressive surgery may also be required when conservative measures do not suffice.

4.3. Dystonic Pain

4.3.1. Characterization of Dystonia

Dystonia is characterized by sustained and forceful twisting movement that leads to abnormal postures and deformities. Dystonic spasms are among the most painful symptoms that a patient with PD may experience. Spasms may be spontaneous or triggered by movement or activity; they may be brief (lasting minutes), prolonged (lasting hours), or even continuous. Dystonia in PD can affect any limb, trunk, neck, face, tongue, jaw, pharynx, and vocal cords, usually developing in sites most severely affected by Parkinsonism. Dystonia may precede the development of Parkinsonism, develop as a late feature, appear after the onset of dopaminergic therapy, follow stereotactic neurosurgery, or be induced by deep-brain stimulation. The pattern of dystonia in PD may be classified as focal, cranial, segmental, or generalized. Dystonia developing during "off" periods most often involves the feet, whereas drug-induced dystonia has a predilection for the neck, trunk, and cranial distribution *(37)*.

The evaluation of dystonia requires especially careful consideration of its relationship to dopaminergic medication. Dystonia may occur as an early morning manifestation of dopaminergic deficiency or as a wearing-off phenomenon later in the day or in the middle of the night. In some patients, dystonia is a painful beginning-of-dose or end-of-dose phenomenon; in others, it develops at the peak of response to a dose of dopaminergic medication. The classic flowing, writhing, choreoathetotic dyskinesias induced by dopaminergic medication are not sustained or painful and are generally not considered to be dystonic. However, drug-induced dystonia may occur, which is characterized by sustained and twisting postures that can be very painful. When the timing of the dystonia is uncertain, it may be helpful to observe the patient in the office for several hours to appreciate the association of dystonia to the medication dose cycle. Classifying dystonia in relation to the levodopa-dosing schedule provides a useful and rational framework for evaluating and treating painful dystonia in PD *(38,39)*.

4.3.2. Early Morning Foot Dystonia

The most thoroughly studied presentation of dystonia in PD is early morning foot dystonia, which develops in approximately 16% of patients with PD and is defined by foot or toe cramping and posturing *(40)*. Every variety of foot posture is possible: plantar flexion, dorsiflexion, foot inversion, curling of the toes, or forced extension of the great toe ("striatal toe"). Foot dystonia is often accompanied by stiffness of the calf muscles.

It has been argued that early morning dystonia is a complication of long-term levodopa therapy because it takes place usually in patients with longer disease duration and in individuals in whom dyskinesias are present *(40–44)*. In a study of 42 patients with PD and foot dystonia, 41 (97.5%) individuals experienced early morning foot dystonia before the first levodopa dose with subsequent milder attacks during the late evening or during the night, suggesting that dystonia is intrinsic to the Parkinsonism in most cases, representing a wearing-off phenomenon *(45)*. However, painful foot dystonia in PD was described long before the advent of levodopa *(46)*. It may also precede the other manifestations of the disorder *(47)*.

4.3.3. *Treatment of Dystonia*

Early morning dystonia is typically relieved by activity, or it resolves shortly following the first dose of dopaminergic medication during the day. In some patients, early morning dystonia is so severe that subcutaneous injections of apomorphine, with its onset of action within minutes, can be justified *(48)*. When dystonia occurs as a wearing-off effect during the day, appropriate treatment is analogous to the treatment of wearing-off motor fluctuations and is aimed at reducing the duration of the "off" period. More frequent levodopa dosing, use of controlled-release levodopa preparations, levodopa supplementation with a catechol-*O*-methyltransferase inhibitor, use of dopamine agonists as adjunctive or monotherapy, or use of apomorphine as a "rescue" agent can all be effective. Although dopaminergic drugs are usually first-line therapy for off-period dystonia in PD, anticholinergic drugs *(41,45)*, baclofen, *(49)*, and lithium *(50)* have also been used successfully. In patients with levodopa-induced dystonia, treatment typically consists of reducing dopaminergic stimulation by decreasing levodopa dosage or by reducing its absorption; substituting a less potent agonist may also be effective.

Injections of botulinum toxin may be beneficial treatment for focal dystonia in PD. In an open-label study of 30 patients with painful foot dystonia, where dystonia was severely or completely disabling in 23 (77%), injections of botulinum toxin A produced dramatic relief of pain and disability *(51)*. Injections were accomplished under electromyographic guidance and tailored to the specific appearance of the dystonic foot. The median dosage was 70 U (range of 40–100 U).

As noted earlier, the clenched fist seen in patients with PD may begin as a dystonic posture, but it can evolve into a sustained contracture relatively quickly. Treatment with intramuscular botulinum toxin injections, given to the flexor digitorum superficialis or lumbricals, can relieve the dystonic component of the process, sometimes for 4 months *(32)*. Active muscular contractions, as documented by electromyography, are associated with good result from botulinum toxin injections, whereas an absence of electromyographic activity, denoting contractures, predicts treatment failure *(32)*. The flexed neck posture that occurs in PD also responds poorly to botulinum toxin injections.

Advanced neurosurgical techniques may also decrease painful dystonia associated with PD. Pallidotomy has been reported to relieve this condition *(18,52)*. Painful off-period dystonia, present in 20 patients who underwent bilateral subthalamic nucleus stimulation, was completely alleviated in 12 individuals, and considerably improved in 4 *(53)*. In a recent study that examined the effect of globus pallidus stimulation on parkinsonian pain *(54)*, all types of off-period painful sensations were markedly reduced: dystonic pain, muscle cramping, dysesthesias, and "global pain," as measured using a rating scale. Benefit developed quickly after surgery and remained stable through the 1-year follow-up interval. Patients with unilateral globus pallidus stimulation experienced pain reduction primarily on the contralateral body side, whereas bilateral stimulation produced bilateral reduction in pain.

Deep-brain stimulation in the subthalamic nucleus or globus pallidus can also induce acute painful, dystonic spasms, possibly owing to the spread of current to the internal capsule. The necessary intervention in this situation is a change in stimulator parameters, usually a reduction in voltage or pulse width, which promptly reverses the muscle spasms. Intrathecal baclofen, effective for spasticity of spinal or cerebral origin, has shown little effect on the dystonia associated with Parkinsonism *(55)*.

4.4. Primary (Central) Pain

4.4.1. Characterization of Central Pain

Perhaps the most striking pain syndromes in patients with PD are those of central origin. Central pain is defined as pain produced directly by a lesion or abnormal function within the central nervous system. Current concepts hold that central pain is generated by the brain and requires the presence of a lesion in the thalamus, its afferent or efferent pathways *(56)*. Most clinical literature implicates the thalamus as the source of central pain, specifically a lesion of the ventroposterior thalamus *(57)*.

Primary (central) parkinsonian pain was outlined in the seminal description of Souques in 1921 *(18)*, in which he described 17 patients with PD or Parkinsonism, some of whom were afflicted with pain syndromes that he believed were intrinsic to PD. He listed many characteristics of his patients' pain: bizarre unexplained sensations of stabbing, burning, scalding, and formication—all descriptions associated with "neuropathic" pain originating in the central or peripheral nervous systems. Souques noted that the presumed central pain syndromes in his patients typically afflicted the side of the body most affected by Parkinsonism and could precede, even by years, the motor manifestations of the disorder. Using a conceptual framework outlined earlier by Dejerine *(58)*, Souques postulated a central origin of pain in PD caused by a disturbance in signaling between the corpus striatum and thalamus.

The argument for a separate central pain syndrome in PD finds support in several unusual case descriptions. In contrast to musculoskeletal conditions, which tend to affect the limbs, muscles, and joints most afflicted with Parkinsonism, reports exist of unusual pain syndromes involving the face, head, epigastrium, abdomen, pelvis, rectum, and genitalia *(6,21,38,59)*, all areas in which painful dystonia or musculoskeletal conditions are unlikely or implausible. Sigwald and Solignac *(21)* described patients with pharyngeal, epigastric, and abdominal pain. In a series of eight patients with Parkinsonism (7 with PD; 1 with atypical Parkinsonism) and oral or genital pain *(59)*, oral pain affected the gums, teeth, tongue, inner cheek, face, and jaw. These oral pain syndromes, resembling the idiopathic "burning mouth syndrome" *(60)*, were described as burning, pulsating sensations often strikingly lateralized within the oral cavity. The pain tended to correlate with "off" periods, but it was not necessarily abolished by dopaminergic therapy. Genital pain occurred in three of the eight individuals—all women—and consisted of burning, numbness, or vibrating sensations. In all patients, the pain had a relentless, obsessional, distressing quality that overshadowed other Parkinsonian symptoms *(59)*.

Consistent with its presumed origin within the central nervous system, peripheral nerve blockade does not abolish central pain in PD, as illustrated by a patient whose oral pain was unaffected by a complete dental nerve block *(59)*. In a similar vein, Sage and colleagues describe a patient with Parkinsonism, dystonia, and severe leg pains, in whom epidural anesthesia with chlorprocaine sufficient to produce complete sympathetic, sensory, and motor blockade, relieved the dystonia but not all elements of the patient's pain, suggesting the presence of a central component to the pain, possibly from deafferentation *(61)*.

Classic central pain is postulated to involve a lesion of the thalamus, but primary Parkinsonian pain may be the consequence of an abnormality of sensory pathways within the basal ganglia. Somatosensory processing within the basal ganglia takes place within the substantia nigra, caudate, putamen, globus pallidus, thalamus, and their interconnections *(62)*. The basal ganglia may perform an important gating role for nociceptive information before it reaches consciousness *(63)*. The fact that 6-hydroxydopamine lesions in the striatum or ventral tegmental area decrease the latencies of nociceptive reflexes in rats suggests that the dopaminergic system has a role in modulating nociceptive information in the striatum and limbic system *(64)*. Battista and Wolff noted that levodopa administration increased the heat-pain threshold and tolerance in patients with PD and speculated that dopamine, presumably acting through striatothalamic projections, modulates the peripheral inputs to the thalamus *(65)*.

4.4.2. Treatment of Primary (Central) Pain

Treatment of presumed central pain in PD is challenging, especially if dopaminergic agents, the first-line therapy for this disabling problem, are not effective. Conventional analgesics, opiates, tricyclics, and atypical neuroleptics (e.g., clozapine) may be helpful *(59)*. In one report of a patient with intractable, recurrent, and severe painful fluttering sensations in her left-thoracic region, subcutaneous injections of apomorphine provided complete relief after all other classes of medication—dopaminergic, benzodiazepines, tricyclic antidepressants, opiates, baclofen, clozapine, and intercostal nerve blocks—had failed *(66)*.

With the increased application of deep-brain stimulation in advanced PD, it is possible that unusual painful or uncomfortable sensations of central origin may be reported. Stimulators can induce a variety of unpleasant sensations, such as the jolting dysesthesias that transiently occur during stimulator-programming sessions, and are reported in up to 70% of patients.

4.5. Akathisia

4.5.1. Characteristics of Restlessness or Akathisia

Restlessness is a frequent and potentially disabling complaint indicated by individuals with PD. Parkinsonian akathisia is characterized by subjective inner restlessness, producing an intolerance of remaining still and manifesting as a constant need to move or change position. In evaluating a complaint of restlessness, it is important to establish that the need to move is not caused by other factors, such as the primary symptoms of Parkinsonism, other somatic complaints or urges, dyskinesias, anxiety, depression, or claustrophobia.

The definition of pure akathisia is meant to exclude additional neuropathic symptoms, but patients with akathisia often describe crawling sensations, burning, or tingling *(67,68)*. Parkinsonian akathisia can be severe: patients may be unable to sit, drive a car, eat at a table, or attend social gatherings. Some patients remain in constant motion. In extreme cases, Parkinsonian akathisia has driven individuals to suicide *(19)*. In about half of the reported cases of Parkinsonian akathisia, symptoms have been noted to fluctuate with levodopa-dosing schedules and to improve with adjustment of dopaminergic medication *(68)*.

4.5.2. Frequency of Akathisia

Like many pain syndromes that occur in PD, restlessness is probably under-recognized and, if specifically inquired about, present more frequently than expected. Gowers provided an early description of this symptom in PD in his 1888 textbook, *Diseases of the Nervous System (5)*. In one survey of 100 patients with PD, 68 (68%) complained of a periodic need to move *(67)*. In 26 of these individuals (26%), restlessness represented genuine Parkinsonian akathisia. Comella and colleagues studied 56 patients with PD; 25 (45%) acknowledged the presence of akathitic movements *(68)*. The movements usually involved the legs and correlated with patients' own subjective descriptions of inner restlessness.

4.5.3. Akathisia and Dopamine

The appearance of Parkinsonian akathisia as a wearing-off phenomenon and its levodopa responsiveness suggest that akathisia is related to impaired dopaminergic neurotransmission. The fact that two other major causes of the syndrome—postencephalitic Parkinsonism and neuroleptic-induced akathisia—are also characterized by dopaminergic dysfunction strengthens the association. Akathisia is suggested to result from dopaminergic deficiency involving the mesocortical pathway, which originates in the ventral tegmental area and is known to be affected in PD *(69)*. Some indirect support for this is provided by the observation that clozapine, which has a high affinity for D4 receptors and preferentially affects the mesocortical and mesolimbic dopaminergic systems, can be remarkably effective in treating akathisia *(70–72)*.

4.5.4. Akathisia and Restless Legs Syndrome

Restlessness is also a core element of the restless legs syndrome (RLS), a disorder of unknown cause in which patients experience an intense and irresistible urge to move the legs, accompanied by sensory complaints and motor restlessness. Characteristically, the symptoms are worse at rest, relieved with motion, and increase in severity in the evening or at night. The possibility that RLS can be dramatically relieved by levodopa or dopamine agonists implies it is a disorder of altered dopaminergic transmission *(73)*. The relationship of RLS to, and its distinction from, akathisia in patients with PD is not always clear.

5. HEADACHE

Headache is an important symptom that may occur in PD, but its relationship to the disease is uncertain. It does not fit into the pain categories already described, but instead represents a painful symptom that often requires its own specific evaluation and treatment. In a survey of 71 patients with PD, 25 individuals (35%) acknowledged headache *(74)*. Headaches were generally located in the nuchal region, but they did not correlate with a clinical assessment of nuchal rigidity. Headaches ranged from dull aching discomfort to sharp squeezing or pulsatile pain. In a subsequent report, a specific early morning headache was described in three individuals, relieved within 2 hours of the first levodopa dose *(75)*. In another report, patients who have PD with headache scored significantly higher on measures of depression and anxiety than those without headache *(76)*. Medication, especially the dopaminergic ergot alkaloids, pergolide and bromocriptine, may also be a source of headache in patients with PD. A severe or unusual headache accompanied by neurological signs can never be attributed to PD and requires thorough neurological evaluation, usually with neuroimaging.

6. DEPRESSION AND PAIN

Depression may alter the interpretation of painful symptoms in PD. Goetz and colleagues *(77)* found that depression is more severe in patients with PD who experience pain than among those who do not. Although there are no systematic data to guide the clinician, it is important that any pain assessment in an individual with PD considers the potential contributing role of depression, which itself may require specific treatment.

7. CONCLUSION

Pain is not regarded as a cardinal feature of PD, but it can be an important complication of the disease and presents a diagnostic and therapeutic challenge to the treating physician. It is vitally important to differentiate Parkinsonian pain from pain produced by other coincident medical conditions. The nature of modern medical practice is that a physician caring for a patient with PD may be the first to evaluate a new or unusual painful complaint; defining the boundaries of neurological inquiry may not be simple. For example, chest pain and abdominal pain may be a result of PD but are best approached from a larger perspective, where appropriate referrals and testing may be necessary.

Approximately 40 to 50% of patients with PD experience pain, and in a minority of these individuals, the problem is so distressing that it overshadows the motor symptoms. Most Parkinsonism-related pain can be assigned to one or more of five categories: musculoskeletal pain, neuritic or radicular pain, dystonia-associated pain, primary or central pain, and akathitic discomfort. There are no diagnostic tests to guide the clinician, but the patients' own descriptions of pain and associated clinical features should enable an accurate diagnosis of pain in most individuals.

REFERENCES

1. Parkinson J. An essay on the shaking palsy. Sherwood, Neely, Jones, London, 1817.
2. Koller WC. Sensory symptoms in Parkinson's disease. Neurology 1984;34:957–959.
3. Hammond WA. A Treatise on Diseases of the Nervous System. Appleton, New York, 1871.
4. Charcot JM. Lectures on the Diseases of the Nervous System. The New Sydenham Society, London, 1877.
5. Gowers WR. A Manual of Diseases of the Nervous System (American Edition). Blakiston, Philadelphia, 1888.
6. Snider SR, Fahn S, Isgreen WP, Cote LJ. Primary sensory symptoms in Parkinsonism. Neurology 1976;26:423–429.
7. Pratorius B, Kimmeskamp S, Milani TL. The sensitivity of the sole of the foot in patients with Morbus Parkinson. Neurosci Lett 2003;346:173–176.

8. Zia S, Cody F, O'Boyle D. Joint position sense is impaired by Parkinson's disease. Ann Neurol 2000;47:218–228.
9. Weder BJ, Leenders KL, Vontobel P, et al. Impaired somatosensory discrimination of shape in Parkinson's disease: association with caudate nucleus dopaminergic function. Hum Brain Mapp 1999;8:1–12.
10. Zia S, Cody FW, O'Boyle DJ. Discrimination of bilateral differences in the loci of tactile stimulation is impaired in subjects with Parkinson's disease. Clin Anat 2003;16:241–247.
11. Schneider JS, Diamond SG, Markham CH. Parkinson's disease: sensory and motor problems in arms and hands. Neurology 1987;37:951–956.
12. Klockgether T, Borutta M, Rapp H, et al. A defect of kinesthesia in Parkinson's disease. Mov Disord 1995;10:460–465.
13. Jobst EE, Melnick ME, Byl NN, et al. Sensory perception in Parkinson disease. Arch Neurol 1997;54:450–454.
14. Rickards C, Cody FWJ. Proprioceptive control of wrist movements in Parkinson's disease. Reduced muscle vibration-induced errors. Brain 1997;120:977–990.
15. Khudados E, Cody FWJ, O'Boyle DJ. Proprioceptive regulation of voluntary ankle movements, demonstrated using muscle vibration, impaired by Parkinson's disease. J Neurol Neurosurg Psychiatry 1999;67:504–510.
16. Rossini PM, Filippi MM, Vernieri F. Neurophysiology of sensorimotor integration in Parkinson's disease. Clin Neurosci 1998;5:121–130.
17. Witjas T, Kaphan E, Azulay JP, et al. Nonmotor fluctuations in Parkinson's disease: frequent and disabling. Neurology 2002;59:408–413.
18. Souques MA. Des douleurs dans la paralysie agitante. Rev Neurol (Paris) 1921;37:629–633.
19. Lewy FH. Die Lehre vom Tonus und der Bewegung Zugleich Systematische Untersuchungen zur Klinik, Physiologie, Pathologie und Pathogenese der Paralysis Agitans. Springer, Berlin, 1923.
20. Wilson SAK. Neurology. Hafner Publishing, New York, 1940.
21. Sigwald J, Solignac J. Manifestations douloureuses de la maladie de Parkinson et paresthesies provoquees par les neuroleptiques. Sem Hop Paris 1960;41:2222–2225.
22. Goetz CG, Tanner CM, Levy M, et al. Pain in Parkinson's disease. Mov Disord 1986;1:45–49.
23. Riley D, Lang AE, Blair RD, et al. Frozen shoulder and other shoulder disturbances in Parkinson's disease. J Neurol Neurosurg Psychiatry 1989;52:63–66.
24. Djaldetti R, Mosberg-Galili R, Sroka H, et al. Camptocormia (bent spine) in patients with Parkinson's disease—characterization and possible pathogenesis of an unusual phenomenon. Mov Disord 1999;14:443–447.
25. Wunderlich S, Csoti I, Reiners K, et al. Camptocormia in Parkinson's disease mimicked by focal myositis of the paraspinal muscles. Mov Disord 2002;17:598–600.
26. Duvoisin RC, Marsden CD. Note on the scoliosis of Parkinsonism. J Neurol Neurosurg Psychiatry 1975;38:787–793.
27. Indo T, Ando K. Studies on the scoliosis of Parkinsonism. Rinsho Shinkeigaku 1980;20:40–46.
28. Grimes JD, Hassan MN, Trent G, et al. Clinical and radiographic features of scoliosis in Parkinson's disease. Adv Neurol 1987;45:353–355.
29. Gortvai P. Deformities of the hands and feet in Parkinsonism and their reversibility by operation. J Neurol Neurosurg Psychiatry 1963;26:33–36.
30. Reynolds FW, Petropoulous GC. Hand deformities in Parkinsonism. J Chron Dis 1965;18:593–595.
31. Bissonnette B. Pseudorheumatoid deformity of the feet associated with Parkinsonism. J Rheumatol 1986;13:825–826.
32. Cordivari C, Misra VP, Catania S, Lees AJ. Treatment of dystonic clenched fist with botulinum toxin. Mov Disord 2001;16:907–913.
33. Quinn NP, Ring H, Honavar M, Marsden CD. Contractures of extremities in parkinsonian subjects:a report of three cases with a possible association with bromocriptine treatment. Clin Neuropharmacol 1988;11:268–277.
34. Pullman SL, Elibol B, Fahn S. Modulation of parkinsonian tremor by radial nerve palsy. Neurology 1994;44:1861–1864.
35. Berg D, Becker G, Reiners K. Reduction of dyskinesia and induction of akinesia induced by morphine in two parkinsonian patients with severe sciatica. J Neural Transm 1999;106:725–728.
36. Hillen ME, Sage JI. Nonmotor fluctuations in patients with Parkinson's disease. Neurology 1996;47:1180–1183.
37. Poewe WH, Lees AJ, Stern GM. Dystonia in Parkinson's disease: clinical and pharmacological features. Ann Neurol 1988;23:73–78.
38. Quinn NP, Koller WC, Lang AE, Marsden CD. Painful Parkinson's disease. Lancet 1986;1:1366–1369.
39. Quinn NP. Classification of fluctuations in patients with Parkinson's disease. Neurology 1998;51(Suppl 2):S25–S29.
40. Curry LJ, Harrison MB, Trugman JM, et al. Early morning dystonia in Parkinson's disease. Neurology 1988;51:283–285.
41. Duvoisin RC, Yahr MD, Lieberman J, et al. The striatal foot. Trans Am Neurol Assoc 1972;97:267.
42. Melamed E. Early-morning dystonia. A late side effect of long term levodopa therapy in Parkinson's disease. Arch Neurol 1979;36:308–310.
43. Nausieda PA, Weiner WJ, Klawans HL. Dystonic foot response of Parkinsonism. Arch Neurol 1980;37:132–136.
44. Ilson J, Fahn S, Cote L. Painful dystonic spasms in Parkinson's disease. Adv Neurol 1984;40:395–398.
45. Poewe W, Lees AJ, Steiger D, Stern GM. Foot dystonia in Parkinson's disease: clinical phenomenology and neuropharmacology. Adv Neurol 1987;45:357–360.
46. Stewart P. Paralysis agitans; with an account of a new symptom. Lancet 1898;2:1258–1260.

47. Lees AJ, Hardie RJ, Stern GM. Kinesigenic foot dystonia as a presenting feature of Parkinson's disease. J Neurol Neurosurg Psychiatry 1984;47:885.
48. Pollak P, Tranchant C. Les autres symptomes de la phase evoluee de la maladie de Parkinson. Rev Neurol (Paris) 2000;156(Suppl):165–173.
49. Lees AJ, Shaw KM, Stern GM. Baclofen in Parkinson's disease. J Neurol Neurosurg Psychiatry 1978;41:707–708.
50. Quinn N, Marsden CD. Lithium for painful dystonia in Parkinson's disease. Lancet 1986;1:1377.
51. Pachetti C, Albani G, Martignoni E, et al. "Off" painful dystonia in Parkinson's disease treated with botulinum toxin. Mov Disord 1995;10:333–336.
52. Laitinen LV, Bergenheim AT, Hariz MI. Leksell's posteroventral pallidotomy in the treatment of Parkinson's disease. J Neurosurg 1992;76:53–61.
53. Limousin P, Krack P, Pollak P, et al. Electrical stimulation of the subthalamic nucleus in advanced Parkinson's disease. New Engl J Med 1998;339:1105–1111.
54. Loher TJ, Burgunder J-M, Weber S, et al. Effect of chronic pallidal deep brain stimulation on off period dystonia and sensory symptoms in advanced Parkinson's disease. J Neurol Neurosurg Psychiatry 2002;73:395–399.
55. Ford B, Greene P, Louis ED, et al. Use of intrathecal baclofen in the treatment of patients with dystonia. Arch Neurol 1996;53:1241–1246.
56. Casey KL. Pain and central nervous system disease: a summary and overview. In: Casey KL, ed. Pain and Central Nervous System Disease. Raven Press, New York, 1991, pp. 1–11.
57. Bogousslavsky J, Regli F, Uske A. Thalamic infarcts: clinical syndromes, etiology and prognosis. Neurology 1988;38:837–848.
58. Dejerine J, Roussy G. Le syndrome thalamique. Rev Neurol 1906;14:521–528.
59. Ford B, Louis ED, Greene P, Fahn S. Oral and genital pain syndromes in Parkinson's disease. Mov Disord 1996;11:421–426.
60. Grushka M, Sessle BJ. Burning mouth syndrome. Dent Clin North Am 1991;35:171–184.
61. Sage JI, Kortis HI, Sommer W. Evidence for the role of spinal cord systems in Parkinson's disease-associated pain. Clin Neuropharmacol 1990;13:171–174.
62. Chudler EH, Dong WK. The role of the basal ganglia in nociception and pain. Pain 1995;60:3–38.
63. Lidsky TI, Manetto C, Schneider JS. A consideration of sensory factors involved in motor functions of the basal ganglia. Brain Res 1985;356:133–146.
64. Saadé NE, Atweh SF, Bahuth NB, Jabbur SJ. Augmentation of nociceptive reflexes and chronic deafferentation pain by chemical lesions of either dopaminergic terminals or midbrain dopaminergic neurons. Brain Res 1997;751:1–12.
65. Battista AF, Wolff B. Levodopa and induced-pain response. A study of patients with Parkinsonian and pain syndromes. Arch Intern Med 1973;132:70–74.
66. Factor SA, Brown DL, Molho ES. Subcutaneous apomorphine injections as a treatment for intractable pain in Parkinson's disease. Mov Disord 2000;15:167–169.
67. Lang AE, Johnson K. Akathisia in idiopathic Parkinson's disease. Neurology 1987;477–481.
68. Comella CL, Goetz CG. Akathisia in Parkinson' disease. Mov Disord 1994;9:545–549.
69. Javoy-Agid F, Agid Y. Is the mesocortical dopaminergic system involved in Parkinson's disease? Neurology 1980;30:1326–1330.
70. Van Tol HH, Bunzow JR, Guen HC, et al. Cloning of the gene for a human D4 receptor with a high affinity for the antipsychotic clozapine. Nature 1991;350:610–614.
71. Linazasoro G, Marti Masso JF, Suarez JA. Nocturnal akathisia in Parkinson's disease: treatment with clozapine. Mov Disord 1993;8:171–174.
72. Trosch RM, Friedman JH, Lannon MC, et al. Clozapine use in Parkinson's disease: a retrospective analysis of a large multicentered clinical experience. Mov Disord 1998;13:377–382.
73. Chokroverty S, Jankovic J. Restless leg syndrome: a disease in search of identity. Neurology 1999;52:907–910.
74. Indo T, Naito A, Sobue I. Clinical characteristics of headache in Parkinson's disease. Headache 1983;23:211–12.
75. Indo T, Takahashi A. Early morning headache of Parkinson's disease: a hitherto unrecognized symptom? Headache 1987;27:151–154.
76. Meco G, Frascarelli M, Pratesi L, Linfante I, Rocchi L, Formisano R. Headache in Parkinson's disease. Headache 1988;28:26–29.
77. Goetz CG, Wilson RS, Tanner CM, Garron DC. Relationships among pain, depression, and sleep alterations in Parkinson's disease. Adv Neurol 1987;45:345–347.

V Sensorimotor Dysfunction in Parkinson's Disease

23
Oculomotor Dysfunction

Parashkev Nachev and Christopher Kennard

SUMMARY

The oculomotor system is known to engage key structures within the basal ganglia and respond to dopaminergic stimulation. Therefore, it is unsurprising that Parkinson's disease (PD) should be associated with distinctive abnormalities of eye movement generation and control. Briefly outlined is the functional neuroanatomy of the oculomotor system, then the examination of the abnormalities seen in PD, their value in the differential diagnosis of Parkinsonism, and their response to pharmacological and surgical treatment are discussed. The chapter concludes with a novel hypothesis that attempts to reconcile saccadic hypometria, the most characteristic oculomotor deficit in PD, with current models of basal ganglia function.

Key Words: Saccades; dopamine; basal ganglia; oculomotor dysfunction; Parkinson's disease; saccadic hypometria.

1. INTRODUCTION

The principal neuro-ophthalmological manifestation of Parkinson's disease (PD) is a disturbance of the oculomotor system. Although it rarely gives rise to symptoms, this disturbance is a valuable subject for study because it illuminates two areas of wider interest: (1) the nature of the motor and cognitive dysfunction in PD, and (2) the role of the basal ganglia in oculomotor control. This chapter provides a brief overview of the anatomy and physiology of eye movements before proceeding to a detailed examination of the oculomotor abnormalities in patients with PD.

2. EYE MOVEMENTS: ANATOMY AND PHYSIOLOGY

Only a small region of the visual field, that subserved by the fovea, contains a detailed representation of objects that fall within it. Thus, the eyes must move to acquire and maintain the object of interest in the foveal field of view. The oculomotor system has evolved to make this process as fast and efficient as possible. Saccades are rapid, conjugate eye movements that bring the image of a peripheral object onto the fovea of each eye; vergence movements are disjunctive movements that ensure the image in each eye corresponds to the same region in space; and smooth-pursuit, vestibular, and optokinetic movements lock the image on the fovea when either the object (smooth pursuit) or the entire head or body (vestibular and optokinetic) is in motion. In our survey of the neural mechanisms underlying eye movements, we shall focus on saccades and smooth pursuit because they are the best studied and of the greatest relevance to PD.

2.1. Saccades

It is customary to classify saccades according to the behavioural context in which they are performed. Thus, *spontaneous saccades* are executed at rest when the subject is not attending to any par-

From: *Current Clinical Neurology*
Parkinson's Disease and Nonmotor Dysfunction
Edited by: R. F. Pfeiffer and I. Bodis-Wollner © Humana Press Inc., Totowa, NJ

ticular item in the visual field and not performing any task. *Reflexive saccades* are executed in response to the sudden appearance of a novel stimulus, usually a visual target. *Voluntary saccades* are executed deliberately by the subject in response to some kind of "internal" decision. Voluntary saccades are further divided into four categories largely for the convenience of the paradigms used to study them, but some are valid from an ecological standpoint. A *memory-guided saccade* is made to the location of an eccentrically placed visual target after a period of time that the target has been extinguished. A *predictive saccade* is executed in anticipation of the appearance of a target. An *antisaccade* acts in response to a visual target but to a location equidistant from and in the opposite direction to the target. Finally, an *endogenous saccade* is executed either in the absence of a peripheral target or in response to a stimulus other than the target.

Because few parameters are required to specify an eye movement, saccades are relatively easy to characterize. The metrics that are most commonly used are: (1) latency, the length of time between the onset of the target and onset of saccade; (2) gain, the ratio of the saccade amplitude and target amplitude; (3) peak velocity; and (4) the final eye position (FEP) after the primary saccade and any secondary saccades required finally to foveate the target. These parameters are not independent: there is a strong positive correlation between the peak velocity and the amplitude of a saccade, which may be used to identify an abnormal eye movement as generated by the saccadic system.

The neuronal circuitry responsible for generating saccades is widely distributed within the brainstem. Commands specifying the horizontal component of a saccade originate within the dorsomedial pons in a region known as the *paramedian pontine reticular formation,* whereas those that specify the vertical originate within the rostral midbrain (for reviews, *see* refs. *1–3*). The saccadic generators in the brainstem receive inputs capable of triggering saccades mostly from the superior colliculus (SC), but saccades may also be evoked via direct projections from several cortical and subcortical areas, including the frontal eye field (FEF), supplementary eye field (SEF), and dorsolateral prefrontal cortex (DLPFC) in the frontal lobe; area 7a and the lateral intraparietal area (LIP) in the parietal lobe; and substantia nigra pars reticulata (SNr) and caudate nucleus in the basal ganglia. Extensive reciprocal connections exist between these areas, particularly projections from the basal ganglia to cortical areas, either directly or via the thalamus.

Most of what is known about the role of the basal ganglia in oculomotor control has been derived from studies in monkeys that have focused on the relation between the CN, SNr, and SC (for a detailed review, *see* ref. *4*). A complex perspective of their interconnections has emerged (*see* Fig. 1).

Neurons in the SC that are capable of generating saccades are found within its intermediate layer. It has been shown that these cells are under tonic inhibition from a population of γ-amino-butyric acid (GABA)ergic cells within the SNr whose firing is transiently suppressed when a saccade is executed, particularly when the saccade is memory-guided. This transient suppression precedes the execution of a saccade—suggesting that it is required for a saccade to be executed—and is mediated through at least three pathways within the basal ganglia. First, a subset of inhibitory neurons within the CN project directly to the SNr. These cells receive rich inputs from the frontal cortex and have highly selective visuomotor responses, including increased activity during memory-guided saccades when compared with other types of saccades *(4)*. Other cells within this population do not project directly to the SNr but instead project to neurons within the globus pallidus externa (GPe), which, in turn, send inhibitory efferents to the SNr, forming a second indirect pathway. The third pathway involves the subthalamic nucleus (STN), which sends excitatory glutaminergic projections to the SNr and receives afferents directly from the cortical eye fields in the frontal lobe and from the striatum via GPe.

The caudate neurons involved in these pathways have been implicated in the control of reward-directed behavior. In modified memory-guided saccade tasks, some of these neurons show anticipatory activity that depends on the association between location of the spatial cue and expectation of reward from executing a saccade to that location *(5)*. This activity may be selective for specific features of the cue *(6)* and may be differentially modulated by the probability of reward *(7)*. Furthermore, saccadic latency and peak velocity (but not other parameters) are significantly influenced by the expectation of reward *(8)*, and latency correlates with the degree of neuronal activity *(7)*.

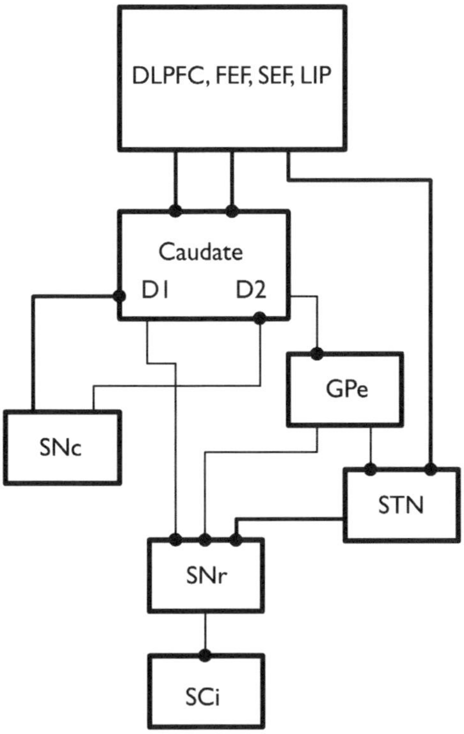

Fig. 1. Oculomotor connections of the basal ganglia. Thick lines denote excitatory connections; thin lines are inhibitory. (Not all known connections are shown. Refer to text for abbreviations.)

The mechanism by which the reward signal is transmitted to the striatum remains obscure, but it is speculated that dopaminergic projections from the substantia nigra pars compacta are critical. Caudate neurons that project directly to the SNr express D1 receptors preferentially, whereas those that project via the GPe express D2 receptors. Some evidence shows that D1-mediated activation may be facilitatory, whereas D2 is inhibitory. If this is indeed the case, dopamine deficiency may produce saccadic abnormalities via dysfunction of either the direct or indirect pathway, and "internally guided" saccades would be expected to be preferentially affected.

In support of this supposition, dopamine depletion following systemic exposure to 1-methyl-4-phenyl-1,2,6-tetrahydropyridine (MPTP) in humans *(9)* and experimental animals *(10,11)* results in infrequent, slow, and hypometric saccades; yet, the systemic manifestations make the study of oculomotor disturbance in these circumstances very difficult. Furthermore, because dopaminergic neurons in the SNc project diffusely to the basal ganglia *(12)*, it is difficult to ascertain the critical locus of dopaminergic action in oculomotor control. However, when MPTP is unilaterally infused directly into the regions of the monkey CN where neurons with oculomotor functions reside, thereby reducing any global effects, specific deficits emerge. These include saccadic hypometria (especially during memory-guided saccades), a marked reduction in the frequency of spontaneous saccades, and a paucity of saccades executed in the contralesional hemifield *(13,14)*. The animals in these experiments also showed evidence of spatial neglect with both a motor and an attentional component.

2.2. *Smooth Pursuit*

The oculomotor system responsible for smooth pursuit is less understood and appears to be segregated from that responsible for saccades, but the degree of segregation is a matter of dispute (for review, *see* ref. *15*). Broadly, the areas involved are the middle temporal and middle superior temporal cortices, FEF, LIP, dorsolateral nuclei in the pons, floccular region of the cerebellum, and the vestibular nuclei.

Smooth pursuit movements are harder to study. The usual parameters of interest are the fidelity with which the eyes can follow a moving target, either a simple-ramp stimulus or a sinusoidally modulated target. This can be expressed by measuring the discrepancy between the eye-pursuit velocity and velocity of the target.

3. OCULOMOTOR ABNORMALITIES IN PD

Although pathologically proven PD can occasionally simulate conditions associated with marked oculomotor disturbance, such as progressive supranuclear palsy *(16)*, gross eye movement abnormalities obvious at the bedside are rarely seen. Their presence should always raise the possibility of another parkinsonian disorder. However, there is no doubt that there are subtle abnormalities, but no clear consensus has emerged as to their precise nature and extent. The major difficulty with existing literature is that there is considerable heterogeneity in the selection of patients and experimental protocols used to study them, particularly the severity and treatment history of the disease and details of the paradigms used to elicit eye movements.

3.1. Saccades

3.1.1. Primary Abnormalities

The most consistent oculomotor abnormality in PD is the saccadic hypometria in which the primary saccade undershoots. This was initially demonstrated in saccades executed to verbal command *(17)*, in the dark *(18,19)*, or to fixed targets *(20)*. Predictive saccades also show hypometria in addition to difficulty in anticipating the stimulus *(21,22)*, and in unilaterally affected patients, the abnormalities were found to be lateralized *(23)*.

In agreement with findings in dopamine-depleted animals, memory-guided saccades are most strikingly affected, regardless of whether the remembered stimulus is visual *(24–27)*, vestibular, or cervical *(28)*. The first question that arises is whether the impaired performance is a consequence of a deficit in spatial-working memory or another resource that is engaged by the memory-guided saccade task. If the former is true, then patients should have difficulty in identifying the target location. In fact, although the primary saccade is hypometric, patients make secondary saccades that produce an accurate FEP when the memory delay is short *(25,26,29,30)* but possibly not when it is longer than 5 seconds *(31)*. Thus, abnormalities of FEP are seen in monkeys with dopaminergic blockade of the DLPFC *(32)*, but if there is a spatial-working memory deficit in PD, it is only revealed by tasks with a high-working memory load. Indeed, an abnormal FEP is found when patients are asked to perform sequences of memory-guided saccades *(27,33)*, and we have shown that this is present only when novel sequences are compared with those rehearsed *(34)*. Furthermore, any deficit in spatial-working memory may be compounded by global abnormalities in executive function interfering with the planning of gaze strategies *(35)*. Nonetheless, these findings do not account for saccadic hypometria of gaze, which occurs equally in the execution of both novel and rehearsed saccadic sequences *(34)*.

Contrary to memory-guided saccades, although some studies have shown mild impairment in reflexive saccades to peripheral stimuli *(20,22)*, most have not *(23–27,29,36,37)*. Two studies have even found a reduction in saccadic reaction time when compared with controls when a "gap" was introduced between the disappearance of the central fixation point and appearance of the peripheral target *(38,39)*. The fact that reflexive saccades should be normal or enhanced when memory-guided saccades are definitely abnormal suggests a dissociation between behavior that is reflexive or exogenously driven and that which is volitional or endogenously driven. There is good evidence from imaging *(40)* and saccadic adaptation *(41)* that this dissociation reflects the operation of separate neural networks in the oculomotor system.

If endogenously and exogenously driven saccades are differentially affected in PD, a task that pits one against the other should demonstrate an impairment. The simplest such task is the antisaccade task, where the subject has to suppress a reflexive saccade to a peripheral target and execute an endogenously driven saccade to the opposite location. Three studies have found no significant impairment in the performance of patients with PD in comparison with age-matched controls *(26,36,37),* and another three have shown impaired performance *(25,42,43).* It is difficult to draw firm conclusions from these studies because of methodological difficulties. However, the one study that employed a "gap" paradigm and tested patients in their "off" state demonstrated more errors, increased latency, and reduced gain in patients with mild-to-moderate PD *(43)* when compared with controls.

3.1.2. Response to Treatment

Although it seems reasonable to suppose that saccadic abnormalities in PD are related to dopaminergic depletion, evidence indicating that they can be reversed with dopaminergic treatment is sparse. Despite that a few studies have shown beneficial effects on the parameters of voluntary saccades *(17,44,45)* and on the ability to perform sequences of memory-guided saccades *(31),* no study has ever demonstrated any improvement in the most characteristic abnormality in PD—the hypometria of memory-guided saccades. By contrast, a study of eight patients who had PD implanted with deep-brain stimulators found that high-frequency stimulation of the STN produced a marked improvement in the gain of memory-guided saccades in the absence of any changes in other saccadic parameters *(46).* Also, there is one case report of similar improvement in memory-guided saccades, as well as antisaccades in a patient with a GPi electrode when the stimulator is turned on *(47).*

3.2. Smooth Pursuit

Abnormalities in smooth pursuit in PD are recognized *(18,20,44,45,48–51),* particularly in smooth-pursuit gain *(45,48),* but these have been less explored. The mechanisms remain uncertain; as with saccades, it is not clear whether the dysfunction is *(44)* or is not *(45,52)* sensitive to dopaminergic replacement. In a recent study, infusion of apomorphine in patients previously untreated with levodopa or dopamine agonists produced an increase in smooth pursuit velocity and gain, but the improvement was not as great as the improvement in limb motor function *(53).*

3.3. Other Abnormalities

Apraxia of eyelid opening usually occurs as an isolated focal dystonia but is occasionally seen in PD *(54).* It may be treated with botulinum toxin injections and may be ameliorated by mechanical stimulation of surrounding skin, such as is produced by wearing goggles *(55).*

Deranged convergence is rarely reported in PD. In one case, it was found to be responsive to levodopa *(56).*

4. DIFFERENTIAL DIAGNOSIS

The oculomotor abnormalities in PD are generally too subtle to detect at bedside. Consequently, their presence or absence is rarely a helpful diagnostic tool in routine clinical practice. In contrast, the presence of marked oculomotor abnormalities is often a helpful guide to another parkinsonian disorder. Clinically obvious impairment in vertical eye movements is characteristic of progressive supranuclear palsy (PSP). But it may be seen in other conditions, such as diffuse Lewy body disease *(57–60)* corticobasal degeneration (CBD; *61*) Guam Parkinson–Dementia Complex *(62),* Whipple's disease *(63),* amyotrophic lateral sclerosis *(64),* postencephalitic Parkinsonism *(65),* and Creutzfeld-Jacob disease *(66,67).* In PSP, slowing of vertical saccades precedes ophthalmoplegia and is probably the earliest sign of oculomotor involvement. A supranuclear gaze palsy may be seen in CBD, but usually only when the disease is advanced *(68).* Eye signs are rarely an early feature of multiple system atrophy (MSA), but may mimic PD in some cases *(69).*

It is uncertain to what extent eye movement recordings are helpful in discriminating between different types of Parkinsonism. One small study has examined simple saccadic metrics in the vertical, horizontal, and diagonal planes in patients with PD, MSA, pure akinesia, PSP, and CBD *(70)*. In comparison to age-matched controls, only patients with PSP had slow saccades (in any direction), and only patients with CBD had increased saccadic latency. Although other parameters (e.g., hypometria, vestibulo-ocular responses, and smooth pursuit) did not discriminate between groups, deviation of oblique saccades toward the horizontal plane was more marked in patients with pure akinesia and PSP. In another study *(36)*, patients with CBD had greater saccadic latency, and those with PSP, more marked hypometria and worse antisaccade performance versus patients with PD, but there were no saccadic criteria by which patients with MSA could be differentiated from those with PD. Thus, detailed eye movement analysis may be helpful in identifying patients with PSP and possibly CBD, but until there is more data on its sensitivity and specificity, it is difficult to recommend it for routine use in the diagnosis of parkinsonian disorders.

5. COMPLICATIONS OF TREATMENT

The oculomotor manifestations of PD do not consistently respond to treatment; yet, treatment is also not associated with any deleterious effects on the oculomotor system.

Generally, the eyes are spared in treatment-induced dyskinesias, but there are isolated reports of patients whose peak-dose dyskinesias have an oculomotor component in the form of large-amplitude oscillations *(71)* or brief tonic deviations of gaze *(72)*.

Pallidotomy produced no improvement in saccadic hypometria in one study of 31 patients with PD and resulted in only slightly reduced-peak velocities in the context of improved peripheral motor function *(73)*. In one small series, an increase in the frequency of square-wave jerks was found in the absence of any change in other saccadic parameters *(74)*. Transient conjugate eye deviation following the implantation of a GPi stimulator has been described in one patient *(75)*, but the deviation was seen only at supratherapeutic voltages and may have resulted from activation of neighboring regions.

6. CONCLUSION

We have seen that the most characteristic oculomotor disturbance in PD is hypometria of voluntary (especially memory-guided) saccades in the context of essentially normal reflexive visual-orienting behavior. Although deficits in spatial working memory and executive function may be contributory, the physiological changes underlying this disturbance remain obscure. Microelectrode recordings in monkeys suggest that caudate neurons may modulate the metrics of saccades in response to the expectation of reward. It is tempting to speculate that similar modulation mediates internally guided behavior in humans, and the saccadic abnormalities in PD are consequent on the dysfunction of these cells within a dopamine-depleted striatum. However, until further evidence is gained, this will have to remain in the realm of speculation.

Even if the role of striatal neurons can be proved, a satisfactory account would need to explain why the abnormalities are largely confined to saccadic gain, and why they are not rapidly responsive to treatment with levodopa. Here we present a hypothetical explanation that addresses these questions.

Saccades in infants are markedly hypometric with a gain of around 0.6. During childhood, saccadic gain increases, but there is always a tendency to undershoot the target even when development is complete; this increase in gain is accompanied by a reduction in saccadic error. Simulations have shown that the relationship between gain and error during development is such that saccadic flight-time is minimized *(76)*. Thus, the larger the saccadic error, the more advantageous it is to undershoot the target because a corrective saccade in the same direction can be executed faster.

Experiments where the saccade target is displaced intrasaccadically to generate error in the saccadic end-position have consistently shown in both monkeys and humans that over numerous trials, a corrective adjustment in gain occurs: this phenomenon is known as *saccadic adaptation*. There is strong lesion *(77)* and imaging *(78,79)* evidence that adaptation relies on the integrity of midline cerebellar structures, at least in adaptation tasks that employ reflexive saccades. Interestingly, in monkey experiments, when the target is shifted to produce a small constant error in the end-position of each saccade, saccadic gain is reduced even when the error is positive, i.e., the saccade is made to undershoot its target *(80,81)*. Hence, the question has not been directly addressed, but it appears that, similar to Harris's prediction *(76)*, the adaptive mechanism responsible for maintaining saccadic accuracy tends to reduce saccadic gain when saccadic error is increased.

A few studies have shown increased variance in the gain of memory-guided saccades in PD *(21,23)* but have not attributed any great significance to it. An increase in variance in these circumstances is also seen in limb movements *(82)* and is predictable from some models of motor dysfunction in PD, where the principal problem is envisaged as a failure to adequately facilitate goal-directed motor plans combined with a failure to inhibit competing ones *(83,84)*. The hypometria may therefore be the consequence of a normal adaptive response to increased variance in saccadic gain produced by a failure to inhibit competing internally guided motor plans. If so, its failure to respond immediately and consistently to treatment with levodopa or to fluctuate in synchrony with "on–off" periods would not be surprising. Such failure of inhibition is paralleled by the well-documented failure of the suppression of antagonist activity in the limbs in PD *(85)*. Furthermore, the importance of inhibition in basal ganglia function has recently been elegantly demonstrated in a neurophysiological study in cats. This study showed that uncrossed nigrocollicular fibers are deactivated ipsilaterally before a saccade is made to release the superior colliculus from inhibition, whereas nigrocollicular fibers that cross to the contralateral colliculus are simultaneously activated, thereby suppressing activity that could have generated a saccade in the opposite direction *(86)*.

Presently, there is no direct empirical support for this hypothesis, but it makes strong predictions about the nature of the oculomotor disturbance in PD, which can be tested experimentally with relative ease. The only study to examine the adaptation of memory-guided saccades in PD has found an increased tendency to hypometria when compared with controls, even during positive adaptation. However, the authors did not report the saccadic gain variance; therefore, its contribution to the difference in adaptation performance cannot be adequately assessed *(87)*.

REFERENCES

1. Sparks DL. The brainstem control of saccadic eye movements. Nat Rev Neurosci 2002;3:952–964.
2. Moschovakis AK, Scudder CA, Highstein SM. The microscopic anatomy and physiology of the mammalian saccadic system. Prog Neurobiol 1996;50:133–254.
3. Tehovnik EJ, Sommer MA, Chou IH, et al. Eye fields in the frontal lobes of primates. Brain Res Brain Res Rev 2000;32:413–448.
4. Hikosaka O, Takikawa Y, Kawagoe R. Role of the basal ganglia in the control of purposive saccadic eye movements. Physiol Rev 2000;80:953–978.
5. Takikawa Y, Kawagoe R, Hikosaka O. Reward-dependent spatial selectivity of anticipatory activity in monkey caudate neurons. J Neurophysiol 2002;87:508–515.
6. Lauwereyns J, Takikawa Y, Kawagoe R, et al. Feature-based anticipation of cues that predict reward in monkey caudate nucleus. Neuron 2002;33:463–473.
7. Lauwereyns J, Watanabe K, Coe B, Hikosaka O. A neural correlate of response bias in monkey caudate nucleus. Nature 2002;418:413–417.
8. Takikawa Y, Kawagoe R, Itoh H, et al. Modulation of saccadic eye movements by predicted reward outcome. Exp Brain Res 2002;142:284–291.
9. Hotson JR, Langston EB, Langston JW. Saccade responses to dopamine in human MPTP-induced Parkinsonism. Ann Neurol 1986;20:456–463.
10. Brooks BA, Fuchs AF, Finocchio D. Saccadic eye movement deficits in the MPTP monkey model of Parkinson's disease. Brain Res 1986;383:402–407.
11. Schultz W, Romo R, Scarnati E, et al. Saccadic reaction times, eye-arm coordination and spontaneous eye movements in normal and MPTP-treated monkeys. Exp Brain Res 1989;78:253–267.
12. Grace AA, Bunney BS. Intracellular and extracellular electrophysiology of nigral dopaminergic neurons—1. Identification and characterization. Neuroscience 1983;10:301–315.

13. Kato M, Miyashita N, Hikosaka O, et al. Eye movements in monkeys with local dopamine depletion in the caudate nucleus. I. Deficits in spontaneous saccades. J Neurosci 1995;15:912–927.
14. Miyashita N, Hikosaka O, Kato M. Visual hemineglect induced by unilateral striatal dopamine deficiency in monkeys. Neuroreport 1995;6:1257–1260.
15. Krauzlis RJ, Stone LS. Tracking with the mind's eye. Trends Neurosci 1999;22:544–550.
16. Seno H, Kobayashi S, Inagaki T, et al. Parkinson's disease associated with argyrophilic grains clinically resembling progressive supranuclear palsy: an autopsy case. J Neurol Sci 2000;178:70–74.
17. Highstein S, Cohen B, Mones R. Changes in saccadic eye movements of patients with Parkinson's disease before and after L-dopa. Trans Am Neurol Assoc 1969;94:277–279.
18. Teravainen H, Calne DB. Studies of parkinsonian movement:1. Programming and execution of eye movements. Acta Neurol Scand 1980;62:137–148.
19. DeJong JD, Jones GM. Akinesia, hypokinesia, and bradykinesia in the oculomotor system of patients with Parkinson's disease. Exp Neurol 1971;32:58–68.
20. Shibasaki H, Tsuji S, Kuroiwa Y. Oculomotor abnormalities in Parkinson's disease. Arch Neurol 1979;36:360–364.
21. Crawford T, Goodrich S, Henderson L, Kennard C. Predictive responses in Parkinson's disease: manual keypresses and saccadic eye movements to regular stimulus events. J Neurol Neurosurg Psychiatry 1989;52:1033–1042.
22. Bronstein AM, Kennard C. Predictive ocular motor control in Parkinson's disease. Brain 1985;108:925–940.
23. Ventre J, Zee DS, Papageorgiou H, Reich S. Abnormalities of predictive saccades in hemi-Parkinson's disease. Brain 1992;115:1147–1165.
24. Crawford TJ, Henderson L, Kennard C. Abnormalities of nonvisually-guided eye movements in Parkinson's disease. Brain 1989;112:1573–1586.
25. Kitagawa M, Fukushima J, Tashiro K. Relationship between antisaccades and the clinical symptoms in Parkinson's disease. Neurology 1994;44:2285–2289.
26. Lueck CJ, Tanyeri S, Crawford TJ, et al. Antisaccades and remembered saccades in Parkinson's disease. J Neurol. Neurosurg Psychiatry 1990;53:284–288.
27. Lueck CJ, Crawford TJ, Henderson L, et al. Saccadic eye movements in Parkinson's disease: II. Remembered saccades—towards a unified hypothesis? Q J Exp Psychol A 1992;45:211–233.
28. Nakamura T, Bronstein AM, Lueck C, et al. Vestibular, cervical and visual remembered saccades in Parkinson's disease. Brain 1994;117:1423–1432.
29. Shaunak S, O'Sullivan E, Blunt S, et al. Remembered saccades with variable delay in Parkinson's disease. Mov Disord 1999;14:80–86.
30. Kimmig H, Haussmann K, Mergner T, Lucking CH. What is pathological with gaze shift fragmentation in Parkinson's disease? J Neurol 2002;249:683–692.
31. Vermersch AI, Rivaud S, Vidailhet M, et al. Sequences of memory-guided saccades in Parkinson's disease. Ann Neurol 1994;35:487–490.
32. Sawaguchi T, Goldman-Rakic PS. The role of D1-dopamine receptor in working memory: local injections of dopamine antagonists into the prefrontal cortex of rhesus monkeys performing an oculomotor delayed-response task. J Neurophysiol 1994;71:515–528.
33. O'Sullivan EP, Shaunak S, Henderson L, et al. Abnormalities of predictive saccades in Parkinson's disease. Neuroreport 1997;8:1209–1213.
34. Hodgson TL, Dittrich WH, Henderson L, Kennard C. Eye movements and spatial working memory in Parkinson's disease. Neuropsychologia 1999;37:927–938.
35. Hodgson TL, Tiesman B, Owen AM, Kennard C. Abnormal gaze strategies during problem solving in Parkinson's disease. Neuropsychologia 2002;40:411–422.
36. Vidailhet M, Rivaud S, Gouider-Khouja N, et al. Eye movements in parkinsonian syndromes. Ann Neurol 1994;35:420–426.
37. Fukushima J, Fukushima K, Miyasaka K, Yamashita I. Voluntary control of saccadic eye movement in patients with frontal cortical lesions and parkinsonian patients in comparison with that in schizophrenics. Biol Psychiatry 1994;36:21–30.
38. Roll A, Wierzbicka MM, Wolf W. The "gap paradigm" leads to express-like saccadic reaction times in Parkinson's disease. Exp Brain Res 1996;111:131–138.
39. Briand KA, Hening W, Poizner H, Sereno AB. Automatic orienting of visuospatial attention in Parkinson's disease. Neuropsychologia 2001;39:1240–1249.
40. Mort DJ, Perry RJ, Mannan SK, et al. Differential cortical activation during voluntary and reflexive saccades in man. Neuroimage 2003;18:231–246.
41. Deubel H. Separate adaptive mechanisms for the control of reactive and volitional saccadic eye movements. Vision Res 1995;35:3529–3540.
42. Crevits L, De Ridder K. Disturbed striatoprefrontal mediated visual behaviour in moderate to severe parkinsonian patients. J Neurol Neurosurg Psychiatry 1997;63:296–299.
43. Briand KA, Strallow D, Hening W, et al. Control of voluntary and reflexive saccades in Parkinson's disease. Exp Brain Res 1999;129:38–48.

44. Gibson JM, Pimlott R, Kennard C. Ocular motor and manual tracking in Parkinson's disease and the effect of treatment. J Neurol Neurosurg Psychiatry 1987;50:853–860.
45. Rascol O, Clanet M, Montastruc JL, et al. Abnormal ocular movements in Parkinson's disease. Evidence for involvement of dopaminergic systems. Brain 1989;112:1193–1214.
46. Rivaud-Pechoux S, Vermersch AI, Gaymard B, et al. Improvement of memory guided saccades in parkinsonian patients by high frequency subthalamic nucleus stimulation. J Neurol Neurosurg Psychiatry 2000;68:381–384.
47. Straube A, Ditterich J, Oertel W, Kupsch A. Electrical stimulation of the posteroventral pallidum influences internally guided saccades in Parkinson's disease. J Neurol 1998;245:101–105.
48. White OB, Saint-Cyr JA, Tomlinson RD, Sharpe JA. Ocular motor deficits in Parkinson's disease. II. Control of the saccadic and smooth pursuit systems. Brain 1983;106:571–587.
49. Corin MS, Elizan TS, Bender MB. Oculomotor function in patients with Parkinson's disease. J Neurol Sci 1972;15:251–265.
50. Gibson JM, Kennard C. Quantitative study of "on-off" fluctuations in the ocular motor system in Parkinson's disease. Adv Neurol 1987;45:329–333.
51. Sharpe JA, Fletcher WA, Lang AE, Zackon DH. Smooth, pursuit during dose-related on-off fluctuations in Parkinson's disease. Neurology 1987;37:1389–1392.
52. Waterston JA, Barnes GR, Grealy MA, Collins S. Abnormalities of smooth eye and head movement control in Parkinson's disease. Ann Neurol 1996;39:749–760.
53. Bares M, Brazdil M, Kanovsky P, et al. The effect of apomorphine administration on smooth pursuit ocular movements in early Parkinsonian patients. Parkinsonism Relat Disord 2003;9:139–144.
54. Krack P, Marion MH. "Apraxia of lid opening," a focal eyelid dystonia: clinical study of 32 patients. Mov Disord 1994;9:610–615.
55. Hirayama M, Kumano T, Aita T, et al. Improvement of apraxia of eyelid opening by wearing goggles. Lancet 2000;356:1413.
56. Racette BA, Gokden MS, Tychsen LS, Perlmutter JS. Convergence insufficiency in idiopathic Parkinson's disease responsive to levodopa. Strabismus 1999;7:169–174.
57. de Bruin VM, Lees AJ, Daniel SE. Diffuse Lewy body disease presenting with supranuclear gaze palsy, Parkinsonism, and dementia: a case report. Mov Disord 1992;7:355–358.
58. Fearnley JM, Revesz T, Brooks DJ, et al. Diffuse Lewy body disease presenting with a supranuclear gaze palsy. J Neurol Neurosurg Psychiatry 1991;54:159–161.
59. Brett FM, Henson C, Staunton H. Familial diffuse Lewy body disease, eye movement abnormalities, and distribution of pathology. Arch Neurol 2002;59:464–467.
60. Lewis AJ, Gawel MJ. Diffuse Lewy body disease with dementia and oculomotor dysfunction. Mov Disord 1990;5:143–147.
61. Cordato NJ, Halliday GM, McCann H, et al. Corticobasal syndrome with tau pathology. Mov Disord 2001;16:656–667.
62. Oyanagi K, Chen KM, Craig UK, et al. Parkinsonism, dementia and vertical gaze palsy in a Guamanian with atypical neuroglial degeneration. Acta Neuropathol. (Berl) 2000;99:73–80.
63. Averbuch-Heller L, Paulson GW, Daroff RB, Leigh RJ. Whipple's disease mimicking progressive supranuclear palsy: the diagnostic value of eye movement recording. J Neurol Neurosurg Psychiatry 1999;66:532–535.
64. Averbuch-Heller L, Helmchen C, Horn AK, et al. Slow vertical saccades in motor neuron disease: correlation of structure and function. Ann Neurol 1998;44:641–648.
65. Wenning GK, Jellinger K, Litvan I. Supranuclear gaze palsy and eyelid apraxia in postencephalitic Parkinsonism. J Neural Transm 1997;104:845–865.
66. Grant MP, Cohen M, Petersen RB, et al. Abnormal eye movements in Creutzfeldt-Jakob disease. Ann Neurol 1993;34:192–197.
67. Zarei M, Nouraei SA, Caine D, et al. Neuropsychological and quantitative oculometric study of a case of sporadic Creutzfeldt-Jakob disease at predementia stage. J Neurol Neurosurg Psychiatry 2002;73:56–58.
68. Rinne JO, Lee MS, Thompson PD, Marsden CD. Corticobasal degeneration. A clinical study of 36 cases. Brain 1994;117:1183–1196.
69. Merchut MP, Brigell M. Olivopontocerebellar atrophy presenting with hemiparkinsonian ocular motor signs. J Clin Neuroophthalmol 1990;10:210–214.
70. Rottach KG, Riley DE, DiScenna AO, et al. Dynamic, properties of horizontal and vertical eye movements in parkinsonian syndromes. Ann Neurol 1996;39:368–377.
71. Shimizu N, Cohen B, Bala SP, et al. Ocular dyskinesias in patients with Parkinson's disease treated with levodopa. Ann Neurol 1977;1:167–171.
72. Linazasoro G, Van Blercom N, Lasa A, et al. Levodopa-induced ocular dyskinesias in Parkinson's disease. Mov Disord 2002;17:186–187.
73. Blekher T, Siemers E, Abel LA, Yee RD. Eye movements in Parkinson's disease: before and after pallidotomy. Invest Ophthalmol Vis Sci 2000;41:2177–2183.
74. Averbuch-Heller L, Stahl JS, Hlavin ML, Leigh RJ. Square-wave jerks induced by pallidotomy in parkinsonian patients. Neurology 1999;52:185–188.
75. Anagnostou E, Sporer B, Steude U, et al. Contraversive eye deviation during deep brain stimulation of the globus pallidus internus. Neurology 2001;56:1396–1399.
76. Harris CM. Does saccadic undershoot minimize saccadic flight-time? A Monte-Carlo study. Vision Res 1995;35:691–701.

77. Straube A, Deubel H, Ditterich J, Eggert T. Cerebellar lesions impair rapid saccade amplitude adaptation. Neurology 2001;57:2105–2108.
78. Desmurget M, Pelisson D, Urquizar C, et al. Functional anatomy of saccadic adaptation in humans. Nat Neurosci 1998;1:524–528.
79. Desmurget M, Pelisson D, Grethe JS, et al. Functional adaptation of reactive saccades in humans: a PET study. Exp Brain Res 2000;132:243–259.
80. Straube A, Fuchs AF, Usher S, Robinson FR. Characteristics of saccadic gain adaptation in rhesus macaques. J Neurophysiol 1997;77:874–895.
81. Robinson FR, Noto CT, Bevans SE. Effect of Visual Error Size on Saccade Adaptation in Monkey. J Neurophysiol 2003;90:1235–1244.
82. Ketcham CJ, Hodgson TL, Kennard C, Stelmach GE. Memory-motor transformations are impaired in Parkinson's disease. Exp Brain Res 2003;149:30–39.
83. Mink JW. The basal ganglia: focused selection and inhibition of competing motor programs. Prog Neurobiol 1996;50:381–425.
84. McAuley JH. The physiological basis of clinical deficits in Parkinson's disease. Prog Neurobiol 2003;69:27–48.
85. Meunier S, Pol S, Houeto JL, Vidailhet M. Abnormal reciprocal inhibition between antagonist muscles in Parkinson's disease. Brain 2000;123:1017–1026.
86. Jiang H, Stein BE, McHaffie JG. Opposing basal ganglia processes shape midbrain visuomotor activity bilaterally. Nature 2003;423:982–986.
87. MacAskill MR, Anderson TJ, Jones RD. Adaptive modification of saccade amplitude in Parkinson's disease. Brain 2002;125:1570–1582.

24
Fatigue

Carol Ewing Garber and Joseph H. Friedman

SUMMARY

Fatigue is a common complaint in patients with Parkinson's disease (PD). More than half of all patients with PD rank fatigue among their three worst symptoms. Fatigue has been variously hypothesized to be caused by dysfunction of the striato–thalamo–cortical loop, abnormalities in the hypothalamic–pituitary–adrenal axis, inflammatory processes, and neurotransmitter abnormalities within the central nervous system. However, there is no firm evidence that any of these proposed etiologies explain the fatigue experienced by patients who have PD or other diseases.

Fatigue may be associated with depression, sleep disorders, and medication-induced adverse effects, but it also remains a distinct symptom that can occur independently from these other disorders and problems. Fatigue is a persistent symptom in individual patients, and it is unrelated to disease severity. Fatigue is difficult to define and even more difficult to measure. Several questionnaires are available to measure fatigue, but many of these are disease-specific and do not apply to patients who have PD. Some questionnaires measure general overall fatigue, whereas others measure different aspects of fatigue, including mental, physical, emotional, motivational, and exertional fatigue. Often fatigue is confused with sleepiness, a related but distinct construct. Clearly, fatigue has a significantly negative impact on the quality of life and physical function of patients with PD. Currently, there is no proven effective treatment for this problematic nonmotor symptom of PD. Additional research is needed to provide a better understanding of this complex problem.

Key Words: Fatigue; central fatigue; motor fatigue; Parkinson's disease (PD); quality of life.

1. INTRODUCTION

Fatigue is a common problem to many neurological, psychiatric, and medical conditions *(1–6)*. For neurologists, the word "fatigue" generally evokes a knee-jerk reaction to "multiple sclerosis," yet fatigue is so much a part of countless disorders that when a patient complains of it, it is impossible to know exactly what to do with the information. Fatigue affects all people at some point. Consider the following:

- Fatigue represents the leading complaint in 4 to 9% of all office visits to internists and family practitioners *(7–9)*.
- A sense of chronic fatigue was reported as a "major problem" by 25% of consecutive patients seen in a primary care clinic; of these, 75% had suffered with it for at least 1 year *(10)*.
- Fatigue was the presenting PD symptom in 2% of newly diagnosed patients in the classic study by Hoehn and Yahr *(11)*.
- Fatigue occurs in 80 to 100% of patients with systemic lupus erythematosus and is among the most commonly reported symptoms *(12,13)*.
- Fatigue has a major impact on quality of life in multiple sclerosis (MS; *14*). One small ($n = 32$) study of MS patients found that fatigue was the worst symptom in 28% *(15)*.

From: *Current Clinical Neurology*
Parkinson's Disease and Nonmotor Dysfunction
Edited by: R. F. Pfeiffer and I. Bodis-Wollner © Humana Press Inc., Totowa, NJ

Table 1
Fatigue Definitions

1. "An overwhelming sense of tiredness, lack of energy and feeling of exhaustion. It is distinguished from symptoms of depression. Fatigue is also distinguished from limb weakness" *(25)*.
2. "A sense of physical tiredness and lack of energy, greater than expected for a usual task" *(146)*.
3. Fatigue Assessment Inventory: "a sense of tiredness, lack of energy, or total body give out" *(27)*.
4. "A condition resulting from previous stress, which leads to reversible impairment of performance and function. Affects the organic interplay of the functions and finally may lead to disturbance of the functional structure of the personality; it is generally accompanied by a reduction in readiness to work and heightened sensation of strain" *(147)*.
5. "A chronic form of tiredness, which is perceived by the patient as being unusual or abnormal and absolutely disproportionate with respect to the amount of exercise or activity he/she has carried out and is not removed by resting or sleeping" *(148)*.
6. "Inability to maintain force" *(149)*. … "Sensation experienced when the effort to perform work, whether physical, mental, or both, seems disproportionate to the task involved *(149)*.
7. "A sense of physical tiredness and lack of energy, interfering with physical functional and social life, distinct from mental exhaustion, sadness, sleepiness, and impaired motor function secondary to PD symptoms" *(61,62)*.
8. "A subjective lack of physical and/or mental energy that is perceived by the individual or caregiver to interfere with usual and desired activities" *(150)*.

Complicating the understanding of fatigue is the difficulty in apprehending its meaning and discrepancies in its use (*see* Table 1). Fatigue is defined as lassitude, overtiredness, and lacking in energy. Synonyms include weariness, debilitation, enervation, languor, listlessness, heaviness, drowsiness, tedium, and overtiredness *(16)*. In physiology, it is used to mean fatigue of a neuron, muscle, or organism. Further complicating comprehension, fatigue is often used as a synonym for sleepiness or tiredness, which are distinct constructs. For example, the *New England Journal of Medicine* published three articles in one issue in 2002 on fatigue in doctors, yet the articles actually focused on sleep deprivation, a related disorder, not physical or mental fatigue *(17–19)*. With so many facets, it is inevitably difficult to interpret the symptom, because it is usually a symptom complex. Grappling with knowledge of this problem is reminiscent of a Bertrand Russel quote, uttered about mathematics, another seemingly straight forward entity: "Mathematics may be defined as the subject in which we never know what we are talking about, nor whether what we are saying is true" *(20)*.

2. MEASURES OF FATIGUE

Attempting to measure a subjective sensation that eludes accurate description is a complex undertaking that will inexorably yield multiple overlapping scales. Such is the case for depression, psychosis, and every other subjective condition. Before the modern era of clinical trials and recent exponential development of rating instruments, concern had been raised that fatigue might not be measurable *(21)*. Since then, many self-report questionnaires have been developed to measure fatigue in a variety of diseases, including neurological, cancer, and immune disorders. These have been developed using inconsistent application of psychometric test development methodologies, and often, small numbers of subjects *(22)*.

Krupp and her collaborators have led the way in measuring fatigue in MS and other disorders, thus shedding light on its appearances in neurological and non-neurological conditions *(23–30)*. The Fatigue Severity Scale (FSS; *26*) is a nine-item questionnaire that employs a seven-point Likert scale response to each of the items. The FSS has been shown to be valid and reliable in a variety of populations *(24–30)* and has been shown to have good discrimination between fatigued and nonfatigued patients with MS *(22)*.

Measures of fatigue that have been used in PD and other neurological disorders consist of: (1) simple visual-analog scales, in which subjects mark a point on a line extending between a point denoted by severe fatigue and another denoted by "not fatigued at all" or "energetic" *(28,31–33);* (2) the Fatigue Assessment Inventory (FAI; *27*); (3) a 30-item self-report scale that contains a 7-item FSS *(26);* (4) the 14-item Fatigue Scale (FS; *34*); and (5) the 21-item Modified Fatigue Impact Scale (MFIS; *35*). All of these have been validated in other diseases. The FS developed by Chalder and colleagues *(34,36)* is a 14-item scale, developed in a community sample, and generally applied to patients with chronic fatigue and CFS *(36,37).* The FibroFatigue Scale *(38)* is a 12-item rating scale utilized to measure fatigue in patients with fibromylagia and chronic fatigue syndrome (CFS).

Several scales have been developed to assess fatigue in cancer patients, including the Multidimensional Fatigue Inventory (MFI; *39*), Schwartz Cancer Fatigue Scale *(40,41),* and the Piper Fatigue Scale (PFS) *(42).* Both the PFS and MFI have been applied to patients with other conditions, including polio, amytrophic lateral sclerosis (ALS), fibromylagia, and chronic fatigue syndrome *(43–46).* The PFS *(42)* consists of a series of 41-item visual-analog scales that address the temporal, visual, affective, intensity, and sensory aspects of fatigue. The MFI is a 20-item self-report scale, which contains the five subsets of general, physical fatigue, mental fatigue, motivation, and activity, being used in many different disorders. The four mental fatigue questions only measure concentration.

Two quality-of-life measures that have been validated in patients with PD—Parkinson's Disease Questionaire 39 (PDQ-39) *(47)* and Parkinson's Disease Questionaire Long Form (PDQL) *(48)*—include fatigue assessments, but the Euro QoL-5 dimension questionnaire (EQ-5D) *(49)* does not. Damiano et al. *(50)* used several PD expert consultants and quality-of-life experts to review the PDQ-39 and PDQL. In doing so, they defined 12 areas that they thought must be covered by a useful quality-of-life scale, including energy/fatigue.

3. FATIGUE IN PD

3.1. *Review of Studies*

Two distinct types of fatigue have been identified: peripheral and central fatigue *(26,51,52).* Peripheral fatigue refers to local muscular fatigue, in which an individual can no longer produce adequate force during repeated muscular contractions *(51,53).* In contrast, central fatigue has both physical and mental components and is characterized by the difficulty in initiating and sustaining mental and physical tasks in the absence of cognitive or motor impairment *(51,53).* Mental fatigue itself may be subdivided into fatigue caused by sustained hyperarousal or hypervigilance (extended hyperarousal or overactivism) versus the fatigue of boredom (extended hypoarousal; *[54]*). Hypovigilance occurs with tedious repetitive tasks. Emotional fatigue can be considered analogous to the sustained hyperarousal of mental fatigue. However, only certain types of inattention might be considered indicative of fatigue; e.g., the inattention of attention deficit disorder would not be an example of fatigue.

Peripheral fatigue is often experienced in patients with sarcopenia that accompanies neuromuscular and rheumatic disorders *(52,55,56),* but the disabling fatigue associated with chronic disorders is central fatigue *(25,51,52).* Central fatigue has generally shown poor associations with other markers of disease *(52).* Fatigue, although a common symptom in multiple neurological disorders, receives little attention in texts (e.g., *see* ref. *57*).

Before considering fatigue in PD, it is useful to review myasthenia gravis (MG) as a paradigmatic illness, because muscle fatigue is its core clinical feature. Weakness is caused by fatigue in muscle contractions. Although the neuropathology of MG is believed to be entirely peripheral, Paul et al. *(58,59)* found high levels of cognitive fatigue in MG patients. Additionally, diminished cognitive performance correlated with self-perception of fatigue *(59).* Other peripheral immune-mediated neuropathic conditions unassociated with muscle fatigue have been related to fatigue *(60).* Interestingly, one study showed that fatigue correlated inversely with the degree of recovery from the Guillain-Barre syndrome *(60),* i.e., the patients who had the best outcome had the most fatigue.

There have been only a few studies of fatigue in PD. Most have discussed phenomenology; a few have looked at treatment. Aside from the report by Hoehn and Yahr *(11),* in which fatigue is listed as a rare-presenting symptom of PD, the first reports focusing on fatigue in PD were published in 1993 *(31,61,62).*

Van Hilten et al. *(62)* compared 65 nondemented patients with PD to 68 age-matched controls. How controls were chosen and whether they were linked by gender was not specified. Their hypothesis was that fatigue would vary over the course of the day. Activity monitors on the nondominant hand were used to assess movements, dyskinetic patients excluded. Fatigue was self-assessed on a five-point scale that asked how often fatigue was present, rather than how severe it was. "Excessive fatigue," defined as fatigue being "often present," "very often present," or "continuously present," was present in 31 patients (48%). In these, 14 did not suffer fatigue at any particular time of day, whereas 2 were most affected in the morning, 5 in mid-day, 5 in the late afternoon, and 5 in the evening. Interestingly, there was no correlation between fatigue and either diurnal motor activity or bedtime, an observation confirmed in a later study *(63).*

In another study *(61),* Van Hilten et al., possibly using some of the same subjects evaluated in the previously cited report *(62),* evaluated both sleep and fatigue in 90 nondepressed nondemented patients with PD (50 men and 40 women). Although this was a case-control study, the control subjects were only compared to patients on sleep disorders measures, not fatigue. Fatigue was measured using the FSS and the seven-point scale, as described previously, where "excess" meant "frequent," "very frequent," or "always present." Fatigue was defined as in definition 7 (Table 1). Excessive daytime fatigue (EDF), defined as fatigue present at least "frequently," afflicted 43% of patients who had PD and had been present for a mean of 8.6 years. However, in half of those affected by EDF, its onset predated the development of PD. Of patients, 15% reported fatigue as their worst symptom of PD; 54% described it as equal to their other PD symptoms; and 31% found it to be their least severe symptom. There was no diurnal aspect to the fatigue and no association with excessive daytime sleepiness (EDS). The lack of a diurnal pattern to the fatigue contrasted with earlier observations based on clinical impression *(64,65).* No relationship was found with medication, and they deduced, as had Schwab *(66),* that fatigue was related to motor dysfunction, a point contested by others.

A survey of fatigue by Friedman and Friedman *(32)* evaluated consecutive nondemented patients who had PD and asked each subject to ask a same-sex friend or relative who was within 5 years of the subject's age and did not have PD to serve as a control. There were 51 of 58 patients with PD and 41 of 58 controls who completed the FSS questionnaire and the Geriatrics Depression Scale *(67).* Patients also scored their fatigue on a visual-analog scale. As expected, patients with PD endorsed significantly greater levels of depression and fatigue than the controls, and one third of patients reported fatigue as the single worst symptom of PD. On a 1 to 7 scale, 58% of all patients with PD scored 5 or greater on the FSS question: "Fatigue is one of the three most disabling symptoms of PD." Most described the fatigue as having a different quality than fatigue experienced prior to the onset of PD; despite that fatigue correlated with depression, it did not correlate with motor dysfunction as hypothesized by previous authors (*see* refs. *61,62,66*). Although fatigue correlated with depression, the authors noted that many nondepressed subjects also suffered from fatigue. Of special note to neurologists was the observation that these patients with PD had a mean score of 4.6 on the FSS, the same instrument used to assess MS patients, whose mean score was 4.8 *(26),* a clinically insignificant difference.

In another study, a convenience sample of 70 patients who had PD living within 30 miles of Duke University *(68)* was evaluated at baseline 1 and 3 years later, and 40% reported fatigue. Fatigue was more prevalent in patients who identified themselves as having "poor health," in contrast to those who identified themselves as being in "good health"; 58.6% of self-characterized "poor health" subjects reported fatigue. Fatigue prevalence increased during the first year in patients who initially thought themselves to be in "good health."

Shilman et al. *(69)* evaluated 99 "selected" nondemented patients who had PD with the FSS (which includes the FAI), Beck Depression Inventory, Beck Anxiety Inventory, and Pittsburgh Sleep Quality Index and used a mean FAI score of 4 or more as the definition for fatigue. Using these criteria, 40% of patients suffered from fatigue. Fatigue correlated with anxiety, but significant associations were not found between fatigue and sleep disorders, gender, age, depression, or motor dysfunction. A positive correlation was found between one measure of activities of daily living (ADL), the Unified Parkinson's Disease Rating Scale (UPDRS) part II, but not with the Schwab and England ADL scale. More than half of the patients scored fatigue as one of their three most disabling symptoms. The lack of correlation between fatigue and motor dysfunction was underscored by the observation that, whereas 37% reported worsened motor function in the morning, only 14% reported fatigue being worse in the morning.

Abe et al. *(70)* studied 26 nondemented patients chosen in a nondisclosed manner (16 men and 10 women) and 26 age- and gender-matched controls with tension or migraine headaches. All patients with PD were on PD medications, but no one was taking antidepressants. Subjects completed the FSS, Zung Self-Assessed Depression Scale, and two neuropsychological measures of frontal lobe function (Go-No-Go task and the Wisconsin Card Sorting Test), a brain magnetic resonance imaging and technicium-99m hexamethyl-proprolene amine oxime (99mTc-HMPAO) single-photon positron emission tomography (SPECT) scan. The patients with PD scored slightly (but not significantly) higher on both fatigue and depression scores than controls. There was no correlation between depression scores and fatigue or motor and fatigue scores for patients who had PD. Interestingly, HMPAO SPECT revealed diminished frontal perfusion in patients who had PD with fatigue. Scores on the neuropsychological tests showed a trend toward a relationship with fatigue. The authors concluded that fatigue in PD may represent frontal lobe dysfunction.

A Norwegian study of fatigue in PD *(71)* reviewed nondemented nondepressed subjects with PD (n = 66) versus those with severe hip arthritis (n = 79) and randomly chosen sex- and age-matched controls (n = 131). The patients comprised almost all eligible patients with PD in four municipalities. The mean FSS scores were 4.1 for PD, 2.9 for arthritics, and 2.7 for controls. When compared to only 25% of the other groups, 50% of patients with PD scored 4 or greater on the FSS. On a univariate analysis, fatigue in patients with PD related to motor dysfunction, but not disease duration or sleep dysfunction; multivariate analysis revealed no factors associated with fatigue. The authors concluded that fatigue in nondepressed patients who had PD did not correlate with any motor or nonmotor factors they could identify.

Lou et al. *(53)* compared 39 patients with mild-to-moderate PD with 32 age-matched controls. How subjects were chosen was not stated. Controls were spouses or friends. The behavioral measures employed were the MFI *(72)*, Fatigue Severity Inventory (a modified form of the FSS), Profiles of Mood States, and two depression scales. Patients scored significantly higher than controls on all five sections of the MFI: general fatigue, physical fatigue, mental fatigue, reduced activity, and reduced motivation. None of the five measures correlated with disease severity (Hoehn and Yahr, stages 1–3 only), and mental fatigue correlated with reduced motivation.

Tolson et al. *(73)*, reporting on a convenience sample of 17 women with PD, found that menstruation was associated with exaggerated PD symptoms, reduced medication effectiveness, increased when "off," and increased fatigue.

A recent study by Garber and Friedman *(63)* characterized the relationships between symptoms of fatigue, physical activity, physical function, and functional capacity in a convenience sample of 37 patients with idiopathic PD. Standard questionnaires were used to measure physical activity (Godin Leisure Activity Questionnaire, Yale Physical Activity Questionnaire), and fatigue (FSS). The Up and Go and Six-Minute Walk Test were used to assess physical function, and functional capacity was measured by a maximal oxygen-uptake exercise test (VO_{2max}). Significant inverse relationships were detected between fatigue severity and leisure activity levels, frequency of vigorous physical activity, time spent performing daily tasks each day, diastolic blood pressure, and VO_{2max}. Fatigue correlated positively with the Up and Go and carbidopa/levodopa (CL) use. A multiple regression analysis was performed with the FSS as the dependent variable and Up and Go, Leisure Activity Score, CL use, VO_{2max}, and diastolic blood pressure as the independent variables. Of these variables, Up and Go and CL use contributed significantly to the predictive model of fatigue, whereas the other variables appeared to be moderator variables that affect the relationships between the variables of interest. The study demonstrated that patients who had PD with more severe fatigue are more sedentary. They also have poorer functional capacity and physical function in comparison to patients with less fatigue, but these results do not imply causality.

3.2. Course of Fatigue

Little is known regarding the natural course of fatigue in PD. The first follow-up study addressing this issue looked retrospectively at patients initially studied 9 years earlier and found that fatigue was a persistent problem *(31)*. Not only did mean fatigue scores worsen, but all subjects who strongly endorsed fatigue as a prominent symptom in the original study remained fatigued 9 years later. Only 2 of 13 subjects who strongly endorsed fatigue as a major symptom at the 9-year mark had not been fatigued earlier. In short, fatigue in this small study generally appeared early and tended to be persistent. Few patients either fell into or out of the fatigued group. The authors had attempted a variety of treatments for most of these subjects, including sedatives at night, antidepressants, stimulants, and exercise, but these were neither systematically administered nor discussed. Fatigue did not predict mortality, dementia, or later alteration of diagnosis (to an alternative Parkinsonian condition). In contrast, Schenkman et al. *(68)* reported an increase in fatigue prevalence in their self-reported "good health" group of patients with PD during the first year of their studies, implying a decline over time. The authors could not locate any other longitudinal studies of fatigue in PD.

3.3. Fatigue and Depression

Estimates of the incidence of depression in patients with PD range from 2% to 70% *(74–77)*. However, depression is often unrecognized in PD *(74,78)*. Depression has been associated with the neurochemical changes occurring in PD; yet, it is not understood why some patients are depressed and others are not *(79–81)*.

Depression is often associated with general feelings of tiredness and malaise, often mistaken for fatigue *(76,79)*. The link between depression and fatigue is complex. For example, fatigue is a major limitation even among those patients with PD who are not depressed *(82)*. A study by Abe and colleagues *(70)* compared patients who had PD with age-matched healthy controls and found no significant relationship between the fatigue and depression, although a notable association was observed between depression and fatigue in the control subjects.

Depression has been related to many dimensions of fatigue, such as mental fatigue and reduced activity, but it has not been shown to correlate with physical fatigue *(44,70,83)*. Cognitive and behavioral factors have been implicated in the persistence of fatigue in patients with other neurological disorders. A study of fatigue in chronic fatigue syndrome patients and MS patients found that perceptions of control were important predictors of fatigue—depression did not explain fatigue *(83,84)*.

3.4. Etiology of Fatigue

Fatigue's etiology in PD and other neurological disorders is unknown *(55)*. In chronic diseases, several mechanisms for fatigue have been hypothesized *(52)*. Theories are (1) a heightened stress response results in altered activation of the hypothalamic–pituitary–adrenal axis; (2) fatigue results from inflammatory processes; and (3) there are alterations in neurotransmission within the central nervous system. None of these proposed theories for the pathology of fatigue have been carefully evaluated for validity in other patients with chronic fatigue, and none have been studied in PD. One fundamentally untested hypothesis proposes that fatigue in PD is the result of disruption of nonmotor functions in the basal ganglia and dysfunction of the striato–thalamo–cortical loop *(51)*. The loss of the neurotransmitter, dopamine, and alterations in serotonin activity have been proposed as important correlates of this dysfunction *(51)*.

Efforts to link symptoms of fatigue to individual muscle fatigue have not been revealing *(53,56)*. Lou and colleagues *(53)* assessed fatigue in 39 patients with PD and 32 age-matched normal controls using the MFI (five dimensions of fatigue: general fatigue, physical fatigue, reduced motivation, reduced activity, and mental fatigue) and the FSI. The patients with PD scored higher than the control subjects in all of the five dimensions of fatigue on the MFI, and no relationship existed between the severity of physical fatigue and mental fatigue. Ziv et al. *(56),* reporting on 17 patients with PD and 10 age-matched controls, measured muscle fatigue during 30-second maximal, isometric forearm flexion. Patients who had PD experienced a 50% increase in fatigue following the exercise; this response improved after an oral dose of levodopa.

Brain perfusion was evaluated in a small group of patients with PD by Abe et al. *(70),* comparing 26 patients with PD (16 men and 10 women) to 26 age- and sex-matched controls without neurological deficits. All patients underwent SPECT using 99mTc-HMPAO and MRI imaging and measurement of fatigue. A significant correlation was observed between perfusion in the frontal lobe and fatigue, such that poorer perfusion was associated with greater fatigue, but this work has not yet been confirmed.

Proinflammatory activity has been proposed as a pathological mechanism of fatigue in MS; however, this has not been well-supported in the literature. Mainero et al. *(85)* failed to show any abnormalities in the blood-brain barrier in patients with MS, which has been thought to reflect damage that results from proinflammatory cytokine activity. A study by Giovannoni et al. *(86)* found no relationship between FSS score and several markers of inflammation, including a marker of interferon-γ-activated macrophage activity, serum C-reactive protein, and soluble intercellular adhesion molecule-1 levels.

Studying MS patients, Roelcke et al. *(87)* found that patients with higher levels of fatigue assessed by the FSS had reduced glucose metabolism bilaterally in the prefrontal area, premotor cortex, putamen, and in the right supplementary motor area. Filippi et al. *(88)* observed that fatigued patients with MS had impaired interactions between functionally related cortical and subcortical areas, whereas Colombo et al. *(89)* reported a significant association between FSS scores and lesions in the parietal lobe, internal capsule, and periventricular trigone in patients with MS. Other studies (*see* refs. *90* and *91*) suggest that pathological changes evident with MRI cannot fully explain fatigue in MS.

4. CENTRAL FATIGUE IN EXERCISE: A POTENTIAL MODEL OF MECHANISMS FOR FATIGUE

During long-duration endurance exercise, such as ultramarathons, where both central and peripheral fatigue occurs, byproducts of the hydrolysis of adenosine triphosphate (ATP), particularly inorganic phosphate, in the muscle have been related to fatigue *(92).* These byproducts are believed to cause fatigue as they accumulate and interfere with transmission of the excitatory impulse across the neuromuscular junction, impair calcium release by the sarcoplasmic reticulum, and prevent muscle cross-bridge formation *(92).* Although not studied in relationship to fatigue symptoms in PD, abnormalities of the function of the mitochondrial respiratory chain in the substantia nigra, including ATP, have been described in patients who have PD *(93,94).* Some studies (but not all) have identified similar abnormalities in the skeletal muscles of patients with PD *(95).* Thus, it is possible that mitochondrial dysfunction, and its subsequent effects on cellular metabolic activity, are related to the symptoms of fatigue experienced by patients who have PD. Whether these reported abnormalities are the cause or effect of the disease is controversial. For instance, it is well-known that mitochondrial density and function in skeletal muscle reflects the participation level in regular physical activity, resulting from alterations in genetic transcription in the sarcomere *(96).*

Some investigations have supported a physiological cause for fatigue in PD. A decline in acute muscle fatigue was observed after an oral dose of levodopa in one study *(56),* suggesting a relationship between muscle fatigue and dopamine deficiency. Another study documented a delay in the anaerobic threshold during exercise after a dose of levodopa in subjects with PD, reflecting improved aerobic metabolism and exercise capacity *(55).* These studies indicate that the dopamine deficiency associated with PD can affect peripheral fatigue, but the effects on central fatigue have been mostly untested.

Studies of endurance athletes *(97,98)* have identified potential roles of several neurotransmitters in central fatigue, including serotonin, dopamine, and acetylcholine. Serotonin has been studied most extensively, and increases in serotonin activity during prolonged exercise have been found to accelerate fatigue, and decreases appear to delay the onset of fatigue *(97,98)*. Known neuromodulators—cytokines and ammonia—may also affect central fatigue during exercise *(98)*.

Possible effects of regular physical activity and exercise on fatigue have been explored in both animal and human models. Interestingly, studies of rats following exercise training have reported increases in the number of D2 dopamine receptors, improved dopamine uptake in the striatum, and reversal of oxidative stress induced by immobilization *(99,100)*. Studies in athletes *(101)* have documented that increased serotonin concentrations from exercise training are related to improved mood and physical efficiency, whereas overtraining results in disruptions in serotonin biosynthesis that appear to be related to mental (central) fatigue.

Whether the mechanisms of central fatigue during exercise have any implications for fatigue in PD is unknown. However, in light of the suspected role of the ATP byproducts and several neurotransmitters (particularly dopamine) in central fatigue, the exercise model may help to expand the understanding of this subject.

5. *Resting Energy Expenditure and Fatigue*

Patients with PD have been reported in several studies to have a higher resting metabolic rate when compared with healthy control subjects *(102,103)*. Markus et al. *(103)* found that levodopa treatment resulted in a reduction in energy expenditure only in patients with rigidity in the untreated state. These findings imply that muscle rigidity is responsible for an increased resting metabolic rate in patients who have PD. However, although it is possible that a higher resting metabolic rate could contribute to fatigue associated with PD, it cannot explain why some, but not all, patients report feeling fatigued.

Complicating the influence of fatigue to the disease process is the observation that pramipexole, used to improve tremors in patients with PD who are already taking levodopa, worsened fatigue *(104)*. A study showed 10 of 34 pramipexole-treated subjects versus 4 of 35 placebo-treated subjects developed fatigue as an adverse effect. There was no correlation between fatigue and tremor reduction. However, fatigue was not assessed with a standard questionnaire in this study, and it may have been sleepiness that patients were actually reporting. Pramipexole is well-known to induce sleepiness *(105)*. In contrast, Abe et al. *(106)* reported that patients with PD using pergolide showed significant improvement in the FSS (from 5.1 to 4.4), and patients taking bromocriptine did not have any change in fatigue (from 4.8 to 4.7).

6. FATIGUE AND RESPIRATORY FUNCTION

Patients with PD have been reported to have inefficient breathing patterns, which could produce a perception of fatigue, particularly during exertion. However, this has not actually been evaluated in any study. Patients with PD have been shown to have a restrictive pattern of flow-volume loops both in "on" and "off" states, and a significant reduction in both forced expiratory volume in 1 second (FEV1) and forced vital capacity (FVC) was noted during the "off" state by De Pandis et al. *(107)* These results have been confirmed by other investigators *(108,109)*.

Weiner et al. *(110)* studied 20 patients with PD and the perception of dyspnea. Perception increased during "off" periods and decreased when "on." These changes were not related to those in respiratory muscle performance or pulmonary function.

Respiratory muscle efficiency is reduced during inspiratory resistive-loaded breathing tasks in PD *(111)*. In a recent report, Masoudi et al. *(112)* studied subjects performing submaximal exercise and found that the ventilatory equivalent, a measure of respiratory efficiency, was abnormally elevated in patients with PD, suggesting inefficient breathing mechanics in patients who had PD. Furthermore, the minute ventilation during exercise was at a greater proportion of the maximum voluntary ventilation, showing that patients with PD encroach on their ventilatory reserve, even at low exertion levels. These results may be caused by ineffective breathing patterns or respiratory muscle inefficiency and may contribute to exercise limitation and possible fatigue in patients with PD.

Recent work by Garber and Friedman *(63)* found that fatigue is associated with reduced levels of physical activity and poorer levels of physical function and exercise capacity in patients with mild-to-moderate idiopathic PD. Patients with more fatigue moved less as part of their daily activities versus patients reporting little fatigue, and they were less likely to engage in regular exercise of any type. Sedentary patients with fatigue had poorer physical capacity and function, both of which reflect probable limitations of the ability to perform ADL. These results demonstrate that fatigue, whether the cause or result of a sedentary lifestyle, is an important negative factor in physical function and quality of life of patients with PD. Similar relationships between fatigue and physical activity have been reported in patients with SLE *(113)*.

7. EFFECTS OF EXERCISE ON FATIGUE

An active lifestyle results in numerous physiological and psychological alterations that have the potential to affect fatigue and physical and mental well being. Some effects of regular exercise include: (1) improvements in exercise capacity and vascular transport capacity; (2) increased myocardial oxygen delivery with reduced demand; (3) increased muscle fiber size, mitochondrial density and activity; (4) improved motor unit recruitment; (5) alterations in endocrine responses and neurotransmitter activity; and many other physiological changes *(114–117)*. Exercise has also been reported to have a positive impact on mood and decreases depression and anxiety in healthy middle-aged and older adults *(117,118)*.

Studies of patients with PD have demonstrated exercise-related improvements in functional mobility, perception of illness, and quality of life *(119–126)*. Although regular exercise has been shown to benefit patients with PD, there have been no studies (to our knowledge) that have used exercise as a therapy for fatigue in patients who have PD. Regular exercise has the potential to alter both the physiology and perceptions of fatigue in patients with PD. Fatigue has been shown to decrease following exercise training in sedentary older *(127)* and obese *(128)* adults.

Several studies of chronic illnesses lend support for the potential beneficial role of exercise as an adjunctive treatment for fatigue in PD. Some studies of MS have reported reduced fatigue, anger, and depression after exercise training *(129,130)*, but others detected no differences in fatigue *(129)*. Reduced fatigue with exercise has also been found in patients with fibromayalgia *(130)*, chronic fatigue syndrome *(131)*, and SLE *(132)*. Yet, it is difficult to exclude the possibility that the reported fatigue was secondary to mood disturbances in these studies.

Exercise has been recommended as a nonpharmacological therapy for fatigue in cancer patients *(133–135)*. Although further study elucidating the effects of exercise on fatigue in cancer has been recommended *(136)*, several studies demonstrate that notable reduction in fatigue in patients with breast and other cancers following exercise, even in patients undergoing chemotherapy *(137–144)*. Schwartz has suggested that the beneficial effects of exercise on fatigue mediate the improvements in quality of life reported with exercise training in cancer patients *(145)*.

Fatigue in MS, cancer, or other chronic conditions is not necessarily the same as fatigue in PD, despite that all contain elements of central and peripheral fatigue. However, the efficacy of exercise as a treatment approach in MS and cancer patients supports the possible effect in patients with PD.

8. CONCLUSION

Fatigue is a common and often debilitating facet of PD with both mental and physical components and is poorly understood. Fatigue is not associated with motor disability. This counter-intuitive observation, in turn, suggests that studies attempting to link muscle fatigue to lassitude are inevitably fruitless to understand the condition and to treat it. Contributing factors, such as sleep dysfunction, depression, and treatable medical conditions, must be assessed and dealt with when possible. Endurance training, rarely harmful, has appeal as an unproven intervention that has been beneficial in most medical disorders and all fatigued populations in which it has been employed.

REFERENCES

1. Taylor RR, Jason LA, Curie CJ. Prognosis of chronic fatigue in a community-based sample. Psychosom Med 2002;64:319–327.
2. Ridsdale L, Evans A, Jerrett W, et al. Patients with fatigue in general practice: a prospective study. BMJ 1993;307:103–106.
3. Comi G, Leocani L, Rossi P, Colombo B. Physiopathology and treatment of fatigue in multiple sclerosis. J Neurol 2001;248:174–179.
4. Tavio M, Milan I, Tirelli U. Cancer-related fatigue. Int J Oncol 2002;21:1093–1099.
5. McCann K, Boore JRP. Fatigue in persons with renal failure who require maintenance hemodialysis. J Adv Nurs 2000;32:1132–1142.
6. McCrone P, Darbishire L, Ridsdale L, Seed P. The economic cost of chronic fatigue and chronic fatigue in UK primary care. Psychol Med 2000;33:253–261.
7. French MA. The clinical significance of tiredness. Can Med Assoc J 1960;82:665–671.
8. Norrelund N, Holnagel H. Fatigue among 40 year olds. Ugeskn Laeger 1979;141:1425–1429.
9. Buchwald D, Sullivan JL, Komaroff AL. Frequency of chronic active Epstein Barr Virus infection in a general medical practice. JAMA 1987;25:2303–2307.
10. Kroenke K, Wood DR, Mangelsdorff E, et al. Chronic fatigue in primary care: prevalence, patient characteristics and outcome. JAMA 1988;260:929–934.
11. Hoehn MM, Yahr MD. Parkinsonism: onset, progression and mortality. Neurology 1967;17:427–442.
12. Liang MH, Rogers M, Larson M, et al. The psychosocial impact of systemic lupus erythematosus and rheumatoid arthritis. Arthritis Rheum 1984;27:13–19.
13. Wang B, Gladman DD, Urowitz MB. Fatigue in lupus is not correlated with disease activity. J Rheumatol 1998;25:892–895.
14. Ford H, Tennant A, Johnson MH. The Leeds MSQOL scale: a disease specific measure of quality of life in multiple sclerosis. J Neurol Neurosurg Psychiatry 1997;62:210.
15. Ford H, Trigwell P, Johnson M. The nature of fatigue in multiple sclerosis. J Psychosom Res 1998;45:33–38.
16. Stein J, Flexner SB, eds. The Random House Thesaurus, College Edition. Random House, New York, 1984.
17. Gaba DM, Howard SK. Patient safety: fatigue among clinicians and the safety of patients. N Engl J Med 2002;347:1249–1255.
18. Weinstein DF. Duty hours for resident physicians-tough choices for teaching hospitals. N Engl J Med 2002;347: 1275–1278.
19. Seinbrook R. The debate over residents working hours. N Engl J Med 2002;347:1296–1302.
20. Russel B. Recent work on the principles of mathematics. International Monthly 1901;4:84.
21. Muscio B. Is a fatigue test possible? Br J Psychol 1921;12:31–46.
22. Flachenecker P, Kumpfel T, Kallmann B, et al. Fatigue in multiple sclerosis: a comparison of different rating scales and correlation to clinical parameters. Mult Scler 2002;8:523–526.
23. Krupp LB, Christodoulou C. Fatigue in multiple sclerosis. Curr Neurol Neurosci Rep 2001;1:294–298.
24. Elkins LE, Krupp LB, Scherl W. The measurement of fatigue and contributing neuropsychiatric factors. Semin Clin Neuropsychiatry 2000;5:58–61.
25. Krupp LB, Pollina DA. Mechanisms and management of fatigue in progressive neurological disorder. Curr Opin Neurol 1996;9:456–460.
26. Krupp LB, LaRocca NG, Muir-Nash J, Steinberg AD. The fatigue severity scale. Application to patients with multiple sclerosis and systemic lupus erythematosus. Arch Neurol 1989;46:1121–1123.
27. Schwartz JE, Jandorf L, Krupp LB. The measurement of fatigue: a new instrument. J Psychosom Res 1993;37:753–762.
28. Krupp LB, Alvarez LA, LaRocca NG, Scheinberg LC. Fatigue in multiple sclerosis. Arch Neurol 1988;45:435–437.
29. Krupp LB, Elkins LE. Fatigue and declines in cognitive functioning in multiple sclerosis. Neurology 2000;55:934–939.
30. Kleinman L, Zodet MW, Hakim Z, et al. Psychometric evaluation of the fatigue severity scale for use in chronic hepatitis C. Qual Life Res 2000;9:499–508.
31. Friedman JH, Friedman H. Fatigue in Parkinson's disease: a nine-year follow-up. Mov Disord 2001;16:1120–1122.
32. Friedman J, Friedman H. Fatigue in Parkinson's disease. Neurology. 1993;43:2016–2018.
33. Lee KA, Hicks G, Nino-Murcia G. Validity and reliability of a scale to assess fatigue. Psychiatry Res 1991;36:291–298.
34. Chalder T, Berelowitz G, Pawlikowska T, et al. Development of a fatigue scale. J Psychosom Res 1993;37:147–153.
35. Multiple Sclerosis Council for Clinical Practice Guidelines. Fatigue and multiple sclerosis: evidence-based management strategies for fatigue in multiple sclerosis. Multiple Sclerosis Council for Clinical Practice Guidelines, Multiple Sclerosis Society, New York, 1998.
36. Morriss RK, Wearden AJ, Mullis R. Exploring the validity of the Chalder Fatigue scale in chronic fatigue syndrome. J Psychosom Res 1998;45:411–417.
37. Taylor RR, Jason LA, Torres A. Fatigue rating scales: an empirical comparison. Psychol Med 2000;30:849–856.
38. Zachrisson O, Regland B, Jahreskog M, et al. A rating scale for fibromyalgia and chronic fatigue syndrome (the FibroFatigue scale). J Psychosom Res 2002;52:501–509.
39. Schneider RA. Reliability and validity of the Multidimensional Fatigue Inventory (MFI-20) and the Rhoten Fatigue Scale among rural cancer outpatients. Cancer Nurs 1998;21:370–373.
40. Schwartz AL. The Schwartz Cancer Fatigue Scale: testing reliability and validity. Oncol Nurs Forum 1998;25:711–717.

41. Schwartz AL, Meek PM, Nail LM, et al. Measurement of fatigue. Determining minimally important clinical differences. J Clin Epidemiol 2002;55:239–244.
42. Piper BF, Dibble SL, Dodd MJ, et al. The revised Piper Fatigue Scale: psychometric evaluation in women with breast cancer. Oncol Nurs Forum 1998;25:677–684.
43. Strohschein FJ, Kelly CG, Clarke AG, et al. Applicability, validity, and reliability of the Piper Fatigue Scale in postpolio patients. Am J Phys Med Rehabil 2003;82:122–129.
44. Lou JS, Reeves A, Benice T, Sexton G. Fatigue and depression are associated with poor quality of life in ALS. Neurology 2003;60:122–123.
45. Gowans SE, DeHueck A, Abbey SE. Measuring exercise-induced mood changes in fibromyalgia: a comparison of several measures. Arthritis Rheum 2002;47:603–609.
46. Reyes M, Gary HE. Jr, Dobbins JG, et al. Surveillance for chronic fatigue syndrome—four U. S. cities, September 1989 through August 1993. MMWR CDC Surveill Summ 1997;46:1–13.
47. Peto V, Jenkinson C, Fitzpatrick R, Greenhall R. The development and validation of a short measure of functioning and well being for individuals with Parkinson's disease. Qual Life Res 1995;4:241–248.
48. de Boer AG, Wijker W, Speelman JD, de Haes JC. Quality of life in patients with Parkinson's disease: development of a questionnaire. J Neurol Neurosurg Psychiatry 1996;61:70–74.
49. Schrag A, Selai C, Jahanshahi M, Quinn NP. The EQ-5D—a generic quality of life measure—is a useful instrument to measure quality of life in patients with Parkinson's disease. J Neurol Neurosurg Psychiatry 2000;69:67–73.
50. Damiano AM, Snyder C, Strausser B, William MK. A review of health related quality of life concepts and measures for Parkinson's disease. Qual Life Res 1999;8:235–243.
51. Chaudhuri A, Behan PO. Fatigue and basal ganglia. J Neurol Sci 2000;179:34–42.
52. Swain MG. Fatigue in chronic disease. Clin Sci (Lond) 2000;99:1–8.
53. Lou J-S, Kearns G, Oken B, et al. Exacerbated physical and mental fatigue in Parkinson's disease. Mov Disord 2001; 16:190–196.
54. Marek T, Noworol G, Karwowski W. Mental fatigue at work and pain perception. Work Stress 1988;2:133–137.
55. LeWitt P. A, Bharucha A, Chitrit I, et al. Perceived exertion and muscle efficiency in Parkinson's disease: L-Dopa effects. Clin Neuropharmacol 1994;17:454–459.
56. Ziv I, Avraham M, Michaelov Y, et al. Enhanced fatigue during motor performance in patients with Parkinson's disease. Neurology 1998;51:1583–1586.
57. Rowland LP, ed. Merritt's Neurology, 10th ed. Lippincott, Williams and Wilkins, Philadelphia, PA, 2000.
58. Paul RH, Cohen RA, Gilchrist JM. Ratings of subjective mental fatigue relate to cognitive performance in patients with myasthenia gravis. J Clin Neurosci 2002;9:243–246.
59. Paul RH, Cohen RA, Goldstein JM, Gilchrist JM. Fatigue and its impact on patients with myasthenia gravis. Muscle Nerve 2000;23:1402–1406.
60. Merkies IS, Schmitz PI, Samijn JP, et al. Fatigue in immune-mediated polyneuropathies. European Inflammatory Neuropathy Cause and Treatment (INCAT) Group. Neurology 1999;53:1648–1654.
61. van Hilten JJ, Weggeman M, van der Velde EA, et al. Sleep, excessive daytime sleepiness and fatigue in Parkinson's disease. J Neural Transm Park Dis Dement Sect 1993;5:235–244.
62. van Hilten JJ, Hoogland G, van der Velde EA, et al. Diurnal effects of motor activity and fatigue in Parkinson's disease. J Neurol Neurosurg Psychiatry 1993;56:874–877.
63. Garber CE, Friedman JH. Effects of fatigue on physical activity and function in patients with Parkinson's disease. Neurology 2003;60:1119–1124.
64. Critchley PH, Malcolm GP, Malcolm PN, et al. Fatigue and melatonin in Parkinson's disease. J Neurol Neurosurg Psychiatry 1991;54:91–92.
65. Marsden CD, Parkes JC, Quinn N. Fluctuations of disability in Parkinson's Disease Clinical Aspects. In: Marsden CD, Fain S., eds. Movement Disorders, London: Butterworth's, 1982;96–119.
66. Schwab RS, England AC, Peterson C. Akinesia in Parkinson's disease. Neurology 1959;9:65–72.
67. Yessavage JA, Brink TL, Rose TL, et al. Development and validation of a geriatric depression screening scale: a preliminary report. J Psychiatr Res 1983;17:37–49.
68. Schenkman M, Wei Zhu C, Cutson T. M, Whetten-Goldstein K. Longitudinal evaluation of economic and physical impact of Parkinson's disease. Parkinsonism Relat Disord 2001;8:41–50.
69. Shulman LM, Taback RL, Bean J, Weiner WJ. Comorbidity of the nonmotor symptoms of Parkinson's disease. Mov Disord 2001;16:507–510.
70. Abe K, Takanashi M, Yanagihara T. Fatigue in patients with PD. Behav Neurol 2000;12:103–106.
71. Herlofson K, Larsen JP. Measuring fatigue in patients with Parkinson's disease—the Fatigue Severity Scale. Eur J Neurol 2002;9:595–600.
72. Smets EM, Garssen B, Bonke B, de Haes JC. The Multidimensional Fatigue Inventory (MFI) psychometric qualities of an instrument to assess fatigue. J Psychosom Res 1995;39:315–325.
73. Tolson D, Fleming V, Schartau E. Coping with menstruation: understanding the needs of women with Parkinson's disease. J Adv Nurs 2002;40:513–521.

74. Burn DJ. Beyond the iron mask: towards better recognition and treatment of depression associated with Parkinson's disease. Mov Disord 2002;17:445–454.
75. Friedman JH, Fernandez HH. The nonmotor problems of Parkinson's disease. The Neurologist 2000;6:8–27.
76. Dooneief G, Mirabello E, Bell K, et al. An estimate of the incidence of depression in idiopathic Parkinson's disease. Arch Neurol 1992;49:305–307.
77. Tandberg E, Larsen JP, Aarsland D, Cummings JL. The occurrence of depression in Parkinson's disease. A community-based study. Arch Neurol 1996;53:175–179.
78. Richard IH. Depression in Parkinson's disease. Curr Treat Options Neurol 2000;2:263–274.
79. Schrag A, Jahanshahi M, Quinn NP. What contributes to depression in Parkinson's Disease? Psychol Med 2001;31:65–73.
80. Cummings JL. Depression and Parkinson's disease, A review. Am J Psychiatry 1992;149:443–454.
81. Gotham AM, Brown RG, Marsden CD. Depression in Parkinson's disease: a quantitative and qualitative analysis. J Neurol Neurosurg Psychiatry 1986;49:381–389.
82. Karlsen K, Larsen JP, Trandberg E, Jorgensen K. Fatigue in patients with Parkinson's disease. Mov Disord 1999;14:237–241.
83. Vercoulen JH, Swanink CM, Galama JM, et al. The persistence of fatigue in chronic fatigue syndrome and multiple sclerosis: development of a model. J Psychosom Res 1998;45:507–517.
84. Schwartz CE, Coulthard-Morris L, Zeng Q. Psychosocial correlates of fatigue in multiple sclerosis. Arch Phys Med Rehabil 1996;77:165–170.
85. Mainero C, Faroni J, Gasperini C, et al. Fatigue and magnetic resonance imaging activity in multiple sclerosis. J Neurol 1999;246:454–458.
86. Giovannoni G, Thompson AJ, Miller DH, Thompson EJ. Fatigue is not associated with raised inflammatory markers in multiple sclerosis. Neurology 2001;57:676–681.
87. Roelcke U, Kappos L, Lechner-Scott J, et al. Reduced glucose metabolism in the frontal cortex and basal ganglia of multiple sclerosis patients with fatigue: a 18F-fluorodeoxyglucose positron emission tomography study. Neurology 1997;48:1566–1571.
88. Filippi M, Rocca MA, Colombo B, et al. Functional magnetic resonance imaging correlates of fatigue in multiple sclerosis. Neuroimage 2002;15:559–567.
89. Colombo B, Martinelli-Boneschi F, Rossi P, et al. MRI and motor evoked potential findings in nondisabled multiple sclerosis patients with and without symptoms of fatigue. J Neurol 2000;247:506–509.
90. Codella M, Rocca MA, Colombo B, et al. Cerebral grey matter pathology and fatigue in patients with multiple sclerosis: a preliminary study. J Neurol Sci 2002;194:71–74.
91. van der Werf SP, Jongen PJ, Lycklama a Nijeholt GJ, et al. Fatigue in multiple sclerosis: interrelations between fatigue complaints, cerebral MRI abnormalities and neurological disability. J Neurol Sci 1998;160:164–170.
92. McLester JR, Jr. Muscle contraction and fatigue: the role of adenosine 5′-diphospate and inorganic phosphate. Sports Med 1997;23:287–305.
93. Taylor DJ, Krige D, Barnes PR, et al. A 31P magnetic resonance spectroscopy study of mitochondrial function in skeletal muscle of patients with Parkinson's disease. J Neurol Sci 1994;125:77–81.
94. Schapira AH. Evidence for mitochondrial dysfunction in Parkinson's disease – a critical appraisal. Mov Disord 1994;9:125–138.
95. Reichmann H, Janetzky B. Mitochondrial dysfunction—a pathogenetic factor in Parkinson's disease. J Neurol 2000;247(Suppl 2):1163–1168.
96. Hood DA. Invited review: contractile activity-induced mitochondrial biogenesis in skeletal muscle. J Appl Physiol 2001;90:1137–1157.
97. Davis JM. Central and peripheral factors in fatigue. J Sports Sci 1995;13(Spec No):S49–S53.
98. Davis JM, Bailey SP. Possible mechanisms of central nervous system fatigue during exercise. Med Sci Sports Exerc 1997;29:45–57.
99. Ingram DK. Age-related decline in physical activity: generalization to nonhumans. Med Sci Sports Exerc 2000;32:1623–1629.
100. Radak Z, Sasvari M, Nyakas C, et al. Single bout of exercise eliminates the immobilization-induced oxidative stress in rat brain. Neurochem Int 2001;39:33–38.
101. Weicker H, Struder HK. Influence of exercise on serotonergic neuromodulation in the brain. Amino Acids 2001;20:35–47.
102. Levi S, Cox M, Lugon M, et al. Increased energy expenditure in Parkinson's disease. BMJ 1990;301:1256–1257.
103. Markus HS, Cox M, Tomkins AM. Raised resting energy expenditure in Parkinson's disease and its relationship to muscle rigidity. Clin Sci 1992;83:1999–2004.
104. Pogarell O, Gasser T, van Hilten JJ, et al. Pramipexole in patients with Parkinson's disease and marked drug resistant tremor: a randomized, double blind, placebo controlled multicenter study. J Neurol Neurosurg. Psychiatry 2002;72:713–720.
105. Schlesinger I, Ravin PD. Dopamine agonists induce episodes of irresistible daytime sleepiness. Eur Neurol 2003;49:30–33.
106. Abe K, Takanashi M, Yanagihara T, Sakoda S. Pergolide mesilate may improve fatigue in patients with Parkinson's disease. Behav Neurol 2001–2002;13:117–121.
107. De Pandis MF, Starace A, Stefanelli F, et al. Modification of respiratory function parameters in patients with severe Parkinson's disease. Neurol Sci 2002;23(Suppl 2):S69–S70.

108. Sabate M, Rodriguez M, Mendez E, et al. Obstructive and restrictive pulmonary dysfunction increases disability in Parkinson disease. Arch Phys Med Rehabil 1996;77:29–34.
109. Polatli M, Akyol A, Cildag O, Bayulkem K. Pulmonary function tests in Parkinson's disease. Eur J Neurol 2001;8:341–345.
110. Weiner P, Inzelberg R, Davidovich A, et al. Respiratory muscle performance and the perception of dyspnea in Parkinson's disease. Can J Neurol Sci 2002;29:68–72.
111. Tzelepis GE, McCool FD, Friedman JH, Hoppin FG Jr. Respiratory muscle dysfunction in Parkinson's disease. Am Rev Respir Dis 1988;138:266–271.
112. Masoudi O, Davis K, Siram A, et al. Ventilation during submaximal exercise in Parkinson's disease. American Thoracic Society (abstract), American Thoracic Society, New York, 2000.
113. Tench C, Bentley D, Vleck V, et al. Aerobic fitness, fatigue, and physical disability in systemic lupus erythematosus. J Rheumatol 2002;29:474–481.
114. Shephard RJ. The scientific basis for exercise prescribing for the very old. J Am Geriatr Soc 1990;38:62–70.
115. American College of Sports Medicine. The recommended quantity and quality for exercise for developing and maintaining cardiorespiratory and muscular fitness in healthy adults. Med Sci Sports Exerc 1998;30:975–991.
116. American College of Sports Medicine. ACSM Position Stand on Exercise and Physical Activity for Older Adults. Med Sci Sports Exerc 1998;30:992–1008.
117. US Department of Health and Human Services, Centers for Disease Control and Prevention, National Center for Chronic Disease Prevention and Health Promotion. Physical Activity and Health: A Report of the Surgeon General. US Department of Health and Human Services, Atlanta, GA, 1996.
118. Babyak M, Blumenthal JA, Herman S, et al. Exercise treatment for major depression: maintenance of therapeutic benefit at 10 months. Psychosomatic Med 2000;62:633–638.
119. Bergen JL, Toole T, Elliott RG III, et al. Aerobic exercise intervention improves aerobic capacity and movement initiation in Parkinson's disease patients. NeuroRehabilitation 2002;17:161–168.
120. Baatile J, Langbein WE, Weaver F, et al. Effect of exercise on perceived quality of life of individuals with Parkinson's disease. J Rehabil Res Dev 2000;37:529–534.
121. Scandalis TA, Bosak A, Berliner JC, et al. Resistance training and gait function in patients with Parkinson's disease. Am J Phys Med Rehabil 2001;80:38–43.
122. de Goede CJ, Keus SH, Kwakkel G, Wagenaar RC. The effects of physical therapy in Parkinson's disease: a research synthesis. Arch Phys Med Rehabil 2001;82:509–515.
123. Stanley RK, Protas EJ, Jankovic J. Exercise performance in those having Parkinson's disease and healthy normals. Med Sci Sports Exerc 1999;31:761–766.
124. Comella CL, Stebbins GT, Brown-Toms N, Goetz CG. Physical therapy and Parkinson's disease. Neurology 1994;44:376–378.
125. Formisano R, Pratesi L, Modarelli FT, et al. Rehabilitation and Parkinson's disease. Scand J Rehab Med 1992;24:157–160.
126. Reuter I, Englehardt M, Stecker K, Baas H. Therapeutic value of exercise training in Parkinson's disease. Med Sci Sports Exerc 1999;31:1544–1549.
127. Pierce EF, Pate DW. Mood alterations in older adults following acute exercise. Percept Mot Skills 1994;79:191–194.
128. Annesi JJ. Effects of minimal exercise and cognitive behavior modification on adherence, emotion change, self-image, and physical change in obese women. Percept Mot Skills 2000;91:322–336.
129. Mostert S, Kesselring J. Effects of a short-term exercise training program on aerobic fitness, fatigue, health perception and activity level of subjects with multiple sclerosis. Mult Scler 2002;8:161–168.
130. Gowans SE, de Hueck A, Voss S, et al. Effect of a randomized, controlled trial of exercise on mood and physical function in individuals with fibromyalgia. Arthritis Rheum 2001;45:519–529.
131. Fulcher KY, White PD. Randomised controlled trial of graded exercise in patients with the chronic fatigue syndrome. BMJ 1997;314:1647–1652.
132. Robb-Nicholson LC, Daltroy L, Eaton H, et al. Effects of aerobic conditioning in lupus fatigue: a pilot study. Br J Rheumatol 1989;28:500–505.
133. Portenoy RK, Itri LM. Cancer-related fatigue: guidelines for evaluation and management. The Oncologist 1999;4:1–10.
134. Mock V, Atkinson A, Barsevick A, et al. NCCN practice guidelines for cancer-related fatigue. Oncology (Huntingt) 2000;14:151–161.
135. Tavio M, Milan I, Tirelli U. Cancer-related fatigue (review). Int. J Oncol 2002;21:1093–1099.
136. Manzullo EF, Escalante CP. Research into fatigue. Hematol Oncol Clin North Am 2002;16:619–628.
137. Schwartz AL, Mori M, Gao R, et al. Exercise reduces daily fatigue in women with breast cancer receiving chemotherapy. Med Sci Sports Exerc 2001;33:718–723.
138. Berger AM. Patterns of fatigue and activity and rest during adjuvant breast cancer chemotherapy. Oncol Nurs Forum 1998;25:51–62.
139. Servaes P, Verhagen CA, Bleijenberg G. Relations between fatigue, neuropsychological functioning, and physical activity after treatment for breast carcinoma: daily self-report and objective behavior. Cancer 2002;95:2017–2026.
140. Servaes P, Prins J, Verhagen S, Bleijenberg G. Fatigue after breast cancer and in chronic fatigue syndrome: similarities and differences. J Psychosom Res 2002;52:453–459.
141. Dimeo F, Rumberger BG, Keul J. Aerobic exercise as therapy for cancer fatigue. Med Sci Sports Exerc 1998;30:475–478.

142. Schwartz AL. Patterns of exercise and fatigue in physically active cancer survivors. Oncol Nurs Forum 1998;25:485–491.
143. Oldervoll LM, Kaasa S, Knobel H, Loge JH. Exercise reduces fatigue in chronic fatigued Hodgkins disease survivors-results from a pilot study. Eur J Cancer 2003;39:57–63.
144. Mock V, Pickett M, Ropka ME, et al. Fatigue and quality of life outcomes of exercise during cancer treatment. Cancer Pract 2000;9:119–127.
145. Schwartz AL. Fatigue mediates the effects of exercise on quality of life. Qual Life Res 1999;8:529–538.
146. Freal JD, Kraft GH, Coryell JK. Symptomatic fatigue in multiple sclerosis. Arch Physical Medical Rehabil 1984;5:135–137.
147. Berrios GE. Feelings of fatigue and psychopathology: a conceptual history. Comp Psychiatry 1990;31:140–151.
148. Tavio M, Milan I, Tirelli U. Cancer-related fatigue (a review). Int J Oncol 2002;21:1093–1099.
149. Lane R. Chronic fatigue syndrome: is it physical? J Neurol Neurosurg. Psychiatry 2000;69:289.
150. Shapiro RT, Schneider DM. Fatigue. In: van den Noort S, Holland N, eds. Multiple Sclerosis in Clinical Practice. Demos, New York, 1999, chapter 3.

Index

O

P

T